Cardiovascular Physiology

Cardiovascular Physiology

TENTH EDITION

ACHILLES J. PAPPANO, PhD

Professor Emeritus
Department of Cell Biology and Calhoun Cardiology Center
University of Connecticut Health Center
Farmington, Connecticut

WITHROW GIL WIER, PhD

Professor
Department of Physiology
University of Maryland School of Medicine
Baltimore, Maryland

ELSEVIER
MOSBY

ELSEVIER
MOSBY

1600 John F. Kennedy Blvd.
Ste 1800
Philadelphia, PA 19103-2899

CARDIOVASCULAR PHYSIOLOGY ISBN: 978-0-323-08697-4

Notice

Knowledge and best practice in this field are constantly changing. As new research and experience broaden our understanding, changes in research methods, professional practices, or medical treatment may become necessary.

Practitioners and researchers must always rely on their own experience and knowledge in evaluating and using any information, methods, compounds, or experiments described herein. In using such information or methods they should be mindful of their own safety and the safety of others, including parties for whom they have a professional responsibility. With respect to any drug or pharmaceutical products identified, readers are advised to check the most current information provided (i) on procedures featured or (ii) by the manufacturer of each product to be administered, to verify the recommended dose or formula, the method and duration of administration, and contraindications. It is the responsibility of practitioners, relying on their own experience and knowledge of their patients, to make diagnoses, to determine dosages and the best treatment for each individual patient, and to take all appropriate safety precautions. To the fullest extent of the law, neither the Publisher nor the authors, contributors, or editors assume any liability for any injury and/or damage to persons or property as a matter of products liability, negligence or otherwise, or from any use or operation of any methods, products, instructions, or ideas contained in the material herein.

Library of Congress Cataloging-in-Publication Data

Pappano, Achilles J.
  Cardiovascular physiology / Achilles J. Pappano, Withrow Gil Wier. -- 10th ed.
    p. ; cm. -- (Mosby physiology monograph series)
  Rev. ed. of: Cardiovascular physiology / Matthew N. Levy, Achilles J. Pappano. 9th ed. c2007.
  Includes bibliographical references and index.
  ISBN 978-0-323-08697-4 (pbk.)
  I. Wier, Withrow Gil. II. Levy, Matthew N., 1922- Cardiovascular physiology. III. Title. IV. Series: Mosby physiology monograph series.
  [DNLM: 1. Cardiovascular Physiological Phenomena. WG 102]
  612.1--dc23   2012032909

Senior Content Strategist: Elyse O'Grady
Content Coordinator: Lee Hood
Publishing Services Managers: Rajendrababu Hemamalini and Anne Altepeter
Senior Project Manager: Douglas Turner
Project Manager: Saravanan Thavamani
Design Manager: Steven Stave

Printed in the United States of America

Last digit is the print number: 9 8 7 6 5 4 3 2 1

To Robert M. Berne and Matthew N. Levy,
whose research and scholarship in cardiovascular physiology
have enriched and inspired generations of students and colleagues

PREFACE

We believe that physiology is the backbone of clinical medicine. In the clinic, the emergency room, the intensive care unit, or the surgical suite, physiological principles are the basis for action. But we also find great intellectual satisfaction in the science of physiology as the means to explain the elegant mechanisms of our bodies. In the tenth edition of Berne and Levy's classic monograph on cardiovascular physiology, we have tried to convey both ideas.

Physiology serves as a foundation that students of medicine must comprehend before they can understand the derangements caused by pathology. This text of cardiovascular physiology emphasizes general concepts and regulatory mechanisms. To present the various regulatory mechanisms clearly, the component parts of the system are first discussed individually. Then, the last chapter describes how various individual components of the cardiovascular system are coordinated. The examples describe how the body responds to two important stresses—exercise and hemorrhage. Selected pathophysiological examples of abnormal function are included to illustrate and clarify normal physiological processes. These examples are distributed throughout the text and are identified by colored boxes with the heading "Clinical Box".

The text incorporates the learning objectives for cardiovascular physiology of the American Physiological Society, except for hemostasis and coagulation. These last-named topics are found in hematology books. The book has been updated and revised extensively. The relation between pressure-volume loops and cardiac function curves, newer aspects of endothelium function, myocardial metabolism and its relation to oxygen consumption and cardiac energetics, and the regulation of peripheral and coronary blood flows have received particular emphasis. Whenever available, physiological data from humans have been included. Some old figures have been deleted and many new figures have been added to aid comprehension of the text. Selected references appear at the end of each chapter. The scientific articles included were chosen for their depth, clarity, and appropriateness.

Throughout the book, *italics* are used to emphasize important facts and concepts, and **boldface** type is used for new terms and definitions. Each chapter begins with a list of objectives and ends with a summary to highlight key points. Case histories with multiple-choice questions are provided to help in review and to indicate clinical relevance of the material. The correct answers and brief explanations for them appear in the appendix.

We thank our readers for their constructive comments. Thanks are also due to the numerous investigators and publishers who have granted permission to use illustrations from their publications. In most cases these illustrations have been altered somewhat to increase their didactic utility. In some cases, unpublished data from investigations by Robert Berne and Matthew Levy and the current authors have been presented.

Achilles J. Pappano
W. Gil Wier

CONTENTS

CHAPTER 4

THE CARDIAC PUMP............55

CHAPTER 5

REGULATION OF THE HEARTBEAT.................91

CHAPTER **9**

THE PERIPHERAL CIRCULATION AND ITS CONTROL............ 171

CHAPTER 13

INTERPLAY OF CENTRAL AND PERIPHERAL FACTORS THAT CONTROL THE CIRCULATION   263

APPENDIX: CASE STUDY ANSWERS 279

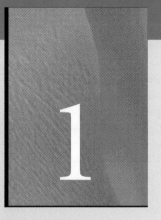

1

OVERVIEW OF THE CIRCULATION AND BLOOD

OBJECTIVES

1. Describe the general structure of the cardiovascular system.

2. Compare the compositions and functions of the blood vessels.

3. Compare the relationship of the vascular cross-sectional area to the velocity of blood flow in the various vascular segments.

4. Indicate the pressure changes and pathways of blood flow throughout the vasculature.

5. Describe the constituents of the blood and explain the functions of the cellular elements of blood.

6. Know the importance of blood group matching before blood transfusions.

The circulatory, endocrine, and nervous systems constitute the principal coordinating and integrating systems of the body. Whereas the nervous system is primarily concerned with communication and the endocrine glands with regulation of certain body functions, the circulatory system serves to transport and distribute essential substances to the tissues and to remove metabolic by-products. The circulatory system also shares in such homeostatic mechanisms as regulation of body temperature, humoral communication throughout the body, and adjustments of O_2 and nutrient supply in different physiologic states.

THE CIRCULATORY SYSTEM

The cardiovascular system accomplishes these functions with a pump (see Chapter 4), a series of distributing and collecting tubes (see Chapter 7), and an extensive system of thin vessels that permit rapid exchange between the tissues and the vascular channels (see Chapter 8). The primary purpose of this text is to discuss the function of the components of the vascular system and the control mechanisms (with their checks and balances) that are responsible for alteration of blood distribution necessary to meet the changing requirements of different tissues in response to a wide spectrum of physiological (see Chapter 9) and pathological (see Chapter 13) conditions.

Before one considers the function of the parts of the circulatory system in detail, it is useful to consider it as a whole in a purely descriptive sense (Figure 1-1). The heart consists of two pumps in series: the right ventricle to propel blood through the lungs for exchange of O_2 and CO_2 (**the pulmonary circulation**) and the left ventricle to propel blood to all other tissues of the body (**the systemic circulation**). The total

1

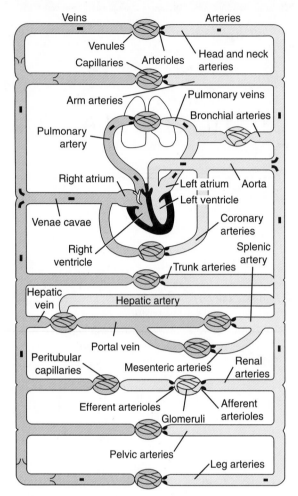

FIGURE 1-1 ■ Schematic diagram of the parallel and series arrangement of the vessels composing the circulatory system. The capillary beds are represented by *thin lines* connecting the arteries (on the *right*) with the veins (on the *left*). The crescent-shaped thickenings proximal to the capillary beds represent the arterioles (resistance vessels). *(Redrawn from Green HD: In Glasser O, editor: Medical physics, vol 1, Chicago, 1944, Mosby-Year Book.)*

flow of blood out of the left ventricle is known as the cardiac output (CO). The rhythmic contraction of the heart is an intrinsic property of the heart whose sinoatrial node pacemaker generates action potentials spontaneously (see Chapter 3). These action potentials are propagated in an orderly manner through the organ to trigger contraction and to produce the cur-

rents detected in the electrocardiogram (see Chapter 3).

Unidirectional flow through the heart is achieved by the appropriate arrangement of effective flap valves. Although the cardiac output is intermittent, continuous flow to the periphery occurs by distention of the aorta and its branches during ventricular contraction (**systole**) and elastic recoil of the walls of the large arteries that propel the blood forward during ventricular relaxation (**diastole**). Blood moves rapidly through the aorta and its arterial branches (see Chapter 7). The branches become narrower and their walls become thinner and change histologically toward the periphery. From the aorta, a predominantly elastic structure, the peripheral arteries become more muscular until the muscular layer predominates at the arterioles (Figure 1-2).

In the large arteries, frictional resistance is relatively small, and mean pressure throughout the system of large arteries is only slightly less than in the aorta. The small arteries and arterioles serve to regulate flow to individual tissues by varying their resistance to flow. The small arteries offer moderate resistance to blood flow, and this resistance reaches a maximal level in the arterioles, sometimes referred to as the stopcocks of the vascular system. Hence *the pressure drop is significant and is greatest in the small arteries and in the arterioles* (Figure 1-3). Adjustments in the degree of contraction of the circular muscle of these small vessels permit regulation of tissue blood flow and aid in the control of arterial blood pressure (see Chapter 9).

In addition to a sharp reduction in pressure across the arterioles, there is also a change from pulsatile to steady flow as pressure continues to decline from the arterial to the venous end of the capillaries (see Figure 1-3). *The pulsatile arterial blood flow, caused by the phasic cardiac ejection, is damped at the capillaries by the combination of distensibility of the large arteries and frictional resistance in the arterioles.*

In a patient with hyperthyroidism **(Graves disease)**, the basal metabolism is elevated and is often associated with arteriolar vasodilation. This reduction in arteriolar resistance diminishes the dampening effect on the pulsatile arterial pressure and is manifested as pulsatile flow in the capillaries, as observed in the fingernail beds of patients with this ailment.

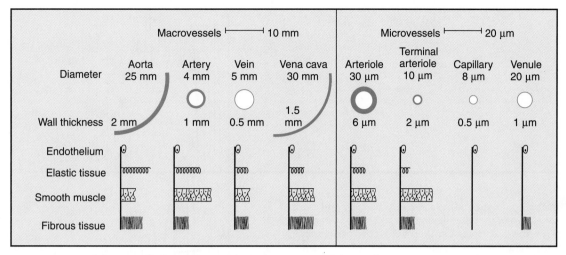

FIGURE 1-2 ■ Internal diameter, wall thickness, and relative amounts of the principal components of the vessel walls of the various blood vessels that compose the circulatory system. Cross-sections of the vessels are not drawn to scale because of the huge range from aorta and venae cavae to capillary. *(Redrawn from Burton AC: Relation of structure to function of the tissues of the wall of blood vessels.* Physiol Rev *34:619, 1954.)*

Many capillaries arise from each arteriole to form the microcirculation (see Chapter 8), so that the total cross-sectional area of the capillary bed is very large, despite the fact that the cross-sectional area of each capillary is less than that of each arteriole. As a result, blood flow velocity becomes quite slow in the capillaries (see Figure 1-3), analogous to the decrease in velocity of flow seen at the wide regions of a river. Conditions in the capillaries are ideal for the exchange of diffusible substances between blood and tissue because the capillaries are short tubes whose walls are only one cell thick and because flow velocity is low.

On its return to the heart from the capillaries, blood passes through venules and then through veins of increasing size with a progressive decrease in pressure until the blood reaches the vena cava (see Figure 1-3). As the heart is approached, the number of veins decreases, the thickness and composition of the vein walls change (see Figure 1-2), the total cross-sectional area of the venous channels diminishes, and the velocity of blood flow increases (see Figure 1-3). Note that the velocity of blood flow and the cross-sectional area at each level of the vasculature are essentially mirror images of each other (see Figure 1-3).

Data indicate that between the aorta and the capillaries the total cross-sectional area increases about 500-fold (see Figure1-3). The volume of blood in the systemic vascular system (Table 1-1) is greatest in the veins and small veins (64%). Of the total blood volume, only about 6% of it is in the capillaries and 14% in the aorta, arteries, and arterioles. In contrast, blood volume in the pulmonary vascular bed is about equal between arteries and capillaries; venous vessels display a slightly larger percentage of pulmonary blood volume. The cross-sectional area of the venae cavae is larger than that of the aorta. Therefore, the velocity of flow is slower in the venae cavae than that in the aorta (see Figure 1-3).

Blood entering the right ventricle via the right atrium is pumped through the pulmonary arterial system at a mean pressure about one seventh that in the systemic arteries. The blood then passes through the lung capillaries, where CO_2 is released and O_2 taken up. The O_2-rich blood returns via the four pulmonary veins to the left atrium and ventricle to complete the cycle. Thus, in the normal intact circulation, the total volume of blood is constant, and an increase in the volume of blood in one area must be accompanied by a decrease in another. However, the *distribution* of the circulating blood to the different body organs is determined by the output of the left ventricle and by the contractile state of the arterioles (resistance vessels) of these organs (see Chapters 9 and 10). In turn, the *cardiac output* is controlled by the rate of heartbeat, cardiac contractility,

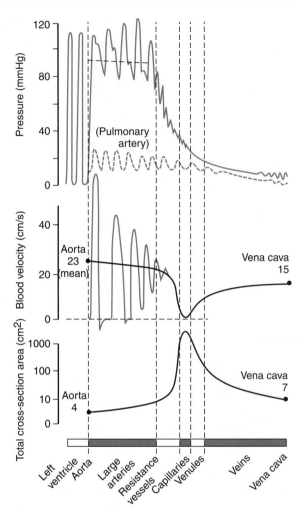

FIGURE 1-3 ▓ Phasic pressure, velocity of flow, and cross-sectional area of the systemic circulation. The important features are the major pressure drop across the small arteries and arterioles, the inverse relationship between blood flow velocity and cross-sectional area, and the maximal cross-sectional area and minimal flow rate in the capillaries. *(From Levick JR: An introduction to cardiovascular physiology, ed 5, London, 2010, Hodder Arnold.)*

venous return, and arterial resistance. The circulatory system is composed of conduits arranged in series and in parallel (see Figure 1-1).

It is evident that the systemic and pulmonary vascular systems are composed of many blood vessels arranged in series and parallel, with respect to blood flow. The total resistance to blood flow of the systemic blood vessels is known as the total peripheral resistance (TPR), and the total resistance of the pulmonary vessels is known as the total pulmonary resistance. Total peripheral resistance and cardiac output determine the mean pressure in the large arteries, though the hydraulic resistance equation (see Chapter 7).

The main function of the circulating blood is to carry O_2 and nutrients to the various tissues in the body, and to remove CO_2 and waste products from those tissues. Furthermore, blood transports other substances, such as hormones, white blood cells, and platelets, from their sites of production to their sites of action. Blood also aids in the distribution of fluids, solutes, and heat. Hence, blood contributes to **homeostasis,** the maintenance of a constant internal environment.

A fundamental characteristic of normal operation of the cardiovascular system is the maintenance of a relatively constant mean (average) blood pressure within the large arteries. The difference between mean arterial pressure ($\overline{P}_a$) and the pressure in the right

TABLE 1-1

Distribution of Blood Volume*

	ABSOLUTE VOLUME (mL)		RELATIVE VOLUME (%)	
Systemic circulation:		4200		84
Aorta and large arteries	300		6.0	
Small arteries	400		8.0	
Capillaries	300		6.0	
Small veins	2300		46.0	
Large veins	900		18.0	
Pulmonary circulation:		440		8.8
Arteries	130		2.6	
Capillaries	110		2.2	
Veins	200		4.0	
Heart (end-diastole)	360	360	7.2	7.2
Total	5000	5000	100	100

*Values apply to a 70-kg woman; increase values by 10% for a 70-kg man.

Data from Boron WF, Boulpaep EL: *Medical physiology*, ed 2, Philadelphia, 2009, Elsevier Saunders.

atrium (P_{ra}) provides the driving force for flow through the resistance (R) of blood vessels of the individual tissues. Thus, when the circulatory system is in steady-state, total flow of blood from the heart (cardiac output, CO) equals total flow of blood returning to the heart. The relation among these variables is described in the following hydraulic equation:

$$\overline{P}_a - P_{ra} = CO \times R$$

The cardiovascular system, together with neural, renal, and endocrine systems, maintains $\overline{P}_a$ at a relatively constant level, despite the large variations in cardiac output and peripheral resistance that are required in daily life. *If the $\overline{P}_a$ is maintained at its normal level under all circumstances, then each individual tissue will be able to obtain the necessary blood flow required to sustain its functions. Because blood flow to the brain and the heart cannot be interrupted for even a few seconds without endangering life, maintenance of the $\overline{P}_a$ is a critical function of the cardiovascular system.*

BLOOD

Blood consists of red blood cells, white blood cells, and platelets suspended in a complex solution (plasma) of various salts, proteins, carbohydrates, lipids, and gases. The circulating blood volume accounts for about 7% of the body weight. Approximately 55% of the blood is plasma; the protein content is 7 g/dL (about 4 g/dL of albumin and 3 g/dL of plasma globulins).

Erythrocytes

The erythrocytes (red blood cells) are flexible, biconcave disks that transport oxygen to the body tissues (Figure 1-4). Mammalian erythrocytes are unusual in that they lack a nucleus. The average erythrocyte is 7 μm in diameter, and these cells arise from **pluripotential stem cells** in the bone marrow. All of the cells in the circulating blood are derived from these stem cells. Most of these immature cells develop into various forms of mature cells, such as **erythrocytes, monocytes, megakaryocytes,** and **lymphocytes.** The erythrocytes lose their nuclei before they enter the circulation, and their average life span is 120 days. Approximately 5 million erythrocytes are present per microliter of blood. However, a small fraction of the pluripotential stem cells remains in the undifferentiated state.

Hemoglobin (about 15 g/dL of blood) is the main protein in the erythrocytes. Hemoglobin consists of **heme,** an iron-containing tetrapyrrole. Heme is linked to **globin,** a protein composed of four polypeptide chains (two α and two β chains in the normal adult). The iron moiety of hemoglobin binds loosely and reversibly to O_2 to form oxyhemoglobin. The affinity of hemoglobin for O_2 is a steep function of the partial pressure of O_2 (Po_2) at Po_2 less than 60 mm Hg (Figure 1-5). This allows ready diffusion of O_2 from hemoglobin to tissue. The binding of O_2 to hemoglobin is affected by pH, temperature, and 2,3-diphosphoglycerate concentration. These factors affect O_2 transport particularly at Po_2 less than 60 mm Hg.

Changes in the polypeptide subunits of globin affect the affinity of hemoglobin for O_2. For example, fetal hemoglobin has two γ chains instead of two β chains. This substitution increases its affinity for O_2. Changes in the polypeptide subunits of globin may induce certain serious diseases, such as **sickle cell anemia** and **erythroblastosis fetalis** (Figure 1-6). Sickle cell anemia is a disorder associated with the presence of **hemoglobin S**, which is an abnormal form of

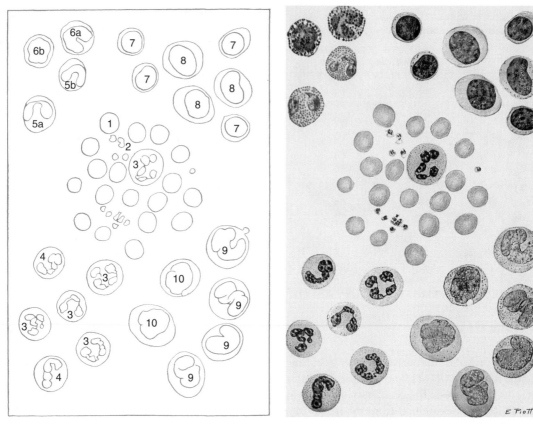

FIGURE 1-4 ■ The morphology of blood cells. 1, Normal red blood cell; 2, platelet; 3, neutrophil; 4, neutrophil, band form; 5a, eosinophil, two lobes; 5b, eosinophil, band form; 6a, basophil, band form; 6b, metamyelocyte, basophilic; 7, lymphocyte, small; 8, lymphocyte, large; 9, monocyte, mature; 10, monocyte, young. *(From Daland GA: A color atlas of morphologic hematology, Cambridge, MA, 1951, Harvard University Press.)*

hemoglobin in the erythrocytes. Many of the erythrocytes in the bloodstream of patients with sickle cell anemia have a sickle-like shape (Figure 1-6). Consequently, many of the abnormal cells cannot pass through the capillaries and, therefore, cannot deliver adequate O_2 and nutrients to the local tissues. **Thalassemia** is also a genetic disorder of the globin genes; α and β forms exist. In either case, the disorder leads ultimately to a **microcytic** (small cell), **hypochromic** (inadequate quantity of hemoglobin) anemia (*upper central panel* of Figure 1-6).

The number of circulating red cells normally remains fairly constant. The production of erythrocytes (**erythropoiesis**) is regulated by the glycoprotein **erythropoietin,** which is secreted mainly by the kidneys. Erythropoietin enhances erythrocyte production

by accelerating the differentiation of stem cells in the bone marrow. This substance is often used clinically to increase red blood cell production in anemic patients.

Leukocytes

There are normally 4000 to 10,000 leukocytes (white blood cells) per microliter of blood. Leukocytes include granulocytes (65%), lymphocytes (30%), and monocytes (5%). Of the granulocytes, about 95% are neutrophils, 4% are eosinophils, and 1% are basophils. White blood cells originate from the primitive stem cells in the bone marrow. After birth, granulocytes and monocytes in humans continue to originate in the bone marrow, whereas lymphocytes originate in the lymph nodes, spleen, and thymus.

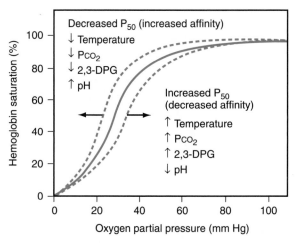

FIGURE 1-5 ■ Oxyhemoglobin dissociation curve showing the saturation of hemoglobin as a function of the partial pressure of O_2 (Po_2) in the blood. Oxygenation of hemoglobin at a given Po_2 is affected by temperature and the blood concentration of metabolites, CO_2, 2,3-diphosphoglyerate (2,3-DPG) and H^+. P_{50}, the partial pressure where hemoglobin is 50% saturated with O_2. *(From Koeppen BM, Stanton BA:* Berne and Levy physiology, *ed 6, Philadelphia, 2008, Mosby Elsevier.)*

Anemia and chronic hypoxia are prevalent in people who live at high altitudes, and such conditions tend to stimulate erythrocyte production and can produce polycythemia (an increased number of red blood cells). When the hypoxic stimulus is removed in subjects with altitude polycythemia, the high erythrocyte concentration in the blood inhibits erythropoiesis. The red blood cell count is also greatly increased in **polycythemia vera,** a disease of unknown cause. The elevated erythrocyte concentration increases blood viscosity, often enough that blood flow to vital tissues becomes impaired.

Granulocytes and monocytes are motile, nucleated cells that contain **lysosomes** that have enzymes capable of digesting foreign material such as microorganisms, damaged cells, and cellular debris. Thus leukocytes constitute a major defense mechanism against infections. Microorganisms or the products of cell destruction release **chemotactic substances** that attract granulocytes and monocytes. When migrating leukocytes reach the foreign agents, they engulf them (**phagocytosis**) and then destroy them through the action of enzymes that form O_2-derived **free radicals** and **hydrogen peroxide**.

Lymphocytes

Lymphocytes vary in size and have large nuclei. Most lymphocytes lack cytoplasmic granules (see Figure 1-5). The two main types of lymphocytes are **B lymphocytes,** which are responsible for **humoral immunity,** and **T lymphocytes,** which are responsible for cell-mediated immunity. When lymphocytes are stimulated by an **antigen** (a foreign protein on the surface of a microorganism or allergen), the B lymphocytes are transformed into **plasma cells,** which synthesize and release antibodies (**gamma globulins**). Antibodies are carried by the bloodstream to a site of infection, where they "tag" foreign invaders for destruction by other components of the immune system.

The main T cells are cytotoxic and are responsible for long-term protection against some viruses, bacteria, and cancer cells. They are also responsible for the rejection of transplanted organs.

Blood Is Divided into Groups by Antigens Located on Erythrocytes

Four principal blood groups, designated O, A, B, and AB, prevail in human subjects. Each group is identified by the type of antigen that is present on the erythrocyte. People with type A blood have A antigens; those with type B blood have B antigens; those with type AB have both A and B antigens, and those with type O have neither antigen. The plasma of group O blood contains antibodies to A, B, and AB.

Group A plasma contains antibodies to B antigens, and group B plasma contains antibodies to A antigens. Group AB plasma has no antibodies to O, A, or B antigens. In blood transfusions, crossmatching is necessary to prevent agglutination of donor red cells by antibodies in the plasma of the recipient. Because plasma of groups A, B, and AB has no antibodies to group O erythrocytes, people with group O blood are called universal donors. Conversely, persons with AB blood are called **universal recipients,** because their plasma has no antibodies to the

GENESIS OF RBC

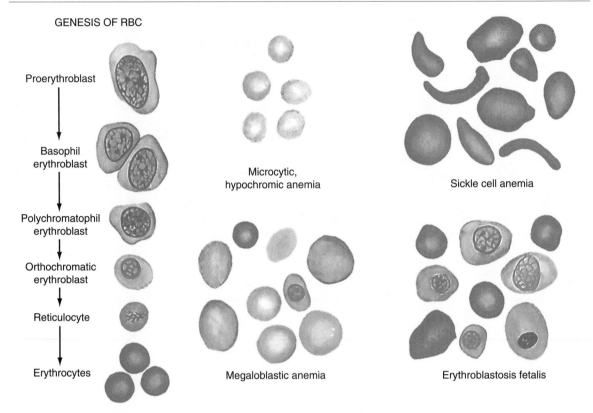

FIGURE 1-6 ■ Genesis of red blood cells (RBCs), and red blood cells in different types of anemias. *(From Guyton AC, Hall JE: Textbook of medical physiology, ed 10, Philadelphia, 2006, WB Saunders.)*

antigens of the other three groups. In addition to the ABO blood grouping, there are **Rh (Rhesus factor)– positive** and **Rh-negative groups**.

An Rh-negative person can develop antibodies to Rh-positive red blood cells if exposed to Rh-positive blood. This can occur during pregnancy if the mother is Rh-negative and the fetus is Rh-positive (inherited from the father). In this case, Rh-positive red blood cells from the fetus enter the maternal bloodstream at the time of placental separation and induce Rh-positive antibodies in the mother's plasma. The Rh-positive antibodies from the mother can also reach the fetus via the placenta and agglutinate and hemolyze fetal red blood cells **(erythroblastosis fetalis,** a hemolytic disease of the newborn). Red blood cell destruction can also occur in Rh-negative individuals who have previously had transfusions of Rh-positive blood and have developed Rh antibodies. If these individuals are given a subsequent transfusion of Rh-positive blood, the transfused red blood cells will be destroyed by the Rh antibodies in their plasma.

SUMMARY

- The cardiovascular system is composed of a heart, which pumps blood, and blood vessels (arteries, capillaries, veins) that distribute the blood to all organs.
- The greatest resistance to blood flow, and hence the greatest pressure drop, in the arterial system occurs at the level of the small arteries and the arterioles.
- Pulsatile pressure is progressively damped by the elasticity of the arteriolar walls and the functional resistance of the arterioles, so that capillary blood flow is essentially nonpulsatile.
- Velocity of blood flow is inversely related to the cross-sectional area at any point along the vascular system.
- Most of the blood volume in the systemic vascular bed is located in the venous side of the circulation.
- Blood consists of red blood cells (erythrocytes), white blood cells (leukocytes and lymphocytes), and platelets, all suspended in a solution containing salts, proteins, carbohydrates, and lipids.
- There are four major blood groups: O, A, B, and AB. Type O blood can be given to people with any of the blood groups because the plasma of all of the blood groups lacks antibodies to type O red cells. Hence people with type O blood are referred to as *universal donors*. By the same token, people with AB blood are referred to as *universal recipients* because their plasma lacks antibodies to red cells of all of the blood groups. In addition to O, A, B, and AB blood groups, there are Rh-positive and Rh-negative blood groups.

ADDITIONAL READING

Adams RH: Molecular control of arterial-venous blood vessel identity, *J Anat* 202:105, 2003.

Christensen KL, Mulvany MJ: Location of resistance arteries, *J Vasc Res* 38:1, 2001.

Conway EM, Collen D, Carmeliet P: Molecular mechanisms of blood vessel growth, *Cardiovasc Res* 49:507, 2001.

Pugsley MK, Tabrizchi R: The vascular system. An overview of structure and function, *J Pharmacol Toxicol Methods* 44:333, 2000.

Secomb TW, Pries AR: The microcirculation: physiology at the mesoscale, *J Physiol* 589:1047, 2011.

Reid ME, Lomas-Francis C: Molecular approaches to blood group identification, *Curr Opin Hematol* 9:152, 2002.

Urbaniak SJ, Greiss MA: RhD haemolytic disease of the fetus and the newborn, *Blood Rev* 14:44, 2000.

CASE 1-1

After a knife wound to the groin, a man develops a large arteriovenous (AV) shunt between the iliac artery and vein.

QUESTION

1. Which of the following changes will occur in his systemic circulation?
   a. Blood flow in the capillaries of the fingernail bed becomes pulsatile.
   b. The circulation time (antecubital vein to tongue) is decreased.
   c. The arterial pulse pressure (systolic minus diastolic pressure) is decreased.
   d. The greatest velocity of blood flow prevails in the vena cava.
   e. Pressure in the right atrium is greater than in the inferior vena cava.

2 EXCITATION: THE CARDIAC ACTION POTENTIAL

OBJECTIVES

1. Characterize the types of cardiac action potentials.
2. Define the ionic basis of the resting potential.
3. Define the ionic basis of cardiac action potentials.
4. Describe the characteristics of the fast- and slow-response action potentials.
5. Explain the temporal changes in cardiac excitability.

Experiments on "animal electricity" conducted by Galvani and Volta two centuries ago led to the discovery that electrical phenomena were involved in the spontaneous contractions of the heart. In 1855 Kölliker and Müller observed that when the nerve of an innervated skeletal muscle preparation contacted the surface of a frog's heart, the muscle twitched with each cardiac contraction.

The electrical events that normally occur in the heart initiate its contraction. Disorders in electrical activity can induce serious and sometimes lethal rhythm disturbances.

CARDIAC ACTION POTENTIALS CONSIST OF SEVERAL PHASES

The potential changes recorded from a typical ventricular muscle fiber are illustrated in Figure 2-1A: When two microelectrodes are placed in an electrolyte solution near a strip of quiescent cardiac muscle, no potential difference (time a) is measurable between the two electrodes. At point b, one microelectrode was inserted into the interior of a cardiac muscle fiber. Immediately the voltmeter recorded a potential difference (V_m) across the cell membrane; the potential of the cell interior was about 90 mV lower than that of the surrounding medium. Such electronegativity of the resting cell interior is also characteristic of skeletal and smooth muscles, nerves, and indeed most cells within the body.

At point c, an electrical stimulus excited the ventricular cell. The cell membrane rapidly depolarized and the potential difference reversed (positive overshoot), such that the potential of the interior of the cell exceeded that of the exterior by about 20 mV. The rapid upstroke of the **action potential** is designated phase 0. Immediately after the upstroke, there was a brief period of partial repolarization (phase 1), followed by a **plateau** (phase 2) of sustained depolarization that persisted for about 0.1 to 0.2 seconds (s). The potential then became progressively more negative (phase 3), until the resting state of polarization was again attained (at point e). **Repolarization** (phase 3) is a much slower process than **depolarization** (phase 0). The interval from the end of repolarization until the

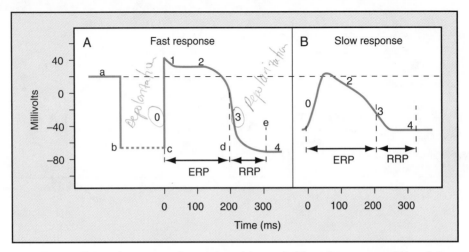

FIGURE 2-1 ■ Changes in transmembrane potential recorded from fast-response (**A**) and slow-response (**B**) cardiac fibers in isolated cardiac tissue immersed in an electrolyte solution from phase 0 to phase 4. **A,** At time a, the microelectrode was in the solution surrounding the cardiac fiber. At time b the microelectrode entered the fiber. At time c an action potential was initiated in the impaled fiber. Time c to d represents the effective refractory period (ERP); time d to e represents the relative refractory period (RRP). **B,** An action potential recorded from a slow-response cardiac fiber. Note that in comparison with the fast-response fiber, the resting potential of the slow fiber is less negative, the upstroke (phase 0) of the action potential is less steep, and the amplitude of the action potential is smaller; also, phase 1 is absent, and the RRP extends well into phase 4, after the fiber has fully repolarized.

beginning of the next action potential is designated phase 4.

The temporal relationship between the action potential and cell shortening is shown in Figure 2-2. Rapid depolarization (phase 0) precedes force development, repolarization is complete just before peak force is attained, and the duration of contraction is slightly longer than the duration of the action potential.

The Principal Types of Cardiac Action Potentials Are the Slow and Fast Types

Two main types of action potentials are observed in the heart, as shown in Figure 2-1. One type, the fast response, occurs in the ordinary atrial and ventricular myocytes and in the specialized conducting fibers (**Purkinje fibers**). The other type of action potential, the **slow response**, is found in the **sinoatrial (SA) node**, the natural pacemaker region of the heart, and in the **atrioventricular (AV) node**, the specialized tissue that conducts the cardiac impulse from atria to ventricles.

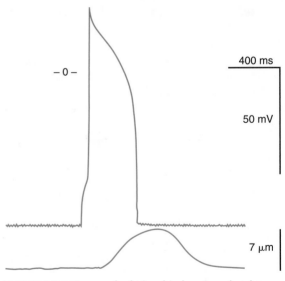

FIGURE 2-2 ■ Temporal relationship between the changes in transmembrane potential and the cell shortening that occurs in a single ventricular myocyte. *(From Pappano A: Unpublished record, 1995.)*

As shown in Figure 2-1, the **membrane resting potential** (phase 4) of the fast response is considerably more negative than that of the slow response. Also, the slope of the upstroke (phase 0), the action potential amplitude, and the overshoot of the fast response are greater than those of the slow response. The action potential amplitude and the steepness of the upstroke are important determinants of propagation velocity, as explained later. Hence, conduction velocity is much slower in slow-response fibers than in fast-response fibers. Slow conduction increases the likelihood of certain rhythm disturbances.

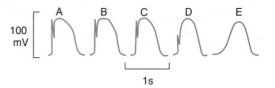

FIGURE 2-3 ■ Effect of tetrodotoxin on the action potential recorded in a calf Purkinje fiber perfused with a solution containing epinephrine and 10.8 mM K^+. The concentration of tetrodotoxin was 0 M in A, 3×10^{-8} M in B, 3×10^{-7} M in C, and 3×10^{-6} M in D and E; E was recorded later than D. *(Redrawn from Carmeliet E, Vereecke J: Adrenaline and the plateau phase of the cardiac action potential. Importance of Ca^{++}, Na^+ and K^+ conductance. Pflügers Arch 313:300, 1969.)*

CLINICAL BOX

Fast responses may change to slow responses under certain pathological conditions. For example, in patients with coronary artery disease, when a region of cardiac muscle is deprived of its normal blood supply, the K^+ concentration in the interstitial fluid that surrounds the affected muscle cells rises because K^+ is lost from the inadequately perfused (**ischemic**) cells. The action potentials in some of these cells may then be converted from fast to slow responses (see Figure 2-18). An experimental conversion from a fast to a slow response through the addition of **tetrodotoxin**, which blocks fast Na^+ channels in the cardiac cell membranes, is illustrated in Figure 2-3.

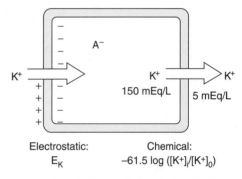

FIGURE 2-4 ■ The balance of chemical and electrostatic forces acting on a resting cardiac cell membrane, based on a 30:1 ratio of the intracellular to extracellular K^+ concentrations and the existence of a nondiffusible anion (A^- inside but not outside the cell.)

The Ionic Basis of the Resting Potential

The various phases of the cardiac action potential are associated with changes in cell membrane **permeability**, mainly to Na^+, K^+, and Ca^{++}. Changes in cell membrane permeability alter the rate of ion movement across the membrane. *The membrane permeability to a given ion defines the net quantity of the ion that will diffuse across each unit area of the membrane per unit concentration difference across the membrane.* Changes in permeability are accomplished by the opening and closing of **ion channels** that are specific for individual ions.

Just as with all other cells in the body, the concentration of K^+ inside a cardiac muscle cell, $[K^+]_i$, greatly exceeds the concentration outside the cell, $[K^+]_o$, as shown in Figure 2-4. The reverse concentration gradient exists for free Na^+ and for free Ca^{++} (not bound to protein). Estimates of the extracellular and intracellular concentrations of Na^+, K^+, and Ca^{++}, and of the

equilibrium potentials (defined later) for these ions, are compiled in Table 2-1.

The resting cell membrane is relatively permeable to K^+ but much less so to Na^+ and Ca^{++}. Hence K^+ tends to diffuse from the inside to the outside of the cell, in the direction of the concentration gradient, as shown on the right side of the cell in Figure 2-4.

Any flux of K^+ that occurs during phase 4 takes place through certain specific **K^+ channels**. Several types of K^+ channels exist in cardiac cell membranes. Some of these channels are controlled (i.e., opened and closed) by the transmembrane voltage, whereas others are controlled by some chemical signal (e.g., a neurotransmitter). The specific K^+ channel through which K^+ passes during phase 4 is a voltage-regulated channel called i_{K1}, which is an **inwardly rectifying K^+ current,** as explained later (Figure 2-5). Many of the

TABLE 2-1

Intracellular and Extracellular Ion Concentrations and Equilibrium Potentials in Cardiac Muscle Cells

ION	EXTRACELLULAR CONCENTRATIONS (mM)	INTRACELLULAR CONCENTRA-TIONS (mM)*	EQUILIBRIUM POTENTIAL (mV)
Na$^+$	145	10	71
K$^+$	4	135	-94
Ca^{++}	2	1×10^{-4}	132

Modified from Ten Eick RE, Baumgarten CM, Singer DH: *Prog Cardiovasc Dis* 24:157, 1981.

*The intracellular concentrations are estimates of the free concentrations in the cytoplasm.

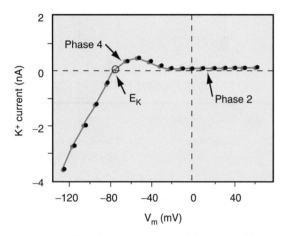

FIGURE 2-5 ■ The K$^+$ currents recorded from a rabbit ventricular myocyte when the potential was changed from a holding potential of –80 mV to various test potentials. Positive values along the vertical axis represent outward currents; negative values represent inward currents. The V$_m$ coordinate of the point of intersection (*open circle*) of the curve with the X axis is the reversal potential; it denotes the Nernst equilibrium potential *(E$_K$)* at which the chemical and electrostatic forces are equal. *(Redrawn from Giles WR, Imaizumi Y: Comparison of potassium currents in rabbit atrial and ventricular cells.* J Physiol [Lond] *405:123, 1988.)*

anions (labeled A$^-$) inside the cell, such as the proteins, are not free to diffuse out with the K$^+$ (see Figure 2-4). Therefore, as the K$^+$ diffuses out of the cell and the A$^-$ remains behind, the cation deficiency causes the interior of the cell to become electronegative.

Therefore, two opposing forces regulate K$^+$ movement across the cell membrane. A chemical force, based on the concentration gradient, results in the net outward diffusion of K$^+$. The counterforce is electrostatic; the positively charged K ions are attracted to the interior of the cell by the negative potential that exists there, as shown on the left side of the cell in Figure 2-4. If the system comes into equilibrium, the chemical and electrostatic forces are equal.

This equilibrium is expressed by the **Nernst equation** for K$^+$, as follows:

$$E_K = 61.5 \log ([K^+]_o / [K^+]_i) \qquad (1)$$

The term to the right of the equals sign represents chemical potential difference at the body temperature of 37° C. The term to the left, E$_K$, called the **potassium equilibrium potential,** represents the electrostatic potential difference that would exist across the cell membrane if K$^+$ were the only diffusible ion.

An experimental disturbance in the equilibrium between electrostatic and chemical forces imposed by **voltage clamping** would cause K$^+$ to move through the K$^+$ channels (see Figure 2-5). If the transmembrane potential (V$_m$) were clamped at a level negative to E$_K$, the electrostatic force would exceed the diffusional force, and K$^+$ would be attracted into the cell (i.e., the K$^+$ current would be **inward**). Conversely, if V$_m$ were clamped at a level positive to E$_K$, the diffusional force would exceed the electrostatic force, and K$^+$ would leave the cell (i.e., the K$^+$ current would be **outward**).

When the measured concentrations of [K$^+$]$_i$ and [K$^+$]$_o$ for mammalian myocardial cells are substituted into the Nernst equation, the calculated value of E$_K$ equals about –94 mV (see Table 2-1). This value is close to, but slightly more negative than, the resting potential actually measured in myocardial cells. Therefore the electrostatic force is slightly weaker than the chemical (diffusional) force, and K$^+$ tends to leave the resting cell.

The balance of forces acting on Na$^+$ is entirely different from that acting on the K$^+$ in resting cardiac cells. The intracellular Na$^+$ concentration, [Na$^+$]$_i$, is much lower than the extracellular Na$^+$ concentration, [Na$^+$]$_o$. At 37° C, the **sodium equilibrium potential**, E$_{Na}$, expressed by the Nernst equation is as follows:

$$E_{Na} = 61.5 \log ([Na^+]_o / [Na^+]_i) \qquad (2)$$

For cardiac cells, E$_{Na}$ is about 70 mV (see Table 2-1). Therefore at equilibrium a transmembrane potential of about +71 mV would be necessary to counterbalance the chemical potential for Na$^+$.

However, the actual voltage of the resting cell is just the opposite. The resting membrane potential of cardiac cells is about −90 mV (see Figure 2-1A). Hence both chemical and electrostatic forces favor entry of extra-cellular Na$^+$ into the cell. The influx of Na$^+$ through the cell membrane is small because the permeability of the resting membrane to Na$^+$ is very low. Nevertheless, it is mainly this small inward current of Na$^+$ that causes the potential of the resting cell membrane to be slightly less negative than the value predicted by the Nernst equation for K$^+$.

The steady inward leak of Na$^+$ would gradually depolarize the resting cell were it not for the metabolic pump that continuously extrudes Na$^+$ from the cell interior and pumps in K$^+$. The metabolic pump involves the enzyme **Na$^+$,K$^+$-ATPase,** which is located in the cell membrane. Pump operation requires the expenditure of metabolic energy because the pump moves Na$^+$ against both a chemical gradient and an electrostatic gradient. Increases in [Na$^+$]$_i$ or in [K$^+$]$_o$ accelerate the activity of the pump. The quantity of Na$^+$ extruded by the pump exceeds the quantity of K$^+$ transferred into the cell by a 3:2 ratio. Therefore, the pump itself tends to create a potential difference across the cell membrane, and thus it is termed an **electrogenic pump**. If the pump is partially inhibited, as by **digitalis**, the resting membrane potential becomes less negative than normal.

The dependence of the transmembrane potential, V$_m$, on the intracellular and extracellular concentrations of K$^+$ and Na$^+$ and on the conductances (g$_K$ and g$_{Na}$, respectively) of these ions is described by the **chord conductance equation,** as follows:

$$V_m = [E_K(g_K/g_{Na} + g_K)] + [E_{Na}(g_{Na}/g_{Na} + g_K)] \quad (3)$$

For a given ion (X), the conductance (g$_x$) is defined as the ratio of the current (i$_x$) carried by that ion to the difference between the V$_m$ and the Nernst equilibrium potential (E$_x$) for that ion; that is,

$$g_x = i_x / (V_m - E_x) \quad (4)$$

The chord conductance equation reveals that the relative, not the absolute, conductances to Na$^+$ and K$^+$ determine the resting potential. In the resting cardiac cell, g$_K$ is about 100 times greater than g$_{Na}$. Therefore the chord conductance equation reduces essentially to the Nernst equation for K$^+$.

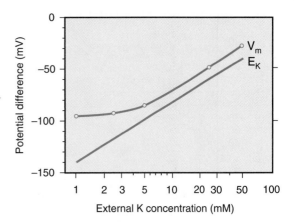

FIGURE 2-6 ■ The transmembrane potential (V$_m$) of a cardiac muscle fiber varies inversely with the potassium (K) concentration of the external medium *(curved line)*. The *straight line* represents the change in transmembrane potential predicted by the Nernst equation for E$_K$. *(Redrawn from Page E: The electrical potential difference across the cell membrane of heart muscle. Biophysical considerations.* Circulation 26:582, 1962.)

When the ratio [K$^+$]$_o$/[K$^+$]$_i$ is increased experimentally by a rise in [K$^+$]$_o$, the measured value of V$_m$ (Figure 2-6) approximates that predicted by the Nernst equation for K$^+$. For extra-cellular K$^+$ concentrations above 5 mM, the measured values correspond closely with the predicted values. The measured levels of V$_m$ are slightly less negative than those predicted by the Nernst equation because of the small but finite value of g$_{Na}$. For values of [K$^+$]$_o$ below 5 mM, the effect of the Na$^+$ gradient on the transmembrane potential becomes more important, as predicted by Equation 3. This increase in the relative importance of g$_{Na}$ accounts for the greater deviation of the measured V$_m$ from that predicted by the Nernst equation for K$^+$ at very low levels of [K$^+$]$_o$ (see Figure 2-6).

The Fast Response Depends Mainly on Voltage-Dependent Sodium Channels

Genesis of the Upstroke

Any process that abruptly depolarizes the resting membrane to a critical potential value (called the **threshold**) induces a propagated action potential. The characteristics of fast-response action potentials are shown in Figure 2-1A. The initial rapid depolarization (phase 0) is related almost exclusively to Na$^+$ influx by

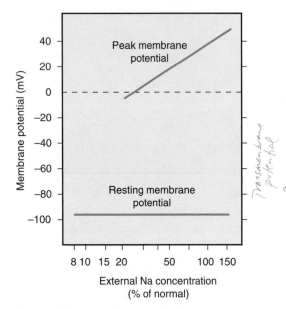

FIGURE 2-7 ■ The concentration of sodium in the external medium is a critical determinant of the amplitude of the action potential in cardiac muscle (*upper line*) but has relatively little influence on the resting potential (*lower line*). *(Redrawn from Weidmann S:* Elektrophysiologie der Herzmuskelfaser, *Bern, 1956, Verlag Hans Huber.)*

virtue of a sudden increase in g_{Na}. The action potential **overshoot** (the peak of the potential during phase 0) varies linearly with the logarithm of $[Na^+]_o$, as shown in Figure 2-7. When $[Na^+]_o$ is reduced from its normal value of about 140 mM to about 20 mM, the cell is no longer excitable.

Specific **voltage-dependent Na^+ channels** (often called **fast Na^+ channels**) exist in the cell membrane. These channels can be blocked selectively by the puffer fish toxin **tetrodotoxin** (see Figure 2-3) and by **local anesthetics**. A voltage-gated Na^+ channel is depicted in Figure 2-8; it contains an α subunit composed of four domains (I-IV) and two β subunits (only one is shown). Each domain has six transmembrane α-helical segments linked by external and internal peptide loops. Transmembrane segment 4 serves as a sensor whose conformation changes with applied voltage and is responsible for channel opening (activation). The intracellular loop that connects domains III and IV functions as the inactivation gate. After depolarization, this loop swings into the mouth of the channel to block ion conductance. The extracellular portions of

the loops that connect helices 5 and 6 in each domain form the pore region and participate in the determination of ion selectivity. The Ca^{++} channels that form the basis of the slow response (see later) are similar in overall structure to Na^+ channels but have a different ion selectivity.

The physical and chemical forces responsible for the transmembrane movements of Na^+ are explained in Figure 2-9. The regulation of Na^+ flux through the fast Na^+ channels can be understood in terms of the "gate" concept. One of these gates, the **m gate**, tends to open as V_m becomes less negative than the threshold potential and is therefore called an **activation gate**. The other, the **h gate**, tends to close as V_m becomes less negative and hence is called an **inactivation gate**. The **m** and **h** designations were originally employed by Hodgkin and Huxley in their mathematical model of ionic currents in nerve fibers.

Panel A in Figure 2-9 represents the resting state (phase 4) of a cardiac myocyte. With the cell at rest, V_m is −90 mV and the **m** gates are closed while the **h** gates are wide open. The electrostatic force in Figure 2-9A is a potential difference of 90 mV, and it is represented by the white arrow. The chemical force, based on the difference in Na^+ concentration between the outside and inside of the cell, is represented by the dark arrow. For an Na^+ concentration difference of about 130 mM, a potential difference of 60 mV (inside more positive than the outside) is necessary to counterbalance the chemical, or diffusional, force, according to the Nernst equation for Na^+ (Equation 2). Therefore we may represent the net chemical force favoring the inward movement of Na^+ in Figure 2-9 (dark arrows) as equivalent to a potential of 60 mV. With the cell at rest, the total electrochemical force favoring the inward movement of Na^+ is 150 mV (panel A). The **m** gates are closed, however, and the conductance of the resting cell membrane to Na^+ is very low. Hence, the **inward Na^+** current is negligible.

Any process that makes V_m less negative tends to open the **m** gates and thereby activates the fast Na^+ channels so that Na^+ enters the cell (Figure 2-9B) *via* the chemical and electrostatic forces. Thus, activation of the fast channels is a **voltage-dependent phenomenon**. The precise potential at which the **m** gates swing open is called the **threshold potential**. The entry of Na^+ into the interior of the cell neutralizes some of the

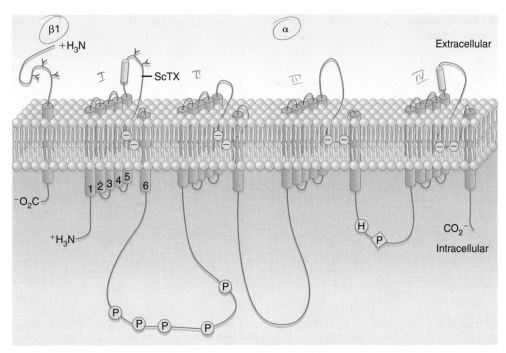

FIGURE 2-8 ■ Schematic structure of a voltage-gated Na^+ channel. The α subunit is composed of 4 domains (I-IV), each of which has 6 transmembrane helices; the N and C termini are cytoplasmic. Transmembrane segment 4 is a voltage sensor whose conformation changes with applied voltage. The 4 domains are arranged around a central pore lined by the extracellular loops of transmembrane segments 5 and 6. The β2 subunit is shown on the left. P, phosphorylation sites; ScTX, scorpion toxin binding site. *(Redrawn from Squire LR, Roberts JL, Spitzer NC, et al: Fundamental neuroscience, ed 2, San Diego, CA, Academic Press, 2002.)*

negative charges inside the cell and thereby diminishes further the transmembrane potential, V_m (Figure 2-9B).

The rapid opening of the **m** gates in the fast Na^+ channels is responsible for the large and abrupt increase in Na^+ conductance, g_{Na}, coincident with phase 0 of the action potential (see Figure 2-12). The rapid influx of Na^+ accounts for the steep upstroke of V_m during phase 0. The maximal rate of change of V_m (dV_m/dt) varies from 100 to 300 V/s in myocardial cells and from 500 to 1000 V/s in Purkinje fibers. The actual quantity of Na^+ that enters the cell is so small and occurs in such a limited portion of the cell's volume that the resulting change in the intracellular Na^+ concentration cannot be measured precisely. The chemical force remains virtually constant, and only the electrostatic force changes throughout the action potential. Hence the lengths of the dark arrows in Figure 2-9 remain constant at 60 mV, whereas the white arrows change in magnitude and direction.

As Na^+ enters the cardiac cell during phase 0, it neutralizes the negative charges inside the cell and V_m becomes less negative. When V_m becomes zero (Figure 2-9C), an electrostatic force no longer pulls Na^+ into the cell. As long as the fast Na^+ channels are open, however, Na^+ continues to enter the cell because of the large concentration gradient. This continuation of the inward Na^+ current causes the cell interior to become positively charged (Figure 2-9D). This reversal of the membrane polarity is the **overshoot** of the cardiac action potential. Such a reversal of the electrostatic gradient tends to repel the entry of Na^+ (Figure 2-9D). However, as long as the inwardly directed chemical forces exceed these outwardly directed electrostatic forces, the net flux of Na^+ is still inward, although the rate of influx is diminished.

The inward Na^+ current finally ceases when the **h** (inactivation) gates close (Figure 2-9E). The opening of the **m** gates occurs very rapidly, in about 0.1 to 0.2 milliseconds [ms], whereas the closure of the **h** gates is slower, requiring 10 ms or more. Inactivation of the fast Na$^+$ channels is completed when the **h** gates close. The **h** gates remain closed until the cell has partially repolarized during phase 3 (at about time d in Figure 2-1A). From time c to time d, the cell is in its **effective refractory period** and does not respond to excitation. This mechanism prevents a sustained, tetanic contraction of cardiac muscle that would interfere with the normal intermittent pumping action of the heart. A period of myocardial relaxation, sufficient to permit the cardiac

ventricles to fill with venous blood during each cardiac cycle, is as essential to the normal pumping action of the heart as is a strong cardiac contraction.

About midway through phase 3 (time d in Figure 2-1A), the **m** and **h** gates in some of the fast Na$^+$ channels resume the states shown in Figure 2-9A. Such channels are said to have **recovered from inactivation**. The cell can begin to respond again to excitation (Figure 2-10). Application of a suprathreshold stimulus to a region of normal myocardium during phase 3

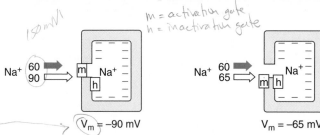
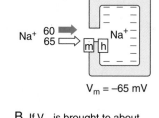
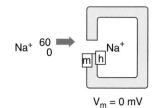

A, During phase 4, the chemical (60 mV) and electrostatic (90 mV) forces favor influx of Na$^+$ from the extracellular space. Influx is negligible, however, because the activation **(m)** gates are closed.

B, If V$_m$ is brought to about −65 V, the m gates begin to swing open, and Na$^+$ begins to enter the cell. This reduces the negative charge inside the cell. The change in V$_m$ also initiates the closure of inactivation **(h)** gates, which operate more slowly than the m gates.

C, The rapid influx of Na$^+$ rapidly decreases the negativity of V$_m$. As V$_m$ approaches 0, the electrostatic force attracting Na$^+$ into the cell is neutralized. Na$^+$ continues to enter the cell, however, because of the substantial concentration gradient, and V$_m$ begins to become positive.

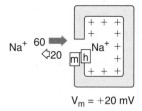
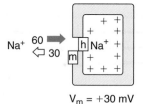

D, When V$_m$ is positive by about 20 mV, Na$^+$ continues to enter the cell, because the diffusional forces (60 mV) exceed the opposing electrostatic forces (20 mV). The influx of Na$^+$ is slow, however, because the net driving force is small, and many of the inactivation gates have already closed.

E, When V$_m$ reaches about 30 mV, the **h** gates have now all closed, and Na$^+$ influx ceases. The **h** gates remain closed until the first half of repolarization, and thus the cell is absolutely refractory during this entire period. During the second half of repolarization, the **m** and **h** gates approach the state represented by panel A, and thus the cell is relatively refractory.

FIGURE 2-9 ■ The gating of a sodium channel in a cardiac cell membrane during phase 4 (**A**) and during various stages of the action potential upstroke (**B** to **E**). The positions of the **m** and **h** gates in the fast Na$^+$ channels are shown at the various levels of V$_m$. The electrostatic forces are represented by the *white arrows,* and the chemical (diffusional) forces by the *dark arrows.*

evokes an action potential. As the stimulus is delivered progressively later during the course of phase 3, the slopes of the action potential upstrokes and the amplitudes of the evoked action potentials progressively increase. Throughout the remainder of phase 3, the cell completes its recovery from inactivation. By time e in Figure 2-1A, the **h** gates have reopened and the **m** gates have reclosed in the remaining fast Na$^+$ channels, as shown in Figure 2-9A.

Statistical Characteristics of the "Gate" Concept
The patch-clamp technique has made it possible to measure ionic currents through single membrane channels. The individual channels open and close repeatedly in a random manner. This process is

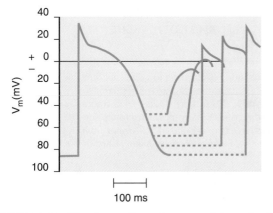

FIGURE 2-10 ■ The changes in action potential amplitude and slope of the upstroke as action potentials are initiated at different stages of the relative refractory period of the preceding excitation. *(Redrawn from Rosen MR, Wit AL, Hoffman BF: Electrophysiology and pharmacology of cardiac arrhythmias. I. Cellular electrophysiology of the mammalian heart. Am Heart J 88:380, 1974.)*

illustrated in Figure 2-11, which shows the current flow through single Na$^+$ channels in a myocardial cell. To the left of the arrow, the membrane potential was clamped at −85 mV. At the arrow, the potential was suddenly changed to −45 mV, at which value it was held for the remainder of the record.

Figure 2-11 indicates that immediately after the membrane potential was made less negative, one Na$^+$ channel opened three times in sequence. It remained open for about 2 or 3 ms each time and closed for about 4 or 5 ms between openings. In the open state, it allowed 1.5 pA of current to pass. During the first and second openings of this channel, a second channel also opened, but for periods of only 1 ms. During the brief times that the two channels were open simultaneously, the total current was 3 pA. After the first channel closed for the third time, both channels remained closed for the rest of the recording, even though the membrane was held constant at −45 mV.

The overall change in ionic conductance of the entire cell membrane at any given time reflects the number of channels that are open at that time. Because the individual channels open and close randomly, the overall membrane conductance represents the statistical probability of the open or closed state of the individual channels. The temporal characteristics of the activation process then represent the time course of the increasing probability that the specific channels will be open, rather than the kinetic characteristics of the activation gates in the individual channels. Similarly, the temporal characteristics of inactivation reflect the time course of the decreasing probability that the channels will be open and not the kinetic characteristics of the inactivation gates in the individual channels.

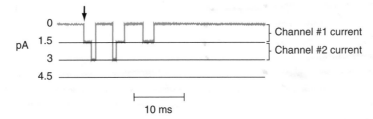

FIGURE 2-11 ■ The current flow (in picoamperes) through two individual Na$^+$ channels in a cultured cardiac cell, recorded by the patch-clamping technique. The membrane potential had been held at −85 mV but was suddenly changed to −45 mV at the *arrow* and held at this potential for the remainder of the record. *(Redrawn from Cachelin AB, DePeyer JE, Kokubun S, et al: Sodium channels in cultured cardiac cells. J Physiol 340:389, 1983.)*

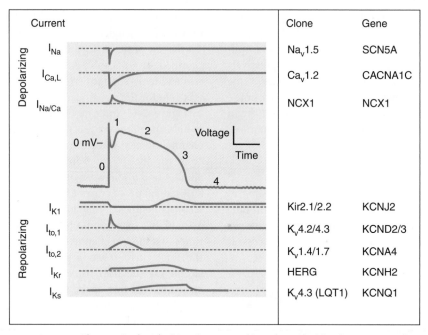

FIGURE 2-12 ■ Changes in depolarizing (*upper panels*) and repolarizing ion currents during the various phases of the action potential in a fast-response cardiac ventricular cell. The inward currents include the fast Na^+ and L-type Ca^{++} currents. Outward currents are I_{K1}, I_{to} and the rapid (I_{Kr}) and slow (I_{Ks}) delayed rectifier K^+ currents. The clones and respective genes for the principal ionic currents are also tabulated. *(Redrawn from Tomaselli G, Marbán E: Electrophysiological remodeling in hypertrophy and heart failure.* Cardiovasc Res *42:270. 1999.)*

Genesis of Early Repolarization

In many cardiac cells that have a prominent plateau, phase 1 constitutes an early, brief period of limited repolarization between the end of the action potential upstroke and the beginning of the plateau (Figure 2-12). Phase 1 reflects the activation of a **transient outward current**, i_{to}, mostly carried by K^+. Activation of these K^+ channels leads to a brief efflux of K^+ from the cell because the interior of the cell is positively charged and because the internal K^+ concentration greatly exceeds the external concentration (see Table 2-1). This brief efflux of K^+ brings about the brief, limited repolarization (phase **1**).

Phase 1 is prominent in Purkinje fibers (see Figure 2-3) and in epicardial fibers from the ventricular myocardium (Figure 2-13); it is much less developed in endocardial fibers. When the basic cycle length at which the epicardial fibers are stimulated is increased from 300 to 2000 ms, phase 1 becomes more pronounced and the action potential duration is increased substantially. The same increase in basic cycle length has no effect on the early portion of the plateau in endocardial fibers, and it has a smaller effect on the action potential duration than it does in epicardial fibers (see Figure 2-13).

Genesis of the Plateau

During the plateau (phase 2) of the action potential, Ca^{++} enters the cell through calcium channels that activate and inactivate much more slowly than do the fast Na^+ channels. During phase 2 (see Figure 2-12), this influx of Ca^{++} is balanced by the efflux of an equal amount of K^+. The K^+ exits through various specific K^+ channels, as described in the next section.

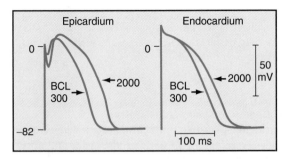

FIGURE 2-13 ■ Action potentials recorded from canine epicardial and endocardial strips driven at basic cycle lengths (BCLs) of 300 and 2000 ms. *(From Litovsky SH, Antzelevitch C: Rate dependence of action potential duration and refractoriness in canine ventricular endocardium differs from that of epicardium: role of the transient outward current* J Am Coll Cardiol 14:1053, 1989.)

Ca⁺⁺ Conductance during the Plateau

The Ca^{++} channels are voltage-regulated channels that are activated as V_m becomes progressively less negative during the upstroke of the action potential. Two types of Ca^{++} channels (**L-type** and **T-type**) have been identified in cardiac tissues. Some of their important characteristics are illustrated in Figure 2-14, which displays the Ca^{++} currents generated by voltage-clamping an isolated atrial myocyte. Note that when V_m is suddenly increased to +30 mV from a holding potential of −30 mV (lower panel), an inward Ca^{++} current (denoted by a downward deflection) is activated. After the inward current reaches maximum (in the downward direction), it returns toward zero very gradually (i.e., the channels inactivate very slowly). Thus, current that passes through these channels is **long lasting**, and they have been designated L-type channels. They are the predominant type of Ca^{++} channels in the heart, and they are activated during the action potential upstroke when V_m reaches about −30 mV. The L-type channels are blocked by Ca^{++} **channel antagonists**, such as verapamil, nifedipine, and diltiazem.

The T-type (transient) Ca^{++} channels are much less abundant in the heart. They are activated at more negative potentials (about −70 mV) than are the L-type channels. Note in Figure 2-14 (upper panel) that when V_m is suddenly increased to −20 mV from a holding potential of −80 mV, a Ca^{++} current is activated and then is inactivated very quickly.

Opening of the Ca^{++} channels is reflected by an increase in Ca^{++} current ($I_{Ca,L}$), that begins during the

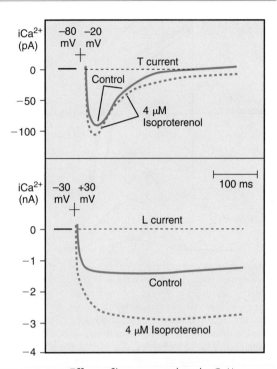

FIGURE 2-14 ■ Effects of isoproterenol on the Ca^{++} currents conducted by T-type (*upper panel*) and L-type (*lower panel*) Ca^{++} channels in canine atrial myocytes. *Upper panel*, Potential changed from −80 to −20 mV; *lower panel*, potential changed from −30 to +30 mV. *(Redrawn from Bean BP: Two kinds of calcium channels in canine atrial cells. Differences in kinetics, selectivity, and pharmacology.* J Gen Physiol 86:1, 1985.)

later phase of the upstroke of the action potential (Figure 2-15). When the Ca^{++} channels open, Ca^{++} enters the cell throughout the plateau because the intracellular Ca^{++} concentration is much less than the extracellular Ca^{++} concentration (see Table 2-1). The Ca^{++} that enters the myocardial cell during the plateau is involved in **excitation-contraction coupling**, as described in Chapter 4.

Neurohumoral factors may influence g_{Ca}. An increase in g_{Ca} by **catecholamines**, such as **isoproterenol** and **norepinephrine**, is probably the principal mechanism by which catecholamines enhance cardiac muscle contractility. Catecholamines interact with β-**adrenergic receptors** located on cardiac cell membranes. This interaction stimulates the membrane-bound enzyme, **adenylyl cyclase**, which raises the intracellular concentration of **cyclic AMP** adenosine monophosphate) (see Figure 4-8). This change enhances the voltage-dependent activation

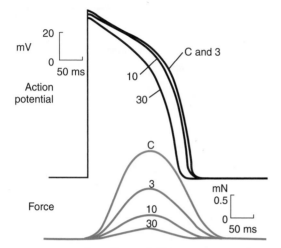

FIGURE 2-15 ■ The effects of diltiazem, a Ca⁺⁺ channel blocking drug, on the action potentials (in millivolts) and isometric contractile forces (in millinewtons) recorded from an isolated papillary muscle of a guinea pig. The tracings were recorded under control conditions (C) and in the presence of diltiazem, in concentrations of 3, 10, and 30 µmol/L. *(Redrawn from Hirth C, Borchard U, Hafner D: Effects of the calcium antagonist diltiazem on action potentials, slow response and force of contraction in different cardiac tissues.* J Mol Cell Cardiol *15:799, 1983.)*

of the L-type Ca⁺⁺ channels in cell membrane (see Figure 2-14, lower panel) and thus augments Ca⁺⁺ influx into the cells from the interstitial fluid. However, catecholamines have little effect on the Ca⁺⁺ current through the T-type channels (see Figure 2-14, upper panel).

The Ca⁺⁺ channel antagonists decrease g_{Ca} during the action potential. By reducing the amount of Ca⁺⁺ that enters the myocardial cells during phase 2, these drugs diminish cardiac contractility and are **negative inotropic agents** (see Figure 2-15). These drugs also diminish the contraction of the vascular smooth muscle by suppressing Ca⁺⁺ entry caused by depolarization or by neurotransmitters such as norepinephrine, and thereby induce arterial vasodilation. This effect reduces the counterforce (**afterload**) that opposes the propulsion of blood from the ventricles into the arterial system, as explained in Chapters 4 and 5. Hence vasodilator drugs, such as the Ca⁺⁺ channel antagonists, are often referred to as **afterload reducing drugs**. This ability to diminish the counterforce

enables the heart to provide a more adequate cardiac output, despite the direct depressant effect that these drugs exert on myocardial fibers.

K⁺ Conductance during the Plateau

During the plateau of the action potential, the concentration gradient for K⁺ between the inside and outside of the cell is virtually the same as it is during phase 4, but the V_m is positive. Therefore the chemical and electrostatic forces greatly favor the efflux of K⁺ from the cell during the plateau (see Figure 2-12). If g_{K1} were the same during the plateau as it is during phase 4, the efflux of K⁺ during phase 2 would greatly exceed the influx of Ca⁺⁺, and a plateau could not be sustained. However, as V_m approaches and attains positive values near the end of phase 0, g_{K1} suddenly decreases as does I_{K1} (see Figure 2-12).

The changes in g_{K1} during the different phases of the action potential may be appreciated through an examination of the current-voltage relationship for the I_{K1} channels (the channels that mainly determine g_K during phase 4). An example of this relationship in an isolated ventricular myocyte is shown in Figure 2-5. Note that the current-voltage curve intersects the voltage axis at a V_m of about −80 mV. The absence of ionic current flow at the intersection indicates that the electrostatic forces must have been equal to the chemical (diffusional) forces (see Figure 2-4) at this potential. Thus in this isolated ventricular cell, the Nernst equilibrium potential (E_K) for K⁺ was −80 mV; in a myocyte in the intact ventricle, E_K is normally about −95 mV.

When the membrane potential was clamped at levels negative to −80 mV in this isolated cell (see Figure 2-5), the electrostatic forces exceeded the chemical forces and an inward K⁺ current was induced (as denoted by the negative values of K⁺ current over this range of voltages). Note also that for V_m more negative than −80 mV, the curve has a steep slope. Thus when V_m equals or is negative to E_K, a small change in V_m induces a substantial change in K⁺ current; that is, g_{K1} is large. During phase 4, the V_m of a myocardial cell is slightly less negative than E_K (see Figure 2-6).

When the transmembrane potential of this isolated myocyte was clamped at levels less negative than −70 mV (see Figure 2-5), the chemical forces exceeded the electrostatic forces. Therefore the net K^+ currents were outward (as denoted by the positive values along the corresponding section of the Y axis).

During phase 4 of the cardiac cycle, the driving force for K^+ (the difference between V_m and E_K) favored the efflux of K^+, mainly through the i_{K1} channels. Note that for V_m values positive to -80 mV, the curve is relatively flat; this is especially pronounced for values of V_m positive to -40 mV. A given change in voltage causes only a small change in ionic current (i.e., g_{K1} is small). Thus g_{K1} is small for outwardly directed K^+ currents but substantial for inwardly directed K^+ currents; that is, the i_{K1} current is **inwardly rectified**. The rectification is most marked over the plateau (phase 2) range of transmembrane potentials (see Figures 2-5 and 2-12). *This characteristic prevents excessive loss of K^+ during the prolonged plateau, during which the electrostatic and chemical forces both favor the efflux of K^+.*

The **delayed rectifier K^+ channels**, which conduct the i_K current, are also activated at voltages that prevail toward the end of phase 0. However, activation proceeds very slowly, over several hundreds of milliseconds. Hence activation of these channels tends to increase I_{Kr} (see next section) slowly and slightly during phase 2. These channels play only a minor role during phase 2, but they do contribute to repolarization (phase 3), as described in the next section. The action potential plateau persists as long as the efflux of charge carried by certain cations (mainly K^+) is balanced by the influx of charge carried by other cations (mainly Ca^{++}). The effects of altering this balance are demonstrated by administration of diltiazem, a calcium channel antagonist. Figure 2-15 shows that with increasing concentrations of diltiazem, the plateau voltage becomes less positive and the duration of the plateau diminishes. Similarly, administration of certain K^+ channel antagonists prolongs the action potential substantially.

Genesis of Final Repolarization

The process of final repolarization (phase 3) starts at the end of phase 2, when the efflux of K^+ from the cardiac cell begins to exceed the influx of Ca^{++}. At least four outward K^+ currents (I_{to}, I_{Kr}, I_{Ks}, and I_{K1}) contribute to the rapid repolarization (phase 3) of the cardiac cell (see Figure 2-12).

The transient outward current (I_{to}) not only accounts for the brief, partial repolarization (phase 1), as previously described, but also helps determine the duration of the plateau; hence it also helps initiate repolarization. For example, the transient outward current is much more pronounced in atrial than in ventricular myocytes. In atrial cells, therefore, the outward K^+ current exceeds the inward Ca^{++} current early in the plateau, whereas the outward and inward currents remain equal for a much longer time in ventricular myocytes. Hence the plateau of the action potential is much less pronounced in atrial than in ventricular myocytes (Figure 2-16).

The delayed rectifier K^+ currents (I_{Kr} and I_{Ks}) are activated near the end of phase 0, but activation is very slow. Therefore these outward I_K currents tend to increase gradually throughout the plateau. Concurrently, the Ca^{++} channels are inactivated after the beginning of the plateau, and therefore the inward Ca^{++} current decreases. As the efflux of K^+ begins to exceed the influx of Ca^{++}, V_m becomes progressively less positive, and repolarization occurs. Two types of delayed rectifier K^+ currents, I_K, are present in cardiac myocytes. The distinction is based mainly on the speed of activation. The currents that activate more rapidly are designated I_{Kr}, whereas the currents that are activated more slowly are designated I_{Ks}. The action potentials recorded from myocytes in the endocardial, central, and epicardial regions of the left ventricle differ substantially in duration. Figure 2-13 illustrates some of the differences that prevail in the epicardial and endocardial layers of the ventricle. Such differences are induced, at least in part, by differences in the distributions of these two types of delayed rectifying I_K channels.

The **inwardly rectified K^+ current** (i_{K1}) contributes substantially to the later repolarization phase. As the net efflux of cations causes V_m to become more negative during phase 3, the conductance of the channels that carry the i_{K1} current progressively increases. This increase is reflected by the hump that is evident in the flat portion of the current-voltage curve at V_m values between -20 and -80 mV in Figure 2-5. Thus as V_m passes through this range of values less negative than E_K, the outward K^+ current increases and thereby accelerates repolarization.

Restoration of Ionic Concentrations

The excess Na^+ that entered the cell rapidly during phase 0 and more slowly throughout the action potential is removed from the cell by the action of the enzyme Na^+,K^+-ATPase. This enzyme ejects Na^+ in exchange for the K^+ that had exited mainly during phases 2 and 3.

Similarly, most of the excess Ca^{++} that had entered the cell during phase 2 is eliminated by a Na^+/Ca^{++} antiporter, which exchanges 3 Na^+ for 1 Ca^{++}. However, a small fraction of the Ca^{++} is eliminated by an adenosine triphosphate (ATP)–driven Ca^{++} pump (see Figure 4-8).

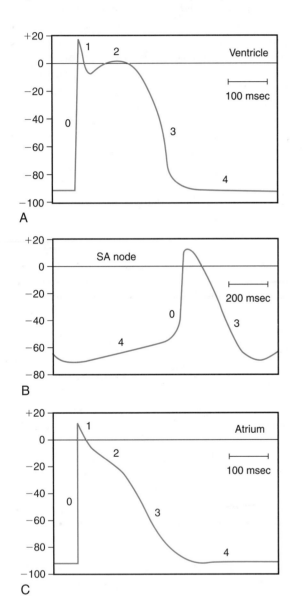

FIGURE 2-16 ▪ Typical action potentials (in millivolts) recorded from cells in the ventricle (**A**), sinoatrial (SA) node (**B**), and atrium (**C**). Note that the time calibration in **B** differs from that in **A** and **C**. *(From Hoffman BF, Cranefield PF: Electrophysiology of the heart, New York, McGraw-Hill, 1960.)*

CLINICAL BOX

The cardiac action potential is generated by the interplay among ionic channels whose currents are produced at appropriate times and voltages (see Figure 2-12). Long QT syndrome (LQTS) is a condition that can lead to cardiac arrhythmias. LQTS can be detected by a prolonged QT interval on an electrocardiogram. Molecular genetic studies show that mutations in genes encoding cardiac ion channels are linked to congenital LQTS. Mutations in *KCNQ1*, *KCNH2*, and *SCN5A* account for most of the inherited forms of LQTS. Mutations in these genes alter the function of the corresponding cardiac ion channel proteins (Kv4.3, hERG, and Nav1.5). Thus, loss-of-function mutation of the *KCNQ1* gene alters the KVLQT1 protein in the K_s channel, resulting in the LQT1 syndrome. A gain-of-function mutation of the *SCN5A* gene that produces the Na_v 1.5 protein for the fast Na^+ channel underlies the LQT3 syndrome. Animal and stem cell models of LQTS based on hERG channel mutations show reduced ionic currents, prolonged action potentials, and early afterdepolarizations. Inherited LQTS is relatively rare, but there is an acquired form of LQTS that is quite common. Acquired LQTS is due to the blockade of hERG potassium channels by drugs.

Ionic Basis of the Slow Response

Fast-response action potentials (see Figure 2-1A) may be considered to consist of four principal components: an upstroke (phase 0), an early repolarization (phase 1), a plateau (phase 2), and a period of final repolarization (phase 3). In the slow response (see Figure 2-1,B), phase 0 is much less steep, phase 1 is absent, phase 2 is brief and not flat, and phase 3 is not separated very distinctly from phase 2. In the fast response, the upstroke is produced by the influx of Na^+ through the fast channels (see Figure 2-12).

When the fast Na^+ channels are blocked, slow responses may be generated in the same fibers under appropriate conditions. The Purkinje fiber action potentials shown in Figure 2-3 clearly exhibit the two response types. In the control tracing (panel A), a prominent notch (phase 1) separates the upstroke from the plateau. Action potential A in Figure 2-3 is a typical fast-response action potential. In action potentials in panels B to E, progressively larger quantities of tetrodotoxin were added to the bathing solution to gradually block the fast Na^+ channels. The sharp upstroke becomes progressively less prominent in action potentials in panels B to D, and it disappears entirely in panel E. Thus, tetrodotoxin had a pronounced effect on the steep upstroke and only a negligible influence on the plateau. With elimination of the steep upstroke (panel E), the action potential resembles a typical slow response.

Certain cells in the heart, notably those in the SA and AV nodes, are normally slow-response fibers. In such fibers, depolarization is achieved by the inward current of Ca^{++} through the Ca^{++} channels. These ionic events closely resemble those that occur during the plateau of fast-response action potentials.

CONDUCTION IN CARDIAC FIBERS DEPENDS ON LOCAL CIRCUIT CURRENTS

The propagation of an action potential in a cardiac muscle fiber by local circuit currents is similar to the process that occurs in nerve and skeletal muscle fibers. In Figure 2-17, consider that the left half of the cardiac fiber has already been depolarized, whereas the right half is still in the resting state. The fluids normally in contact with the external and internal surfaces of the membrane are electrolyte solutions and are good electrical conductors. Hence current (in the abstract sense) flows from regions of higher potential to those of lower potential, denoted by the plus and minus signs, respectively. In the external fluid, current flows from right to left between the active and resting zones, and it flows in the reverse direction intracellularly. In electrolyte solutions, current is caused by a movement of cations in one direction and anions in the opposite direction. At the cell exterior, for example, cations flow from right to left, and anions from left to right (Figure 2-17). In the cell interior, the opposite migrations occur. These local currents tend to depolarize the region of the resting fibers adjacent to the border. Repetition of this process causes propagation of the excitation wave along the length of the cardiac fiber.

For propagation of the impulse from one cell to another, consider the left half of Figure 2-17 a depolarized cell and the right half a cell in the resting state. When the wave of depolarization reaches the end of the cell, the impulse is conducted to adjacent cells through gap junctions or nexuses (see Figures 4-2 and 4-3). Gap junctions are preferentially located at the ends of the cell and are rather sparse along lateral cell borders. Therefore, impulses pass more readily longitudinally (isotropic) than laterally from cell to cell (anisotropic). Gap junction channels are composed of proteins called connexins that form electrical connections between cells. Connexins vary in their composition and in their tissue distribution within the heart. Each cell synthesizes a hemichannel consisting of six connexons arranged like barrel staves. The hemichannel is transported to the gap junction locus on the cell membrane, where it docks with a hemichannel from an adjacent cell to form an ion channel. These channels are rather nonselective in their permeability to ions and have a low electrical resistance that allows ionic current to pass from one cell to another. The electrical resistance of gap junctions is similar to that of cytoplasm. The flow of charge from cell to cell follows the principles of local circuit currents and therefore allows intercellular propagation of the impulse.

Conduction of the Fast Response

In the fast response, the fast Na^+ channels are activated when the transmembrane potential is suddenly brought

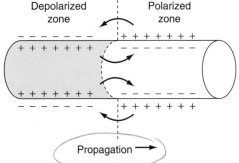

FIGURE 2-17 ■ The role of local currents in the propagation of a wave of excitation down a cardiac fiber.

Higher potential   Lower potential

from a resting value of about −90 mV to the threshold value of about −70 mV. The inward Na^+ current then depolarizes the cell very rapidly at that site. This portion of the fiber becomes part of the depolarized zone, and the border is displaced accordingly (to the right in Figure 2-17). The same process then begins at the new border.

At any given point on the fiber, the greater the **amplitude** and the greater the **rate of change of potential** (dV_m/dt) of the action potential during phase 0, the more rapid is the conduction down the fiber. The amplitude of the action potential equals the difference in potential between the fully depolarized and the fully polarized regions of the cell interior (see Figure 2-17). The magnitude of the local currents is proportional to this potential difference. Because these local currents shift the potential of the resting zone toward the threshold value, they are the local stimuli that depolarize the adjacent resting portion of the fiber to its threshold potential. *The greater the potential difference between the depolarized and polarized regions* (i.e., the greater the amplitude of the action potential), *the more efficacious are the local stimuli, and the more rapidly the wave of depolarization is propagated down the fiber.*

The rate of change of potential (dV_m/dt) during phase 0 is also an important determinant of the conduction velocity. The reason can be appreciated by referring again to Figure 2-17. If the active portion of the fiber depolarized very gradually, the local currents across the border between the depolarized and polarized regions would be very small. Thus the resting region adjacent to the active zone would be depolarized very slowly, and consequently each new section of the fiber would require more time to reach threshold.

The level of the resting membrane potential is also an important determinant of conduction velocity. This factor operates through its influence on the amplitude and maximal slope of the action potential. The resting potential may vary for several reasons: (1) it can be altered experimentally through varying of $[K^+]_o$ (see Figure 2-6); (2) in cardiac fibers that are intrinsically automatic, V_m becomes progressively less negative during phase 4 (see Figure 2-16B); and (3) during a premature excitation, repolarization may not have been completed when the next excitation arrives (see Figure 2-10). In general, the less negative the level of V_m, the less is the velocity of impulse propagation, regardless of the reason for the change in V_m.

The results of an experiment in which the resting V_m of a bundle of Purkinje fibers was varied by altering the value of $[K^+]_o$ are shown in Figure 2-18. When $[K^+]_o$ was 3 mM (panels A and F), the resting V_m was −82 mV and the slope of phase 0 was steep. At the end of phase 0, the overshoot attained a value of 30 mV. Hence the amplitude of the action potential was 112 mV. When $[K^+]_o$ was increased gradually to 16 mM (panels B to E), the resting V_m became progressively less negative. Concomitantly, the amplitudes and durations of the action potentials and the steepness of

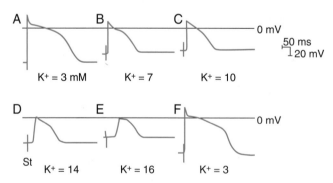

FIGURE 2-18 ■ The effect of changes in external potassium (K^+) concentration on the transmembrane action potentials recorded from a Purkinje fiber. The fiber bundle was stimulated at some distance from the impaled cell, and the stimulus artifact (St) appears as a biphasic spike to the left of the upstroke of the action potential. The time from this artifact to the beginning of phase 0 is inversely proportional to the conduction velocity. The *horizontal lines* near the peaks of the action potentials denote 0 mV. *(From Myerburg RJ, Lazzara R. In Fisch E, editor:* Complex electrocardiography, *Philadelphia, 1973, FA Davis.)*

the upstrokes all diminished. As a consequence, the conduction velocity diminished progressively, as indicated by the distances from the stimulus artifacts to the upstrokes. At the $[K^+]_o$ levels of 14 and 16 mM (panels D and E), the resting V_m had attained levels sufficient to inactivate all the fast Na^+ channels. The action potentials in panels D and E are characteristic slow responses, mediated by the inward Ca^{++} current. When the $[K^+]_o$ concentration of 3 mM was reestablished (panel F), the action potential was again characteristic of the normal fast response (as in panel A).

CLINICAL BOX

Most of the experimentally induced changes in transmembrane potential shown in Figure 2-18 also take place in patients with **coronary artery disease**. When blood flow to a region of the myocardium is diminished, the supply of oxygen and metabolic substrates delivered to the ischemic tissues is insufficient. The Na^+,K^+-ATPase in the membrane of the cardiac myocytes requires considerable metabolic energy to maintain the normal transmembrane exchanges of Na^+ and K^+. When blood flow is inadequate, the activity of the Na^+,K^+-ATPase is impaired, and the ischemic myocytes gain excess Na^+ and lose K^+ to the surrounding interstitial space. Consequently, the K^+ concentration in the extracellular fluid surrounding the ischemic myocytes is elevated, and therefore the myocytes are affected by the elevated K^+ concentration in much the same way as was the myocyte depicted in Figure 2-18. Such changes may lead to serious aberrations of cardiac rhythm and conduction.

Conduction of the Slow Response

Local circuits (see Figure 2-17) are also responsible for propagation of the slow response. However, the characteristics of the conduction process differ quantitatively from those of the fast response. The threshold potential is about −40 mV for the slow response, and conduction is much slower than for the fast response. The conduction velocities of the slow responses in the SA and AV nodes are about 0.02 to 0.1 m/s. The fast-response conduction velocities are about 0.3 to 1 m/s for myocardial cells and 1 to 4 m/s for the specialized conducting fibers in the atria and ventricles. Conduction in slow-response fibers is more likely to be blocked

than conduction in fast-response fibers. Also, impulses in slow-response fibers cannot be conducted at such rapid repetition rates.

CARDIAC EXCITABILITY DEPENDS ON THE ACTIVATION AND INACTIVATION OF SPECIFIC CURRENTS

Detailed knowledge of cardiac excitability is essential because of the rapid development of artificial pacemakers and other electrical devices for correcting serious disturbances of rhythm. The excitability characteristics of cardiac cells differ considerably, depending on whether the action potentials are fast or slow responses.

Fast Response

Once the fast response has been initiated, the depolarized cell is no longer excitable until about the middle of the period of final repolarization (see Figures 2-1A, 2-10). The interval from the beginning of the action potential until the fiber is able to conduct another action potential is called the **effective refractory period.** In the fast response, this period extends from the beginning of phase 0 to a point in phase 3 when repolarization has reached about −50 mV (time c to time d in Figure 2-1A). At about this value of V_m, some fast channels have recovered sufficiently from inactivation to permit a feeble response to stimulation.

Full excitability is not regained until the cardiac fiber has been fully repolarized (time e in Figure 2-1A). During period d to e in the figure, an action potential may be evoked, but only when the stimulus is stronger than one that could elicit a response during phase 4. Period d to e is called the **relative refractory period.**

When a fast response is evoked during the relative refractory period of a previous excitation, its characteristics vary with the membrane potential that exists at the time of stimulation. The nature of this voltage dependency is illustrated in Figure 2-10. As the fiber is stimulated later and later in the relative refractory period, the amplitude of the response and the rate of rise of the upstroke increase progressively. As a consequence of the greater amplitude and upstroke slope of the evoked response, the propagation velocity increases as the cell is stimulated later in the relative refractory period. Once the fiber is fully repolarized, the response is constant no matter what time in phase 4 the stimulus is applied. By the end of phase 3, the fast Na$^+$ channels recover fully from inactivation after several milliseconds in fully repolarized cells. This reflects the fact that recovery from inactivation depends on time as well as voltage.

Slow Response

The relative refractory period during the slow response extends well beyond phase 3 (see Figure 2-1B). Even after the cell has completely repolarized, it may be difficult to evoke a propagated response for some time. This characteristic, called **postrepolarization refractoriness,** arises from the long time constant for recovery from inactivation.

Action potentials evoked early in the relative refractory period are small, and the upstrokes are not very steep (Figure 2-19). The amplitudes and upstroke slopes gradually increase as action potentials are elicited later and later in the relative refractory period. The recovery of full excitability is much slower than for the fast response. Impulses that arrive early in the relative refractory period are conducted much more slowly than those that arrive late in that period. The lengthy refractory periods also lead to conduction blocks. Even when slow responses recur at a low repetition rate, the fiber may be able to conduct only a fraction of those impulses.

Effects of Cycle Length

Changes in cycle length alter the action potential duration of cardiac cells and thus change their refractory periods. Consequently, the changes in cycle length are important factors in the initiation or termination of certain dysrhythmias. Changes in action potential durations produced by stepwise reductions in cycle length from 2000 to 200 ms in a Purkinje fiber are shown in Figure 2-20. Note that as the cycle length is diminished, the action potential duration decreases.

This direct correlation between action potential duration and cycle length is ascribable mainly to changes in g_K that involve the delayed rectifier K$^+$

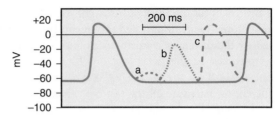

FIGURE 2-19 ■ The effects of excitation at various times after the initiation of an action potential in a slow-response fiber. In this fiber, excitation very late in phase 3 (or early in phase 4) induces a small, nonpropagated (local) response (a). Later in phase 4, a propagated response (b) may be elicited; its amplitude is small and the upstroke is not very steep. This response, which displays postrepolarization refractoriness, is conducted very slowly. Still later in phase 4, full excitability is regained, and the response (c) displays its normal characteristics. *(Modified from Singer DH, Baumgarten CM, Ten Eick RE: Cellular electrophysiology of ventricular and other dysrhythmias: studies on diseased and ischemic heart.* Prog Cardiovasc Dis *24:97, 1981.)*

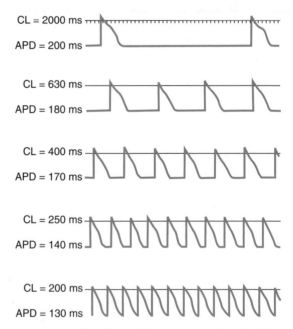

FIGURE 2-20 ■ The effect of changes in cycle length (CL) on the action potential duration (APD) of canine Purkinje fibers. *(Modified from Singer D, Ten Eick RE: Aberrancy: electrophysiologic aspects.* Am J Cardiol *28:381, 1971.)*

channels. The i_{Kr} current activates slowly, remains activated for hundreds of milliseconds before inactivation, and is inactivated very slowly. Consequently, as the basic cycle length is diminished, each action potential tends to occur earlier in the inactivation period of the i_{Kr} current initiated by the preceding action potential. Therefore, the shorter the basic cycle length, the greater the outward K^+ current will be during phase 2. Hence the action potential duration diminishes.

SUMMARY

- The transmembrane action potentials that can be recorded from cardiac myocytes comprise the following five phases (0 to 4):
  - Phase 0, upstroke. A suprathreshold stimulus rapidly depolarizes the membrane by activating the fast Na^+ channels.
  - Phase 1, early partial repolarization. Achieved by the efflux of K^+ through channels that conduct the transient outward current, I_{to}.
  - Phase 2, plateau. Achieved by a balance between the influx of Ca^{++} through Ca^{++} channels and the efflux of K^+ through several types of K^+ channels.
  - Phase 3, final repolarization. Initiated when the efflux of K^+ exceeds the influx of Ca^{++}. The resulting partial repolarization rapidly increases the K^+ conductance and rapidly restores full repolarization.
  - Phase 4, resting potential. The transmembrane potential of the fully repolarized cell is determined mainly by the conductance of the cell membrane to K^+.
- Two principal types of action potentials may be recorded from cardiac cells:
- Fast-response action potentials may be recorded from atrial and ventricular myocardial fibers and from specialized conducting (Purkinje) fibers. The action potential is characterized by a large-amplitude, steep upstroke, which is produced by the activation of the fast Na^+ channels. The effective refractory period begins at the upstroke of the action potential and persists until about midway through phase 3.
- Slow-response action potentials may be recorded from normal sinoatrial (SA) and atrioventricular (AV) nodal cells and from abnormal myocardial cells that have been partially depolarized. The action potential is characterized by a less negative resting potential, a smaller amplitude, and a less steep upstroke than is the fast-response action potential. The upstroke is produced by the activation of Ca^{++} channel.

ADDITIONAL READING

Carmeliet E: Cardiac ionic currents and acute ischemia: from channels to arrhythmias, *Physiol Rev* 79:917, 1999.

Grant AO: Cardiac Ion Channels, *Circ Arrhythmia Electrophysiol* 2:185, 2009.

Noble D: Modeling the heart–from genes to cells to the whole organ, *Science* 295:1678, 2002.

Priori SG: The fifteen years of discoveries that shaped molecular electrophysiology: time for appraisal, *Circ Res* 107:451, 2010.

Sanguinetti MC: HERG1 channelopathies, *Pflügers Arch.* 460:265, 2010.

ten Tusscher KH, Noble D, Noble PJ, Panfilov AV: A model for human ventricular tissue, *Am J Physiol* 286:H1573, 2004.

Zipes DP, Jalife J: *Cardiac electrophysiology: from cell to bedside*, ed 4, Philadelphia, 2004, WB Saunders.

CASE 2-1

HISTORY

A 63-year-old man suddenly felt a crushing pain beneath his sternum. He became weak, he was sweating profusely, and he noticed his heart was beating rapidly. He called his physician, who made the diagnosis of myocardial infarction. The tests made at the hospital confirmed his doctor's suspicion that the patient had suffered a "heart attack"; that is, a major coronary artery to the left ventricle had suddenly become occluded. An electrocardiogram indicated that the SA node was the source of the rapid heart rate. Two hours after admission to the hospital, the patient suddenly became much weaker. His arterial pulse rate was only about 40 beats/min. An electrocardiogram at this time revealed that the atrial rate was about 90 beats/min and that conduction through the AV junction was completely blocked, undoubtedly because the infarct affected the AV conduction system. Electrodes of an artificial pacemaker were inserted into the patient's right ventricle, and the ventricle was paced at a frequency of 75 beats/min. The patient felt stronger and more comfortable almost immediately.

QUESTIONS

1. Soon after coronary artery occlusion, the interstitial fluid K^+ concentration rose substantially in the flow-deprived region. In this region, the high extracellular K^+ concentration:
   a. increased the propagation velocity of the myocardial action potentials.
   b. decreased the postrepolarization refractoriness of the myocardial cells.
   c. changed the resting (phase 4) transmembrane potential to a less negative value.
   d. diminished the automaticity of the myocardial cells.
   e. decreased the likelihood of reentry dysrhythmias.

2. The attending physician was alerted to the possibility of an arrhythmia because the high extracellular K^+ concentration could:
   a. directly increase the entry of Na^+ through fast Na^+ channels.
   b. hyperpolarize the resting membrane.
   c. increase the rate of slow diastolic depolarization in SA node cells.

   d. slow conduction velocity by reducing Na^+ channel availability.
   e. decrease the release of norepinephrine from cardiac sympathetic nerves.

3. The most likely mechanism responsible for the patient's arterial pulse rate of about 40 beats/min after impulse conduction through the AV junction was blocked is:
   a. excitation of the ventricles via an AV bypass tract.
   b. conversion of ventricular myocardial fibers to automatic cells.
   c. firing of ventricular ectopic cells that have the same electrophysiological characteristics as SA node cells.
   d firing of automatic cells (Purkinje fibers) in the specialized conduction system of the ventricles.
   e. excitation of ventricular cells by the rhythmic activity in the autonomic neurons that innervate the heart.

4. While the heart was being paced, the cardiologist discontinued ventricular pacing periodically to test the patient's cardiac status. The cardiologist found that the ventricles did not begin beating spontaneously until about 5 to 10 s after cessation of pacing, because the preceding period of pacing led to:
   a. overdrive suppression of the automatic cells in the ventricles.
   b. release of norepinephrine from the cardiac sympathetic nerves.
   c. release of neuropeptide Y from the cardiac sympathetic nerves.
   d. fatigue of the ventricular myocytes.
   e. release of acetylcholine from the cardiac parasympathetic nerves.

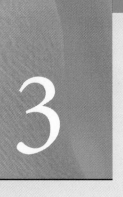

3

AUTOMATICITY: NATURAL EXCITATION OF THE HEART

1. Explain the basis of automaticity.
2. Describe the conduction of excitation through the heart.
3. Explain the basis of reentry.
4. Describe the components of the electrocardiogram.
5. Explain various cardiac rhythm disturbances.

THE HEART GENERATES ITS OWN PACEMAKING ACTIVITY

The nervous system controls various aspects of cardiac function, including the frequency at which the heart beats and the vigor of each contraction. However, cardiac function certainly does not require intact nervous pathways. Indeed, a patient with a completely denervated heart (a cardiac transplant recipient) can adapt well to stressful situations.

Automaticity (the ability of the heart to initiate its own beat) and **rhythmicity** (the regularity of pacemaking activity) are properties intrinsic to cardiac tissue. *The heart continues to beat even when it is completely removed from the body; the vertebrate heartbeat is myogenic.* If the coronary vasculature is artificially perfused, rhythmic cardiac contraction persists for many hours. Apparently, at least some cells in the walls of all four cardiac chambers are capable of initiating beats; such cells reside mainly in the nodal tissues or specialized conducting fibers of the heart.

All cardiac myocytes in the embryonic heart have pacemaker properties. Some myocytes synthesize large amounts of contractile proteins to become "working" myocardium. Others retain pacemaking ability and generate impulses spontaneously; the mammalian heart region that ordinarily generates impulses at the greatest frequency is the sinoatrial (SA) node; it is the **natural pacemaker** of the heart.

Detailed mapping of the electrical potentials on the surface of the right atrium has revealed that two or three sites of automaticity, located 1 or 2 cm from the SA node itself, serve along with the SA node as an **atrial pacemaker complex**. At times, all of these loci initiate impulses simultaneously. At other times, the site of earliest excitation shifts from locus to locus, depending on conditions such as the level of autonomic neural activity.

Ectopic pacemakers may serve as safety mechanisms when the normal pacemaking centers cease functioning. However, if an ectopic center fires while the normal pacemaking center still functions, the ectopic activity may induce either sporadic rhythm disturbances, such as **premature depolarizations**, or continuous rhythm disturbances, such as **paroxysmal tachycardias**. These **dysrhythmias** are discussed later in this chapter.

When the SA node and the other components of the atrial pacemaker complex are excised or destroyed, pacemaker cells in the atrioventricular (AV) node usually become the pacemaker for the entire heart.

Purkinje fibers that constitute the specialized conduction system of the ventricles also possess automaticity. Characteristically, they fire at a very slow rate. When the AV junction is unable to conduct the impulse from the atria to the ventricles, **idioventricular pacemakers** in the Purkinje fiber network initiate ventricular excitation and contractions. Such contractions occur at a frequency of only 30 to 40 beats per minute (beats/min). These low frequencies are usually not sufficient to allow the heart to pump an adequate cardiac output.

> Regions of the heart other than the SA node may initiate beats under special circumstances; such sites are called **ectopic foci**, or **ectopic pacemakers**. Ectopic foci may become pacemakers when (1) their own rhythmicity becomes enhanced; (2) the rhythmicity of the higher-order pacemakers becomes depressed; or (3) all conduction pathways are blocked between the ectopic focus and those regions with greater rhythmicity.

Sinoatrial Node

The SA node is the phylogenetic remnant of the sinus venosus of lower vertebrate hearts. In humans it is about 8 mm long and 2 mm thick. It lies in the groove where the superior vena cava joins the right atrium (Figure 3-1). The sinus node artery runs lengthwise through the center of the node.

The SA node contains two principal cell types of: (1) small, round cells, that have few organelles and myofibrils and (2) slender, spindle-shaped cells that are intermediate in appearance between the round cells and the ordinary atrial myocardial cells. The round cells are probably the pacemaker cells, whereas the transitional cells serve a subsidiary pacemaker role

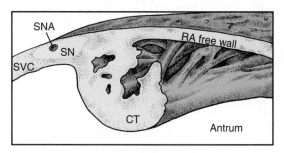

FIGURE 3-1 ■ The location of the SA node (SN) near the junction between the superior vena cava (SVC) and right atrium (RA). CT, crista terminalis; SNA, Sinoatrial artery. *(Redrawn from James TN: The sinus node.* Am J Cardiol *40:965, 1977.)*

and conduct the impulses within the node and to the nodal margins.

A typical transmembrane action potential recorded from a cell in the SA node is depicted in Figure 2-16B. Compared with the transmembrane potential recorded from a ventricular myocardial cell (Figure 2-16A), the maximum diastolic potential of the SA node cell is usually less, the upstroke of the action potential (phase 0) is less steep, a plateau is not sustained, and repolarization (phase 3) is more gradual. These are all characteristic of the slow response described in Chapter 2.

The transmembrane potential (V_m) during phase 4 is much less negative in SA (and AV) nodal automatic cells than in atrial or ventricular myocytes because nodal cells lack the i_{K1} (inward-rectifying) type of K^+ channel. Therefore the ratio of conductances of K^+ (g_K) and Na^+ (g_{Na}), or g_K/g_{Na}, during phase 4 is much less in the nodal cells than in the myocytes. During phase 4, therefore, V_m deviates much more from the K^+ equilibrium potential (E_K) in nodal cells than it does in myocytes.

Although primary SA node pacemaker cells have fast Na^+ channels, their function is suppressed because they are inactivated at the maximum diastolic potential of these cells. Thus, tetrodotoxin has no influence on the action potential (Figure 3-2A) at the primary SA nodal pacemaker site. This fact indicates that the action potential upstroke is not produced by an inward current of Na^+ through the fast channels. However, blockade of Ca^{++} channels by nifedipine suppresses action potential generation in

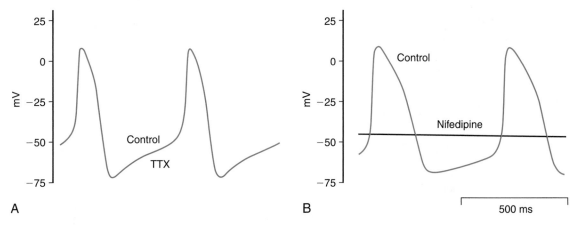

FIGURE 3-2 ■ At the leading pacemaker site in the sinoatrial node, tetrodotoxin (TTX; 20 μM) does not change SA node action potential or frequency (**A**), whereas nifedipine (2 μM) suppresses spontaneous action potentials completely (**B**). *(Redrawn from Boyett MR, Honjo H, Kodama I: The sinoatrial node, a heterogeneous pacemaker structure.* Cardiovasc Res *47:658-687, 2000, with permission from Oxford University Press.)*

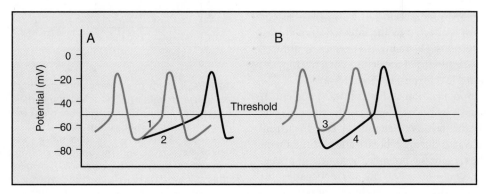

FIGURE 3-3 ■ Mechanisms involved in changes of frequency of pacemaker firing. **A,** A reduction in the slope of the pacemaker potential from 1 to 2 diminishes the frequency. **B,** An increase in the maximum negativity at the end of repolarization (from 3 to 4) also diminishes the frequency.

primary SA node cells (Figure 3-2B). Subsidiary or latent pacemaker cells within the SA node have a more negative maximum diastolic potential that allows some Na^+ channels to recover from inactivation. Tetrodotoxin or local anesthetic drugs can block such channels and impede conduction from primary pacemaker cells to the atrium.

The principal feature that distinguishes a pacemaker fiber from other cardiac fibers resides in phase 4. In nonautomatic cells the potential remains constant during this phase, whereas in a pacemaker fiber there is a slow depolarization, called the **pacemaker potential**, throughout phase 4. Depolarization proceeds at a steady rate until a threshold is attained, and then an action potential is triggered.

The discharge frequency of pacemaker cells may be varied by a change in either the rate of depolarization during phase 4 or the maximal diastolic potential (Figure 3-3). A change of the threshold potential, the voltage at which the action potential is initiated, is another variable that affects pacemaker cell frequency.

Changes in autonomic neural activity often also induce a **pacemaker shift**, in which the site of initiation of the cardiac impulse may shift to a different locus within the SA node or to a different component of the atrial pacemaker complex.

Ordinarily, the frequency of pacemaker firing is controlled by the activity of both divisions of the autonomic nervous system. Increased sympathetic nervous activity, through the release of norepinephrine, raises the heart rate principally by increasing the slope of the pacemaker potential (slope 1 in Figure 3-3A). This mechanism of increasing heart rate operates during physical exertion, anxiety, and certain illnesses, such as **febrile infectious diseases**. Increased vagal activity, through the release of acetylcholine, diminishes the heart rate by hyperpolarizing the pacemaker cell membrane (slope 4 in Figure 3-3B) and by reducing the slope of the pacemaker potential (slope 2 in Figure 3-3A).

Ionic Basis of Automaticity

Several ionic currents contribute to the slow depolarization that occurs during phase 4 in automatic cells in the heart. In SA node pacemaker cells , the diastolic depolarization is affected by the interaction of at least three ionic currents: (1) an inward current, I_f, induced by hyperpolarization; (2) a calcium current, I_{Ca}; and (3) an outward K^+ current, I_K (Figure 3-4).

The hyperpolarization-induced inward current, I_f, is carried mainly by Na^+ through specific channels that differ from the fast Na^+ channels. The I_f current becomes activated during repolarization of the membrane, as the membrane potential becomes more negative than about −60 mV. The more negative the membrane potential becomes at the end of repolarization, the greater the activation of the I_f current.

The second current responsible for diastolic depolarization is the L-type calcium current, I_{Ca}. This current becomes activated toward the end of phase 4, as the transmembrane potential reaches a value of about −55 mV (see Figure 3-4). Once the Ca^{++} channels become activated, the influx of Ca^{++} into the cell increases. The influx of Ca^{++} accelerates the rate of diastolic depolarization, which then leads to the upstroke of the action potential. A decrease in the external Ca^{++} concentration or the addition of a calcium channel antagonist (see Figure 3-2B) reduces the amplitude of the action potential and the slope of the pacemaker potential in SA node cells.

The progressive diastolic depolarization mediated by the two inward currents, I_f and I_{Ca}, is opposed by a third current, an outward K^+ current, I_K. This K^+ efflux

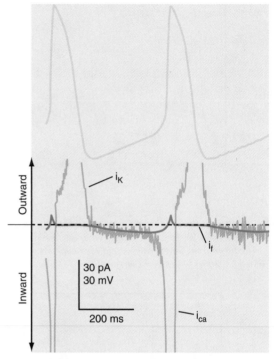

FIGURE 3-4 ■ Transmembrane potential changes (*top half*) that occur in sinoatrial node cells and their relation to three ionic currents (*bottom half*): (1) the current, I_{Ca}; (2) a hyperpolarization-induced inward current, I_f; and (3) an outward K^+ current, I_K. The thin noisy trace shows net membrane current and the approximate time course of repolarizing outward K^+ current, I_K, hyperpolarization-induced inward current, I_f, and the L-type Ca^{++} current, I_{Ca}. The *thick bold line* in the current trace indicates the magnitude and direction of estimated I_f. *(Redrawn from van Ginneken AC, Giles W: Voltage clamp measurements of the hyperpolarization-activated inward current I(f) in single cells from rabbit sino-atrial node.* J Physiol 434:57, 1991.)

tends to repolarize the cell after the upstroke of the action potential. The outward K^+ current continues well beyond the time of maximal repolarization, but it diminishes throughout phase 4 (see Figure 3-4). Hence the opposition of I_K to the depolarizing effects of the two inward currents I_{Ca} and I_f, gradually decreases.

The role of I_f in SA node pacemaking was challenged when agents that block I_f slowed SA node frequency only slightly. On the other hand, drugs that block I_K or I_{Ca} in primary pacemaker cells (Figure 3-2B) suppressed automaticity. However, I_f exerts a greater role in pacemaking in subsidiary pacemaker cells in the SA node. In addition, other ionic currents via T-type Ca channels, the Na^+-Ca^{++} exchanger and a sustained inward Na^+ current were detected in SA node cells. In later studies a timing mechanism composed of ionic channels in the plasma membrane and the sarcoplasmic reticulum (SR) membrane has been proposed. Thus, Ca^{++} entering the cell through L-type channels not only produces I_{Ca} but also releases Ca^{++} from the SR. The released Ca^{++} leaves the cell via the Na^+/Ca^{++} antiporter, generating an inward current during diastolic depolarization. Released Ca^{++} from the SR may participate in diastolic depolarization not only via the Na^+/Ca^{++} antiporter but also by virtue of the depletion of SR Ca^{++}. Store-operated Ca^{++} channels (SOCCs) are activated by Ca^{++} depletion from the SR; entry of Ca^{++} through transient receptor potential (TRP) channels can also assist diastolic depolarization and the regulation of SA node frequency. Several TRP channel isoforms have been detected in the SA node as well as in other cardiac tissues. Overall, the structural complexity of the node, together with the many ionic currents that contribute to pacemaking, allow the SA node to sustain this vital function under a variety of physiological and pathological conditions.

The ionic basis for automaticity in the AV node pacemaker cells appears similar to that in the SA node cells. In cardiac Purkinje fibers, automaticity can be detected at two voltage ranges, from −60 to −100 mV and from −50 to 0 mV. The **slow diastolic depolarization** in the voltage range from −60 to −100 mV is attributed to a voltage- and time-dependent K^+ current. The action potential arises from the fast Na^+ current. Whether the hyperpolarization-induced inward current, I_f, functions physiologically in this voltage range remains to be clarified. Automaticity at −50 to 0 mV depends on I_K and I_{Ca}, but the precise mechanism is not known.

Autonomic neurotransmitters affect automaticity by altering the ionic currents across the cell membranes. The β-adrenergic transmitters increase all three currents involved in SA nodal automaticity. The adrenergically mediated increase in the slope of diastolic depolarization indicates that the augmentations of I_f and I_{Ca} must exceed the enhancement of I_K. Adrenergic transmitters also increase automaticity in Purkinje fibers; this is evident at both voltage ranges.

The hyperpolarization (Figure 3-5) induced by acetylcholine released at the vagus endings in the heart is

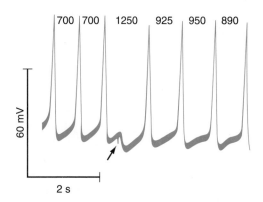

700 | 700 | 1250 | 925 | 950 | 890

60 mV

2 s

FIGURE 3-5 ■ Effect of a brief vagal stimulus (*arrow*) on the transmembrane potential recorded from a sinoatrial node pacemaker cell in an isolated cat atrium preparation. The cardiac cycle lengths, in milliseconds, are denoted by the *numbers* at the top of the figure. *(Modified from Jalife J, Moe GK: Phasic effects of vagal stimulation on pacemaker activity of the isolated sinus node of the young cat.* Circ Res *45:595, 1979.)*

achieved by an increased conductance mediated through activation of specific K^+ channels that are controlled by the cholinergic receptors ($I_{K,ACh}$). Acetylcholine also depresses the I_f and I_{Ca} currents.

Overdrive Suppression

A period of excitation at a high frequency depresses automaticity of pacemaker cells. This phenomenon is known as **overdrive suppression**. The firing of the SA node tends to suppress the automaticity in the other loci because the SA node has a greater intrinsic rhythmicity than the other latent pacemaking sites in the heart.

The mechanism responsible for overdrive suppression appears to be based on the activity of the membrane pump (Na^+,K^+-ATPase) that actively extrudes three Na^+ from the cell, in exchange for two K^+. During each depolarization, a certain quantity of Na^+ enters the cell; therefore the more frequently it is depolarized, the greater the amount of Na^+ that enters the cell per minute. At high excitation frequencies the Na^+ pump becomes more active in extruding this larger quantity of Na^+ from the cell interior. This enhanced pump activity hyperpolarizes the cell through the net loss of cations from the cell interior. Because of the hyperpolarization, the slow diastolic depolarization requires more time to reach the threshold, as shown in Figure 3-3B. Furthermore, when the overdrive

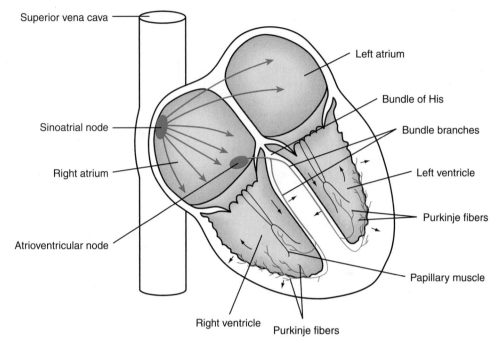

FIGURE 3-6 ■ Schematic representation of the conduction system of the heart.

suddenly ceases, the Na$^+$ pump does not decelerate instantaneously but continues to operate at an accelerated rate for some time. This excessive extrusion of Na$^+$ opposes the gradual depolarization of the pacemaker cell during phase 4 and thereby suppresses its intrinsic automaticity temporarily.

CLINICAL BOX

If an atrial ectopic focus suddenly begins to fire at a high rate (e.g., 150 impulses per minute) in an individual with a normal heart rate of 70 beats per minute, the ectopic center would become the pacemaker for the entire heart. When that rapid ectopic focus suddenly stops firing, the SA node might remain quiescent briefly because of overdrive suppression. The interval from the end of the period of overdrive until the SA node resumes firing is called the **sinus node recovery time**. In patients with the so-called **sick sinus syndrome**, the sinus node recovery time may be markedly prolonged. The resultant period of asystole (cardiac standstill) can cause loss of consciousness.

Atrial Conduction

From the SA node, the cardiac impulse spreads radially throughout the right atrium (Figure 3-6) along ordinary atrial myocardial fibers, at a conduction velocity of approximately 1 m/s. A special pathway, the **anterior interatrial myocardial band** (or **Bachmann's bundle**), conducts the impulse from the SA node directly to the left atrium. Three tracts, the **anterior, middle, and posterior internodal pathways**, have been described. These tracts consist of a mixture of ordinary myocardial cells and specialized conducting fibers. Some investigators assert that these pathways constitute the principal routes for conduction of the cardiac impulse from the SA node to the AV node.

The configuration of the atrial action potential is depicted in Figure 2-16C. Compared with the potential recorded from a typical ventricular fiber (see Figure 2-16A), the plateau (phase 2) is not as well developed, repolarization (phase 3) occurs as a slower rate, and the action potential duration is briefer.

Atrioventricular Conduction

The cardiac action potential proceeds along the internodal pathways in the atrium and ultimately reaches the AV node (see Figure 3-6). This node is approximately 22 mm long, 10 mm wide, and 3 mm thick in adult humans. The node is situated posteriorly on the right side of the interatrial septum and is circumscribed by the ostium of the coronary sins, the tendon of Todaro, and the tricuspid valve. The AV node contains the same two cell types as the SA node, but the round cells are more sparse and the spindle-shaped cells preponderate. Conduction of the impulse from the atrium to the AV node has been described as consisting of fast and slow pathways. There is some anatomical evidence for this well-known observation. The existence of fast and slow conduction paths allows a substrate for reentrant circuits within the AV node. Cells in the inferior portion of the AV node serve as a subsidiary pacemaker.

The AV node is divided into three functional regions: (1) the AN region, the transitional zone between the atrium and the remainder of the node; (2) the N region, the midportion of the AV node; and (3) the NH region, the zone in which nodal fibers gradually merge with the **bundle of His**, which is the upper portion of the specialized ventricular conducting system. Normally, the AV node and bundle of His constitute the only pathways for conduction from atria to ventricles.

Several features of AV conduction are of physiological and clinical significance. The principal delay in the passage of the impulse from the atria to the ventricles occurs in the AN and N regions of the AV node. The conduction velocity is actually less in the N region than in the AN region. However, the path length is substantially greater in the AN region than in the N region. The conduction times through the AN and N regions largely account for the delay between the onsets of the **P wave** (the electrical manifestation of the spread of atrial excitation) and the **QRS complex** (spread of ventricular excitation) in the electrocardiogram (Figure 3-7). *Functionally, this delay between atrial excitation and ventricular excitation permits optimal ventricular filling during atrial contraction.*

In the N region, slow-response action potentials prevail. The resting potential is about −60 mV, the upstroke velocity is very low (about 5 V/s), and the

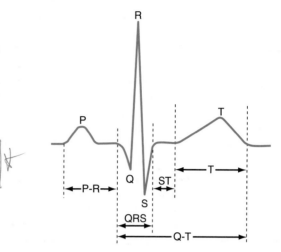

FIGURE 3-7 ▪ Configuration of a typical scalar electrocardiogram, illustrating the important deflections and intervals.

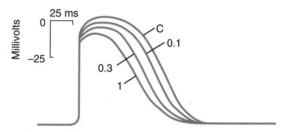

FIGURE 3-8 ▪ Transmembrane potentials recorded from a rabbit atrioventricular node cell under control conditions (C) and in the presence of the calcium channel–blocking drug diltiazem in concentrations of 0.1, 0.3, and 1.0 µmol/L. *(Redrawn from Hirth C, Borchard U, Hafner D: Effects of the calcium antagonist diltiazem on action potentials, slow response and force of contraction in different cardiac tissues. J Mol Cell Cardiol 15:799, 1983.)*

conduction velocity is about 0.05 m/s. Tetrodotoxin, which blocks the fast Na⁺ channels, does not affect the action potentials in this region. Conversely, the Ca⁺⁺ channel antagonists decrease the amplitude and duration of the action potentials (Figure 3-8) and slow AV conduction. The shapes of the action potentials in the AN region are intermediate between those in the N region and the atria. Similarly, the action potentials in the NH region are transitional between those in the N region and the bundle of His. The relative refractory period of the cells in the N region extends well beyond the period of complete repolarization; that is, these cells display postrepolarization refractoriness (see Figure 2-19).

As the repetition rate of atrial depolarizations is increased, conduction through the AV junctions slows. An abnormal prolongation of AV conduction time is called **first-degree AV block** (Figure 3-9A). Most of the prolongation of AV conduction caused by an increase in repetition rate takes place in the N region.

Impulses tend to be blocked in the AV node at stimulus frequencies that are easily conducted in other regions of the heart. If the atria are depolarized at a high frequency, only a fraction (e.g., one half) of the atrial impulses might be conducted through the AV junction to the ventricles. The conduction pattern in which only a fraction of the atrial impulses are conducted to the ventricles is called **second-degree AV block** (see Figure 3-9B). This type of block may protect the ventricles from excessive contraction frequencies,

wherein the filling time between successive ventricular contractions might be inadequate and therefore the ventricles would be unable to deliver an adequate cardiac output.

Retrograde conduction can occur through the AV node. However, the propagation time is significantly longer, and the impulse tends to be blocked at lower repetition rates during retrograde conduction than during antegrade conduction . Finally, the AV node is a common site for reentry, a phenomenon explained later in this chapter.

The autonomic nervous system regulates AV conduction. Weak vagal activity may simply prolong the AV conduction time. Stronger vagal activity may cause some or all of the impulses arriving from the atria to be blocked in the node. The conduction pattern in which none of the atrial impulses reach the ventricles over a substantial number of atrial depolarizations is called

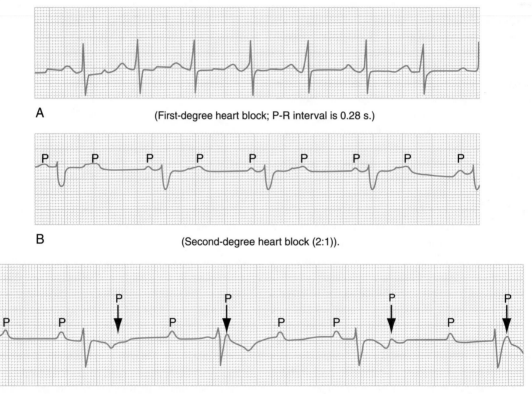

A   (First-degree heart block; P-R interval is 0.28 s.)

B   (Second-degree heart block (2:1)).

C   (Third-degree heart block; note the dissociation between the P waves and the QRS complexes.)

FIGURE 3-9 ■ Atrioventricular (AV) blocks. **A,** First-degree heart block; P-R interval is 0.28 s. **B,** Second-degree heart block (2:1). **C,** Third-degree heart block; note the dissociation between the P waves and the QRS complexes.

third-degree, or **complete, AV block** (see Figure 3-9C). The delayed conduction or block induced by vagal stimulation occurs largely in the N region of the node.

Acetylcholine released by vagus nerve fibers hyperpolarizes the conducting fibers in the N region (Figure 3-10). The greater the hyperpolarization at the time of arrival of the atrial impulse, the more impaired the AV conduction will be. In the experiment shown in Figure 3-10, vagus nerve fibers were stimulated intensely (at St) shortly before the second atrial depolarization (A_2). This atrial impulse arrived at the AV node cell when its cell membrane was maximally

hyperpolarized. The absence of a corresponding depolarization of the bundle of His (H) shows that the second atrial impulse was not conducted through the AV node. Only a small, nonpropagated response to the second atrial impulse is evident in the recording from the conducting fiber.

Cardiac sympathetic nerves, on the other hand, facilitate AV conduction. They decrease AV conduction time and enhance the rhythmicity of the latent pacemakers in the AV junction. The norepinephrine released at the sympathetic nerve terminals increases the amplitude and slope of the upstroke of the AV nodal action potentials, principally in the AN and N regions of the node.

Ventricular Conduction

The bundle of His passes subendocardially down the right side of the interventricular septum for about 1 cm and then divides into the right and left **bundle branches** (Figures 3-6 and 3-11). The right bundle branch is a direct continuation of the bundle of His and proceeds down the right side of the interventricular septum. The left bundle branch, which is considerably thicker than the right, arises almost perpendicularly from the bundle of His and perforates the interventricular septum. On the subendocardial surface of the left side of the interventricular septum, the main left bundle branch splits into a thin **anterior division** and a thick **posterior division.**

The right bundle branch and the two divisions of the left bundle branch ultimately subdivide into a

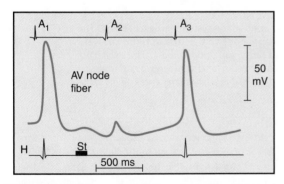

FIGURE 3-10 ■ Effects of a brief vagal stimulus (St) on the transmembrane potential recorded from an atrioventricular (AV) nodal fiber from a rabbit. Note that shortly after vagal stimulation, the membrane of the fiber was hyperpolarized. The atrial excitation (A_2) that arrived at the AV node when the cell was hyperpolarized failed to be conducted, as denoted by the absence of a depolarization in the His electrogram (H). The atrial excitations that preceded (A_1) and followed (A_3), excitation A_2, were conducted to the His bundle region. *(Redrawn from Mazgalev T, Dreifus LS, Michelson EL, et al: Vagally induced hyperpolarization in atrioventricular node. Am J Physiol 251:H631, 1986.)*

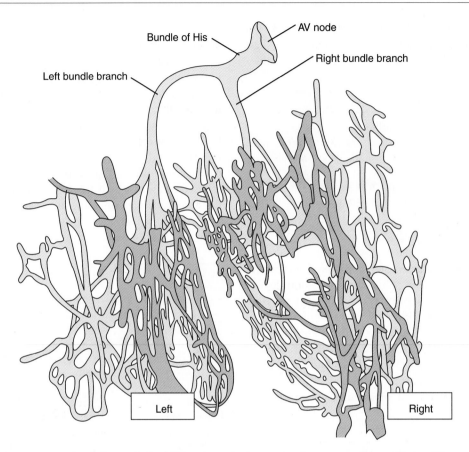

Bundle of His

AV node

Right bundle branch

Left bundle branch

Left

Right

FIGURE 3-11 ▪ Atrioventricular (AV) and ventricular conduction system of the calf heart. The *dark blue arrows* indicate conduction from the sinoatrial node to the atria and the atrioventricular node and then to the bundle branches and terminal Purkinje fibers. The *small black arrows* show conduction within the interventricular septum and the ventricular myocardium. *(Redrawn from DeWitt LM: Observations on the sino-ventricular connecting system of the mammalian heart.* Anat Rec *3:475, 1909.)*

complex network of conducting fibers called *Purkinje fibers*, which ramify over the subendocardial surfaces of both ventricles. In certain mammalian species, such as cattle, the Purkinje fiber network is arranged in discrete, encapsulated bundles (see Figure 3-11).

CLINICAL BOX

Impulse conduction in the right bundle branch, the main left bundle branch, or either division of the left bundle branch may be impaired as a consequence of a degenerative process or of coronary artery disease. Conduction blocks in one or more of these pathways give rise to characteristic electrocardiographic patterns. Block of either of the main bundle branches is known as right or left **bundle branch block.** Block of either division of the left bundle branch is called **left anterior hemiblock** or **left posterior hemiblock.**

Purkinje fibers are the broadest cells in the heart, 70 to 80 μm in diameter, compared with 10 to 15 μm for ventricular myocytes. The large diameter accounts in part for the greater conduction velocity in Purkinje than in myocardial fibers. Conduction of the action potential over the Purkinje fiber system is faster than in any other tissue within the heart; estimates of conduction velocity vary from 1 to 4 m/s. This permits a rapid activation of the entire endocardial surface of the ventricles. Purkinje cells have abundant, linearly arranged sarcomeres, just like myocardial cells. However, the T-tubular system is absent in the Purkinje cells of many species but is well developed in the myocardial cells (see Chapter 4).

The action potentials recorded from Purkinje fibers resemble those of ordinary ventricular myocardial fibers (see Figure 2-16A). In general, phase 1 is more prominent in Purkinje fiber action potentials (see Figure 2-3) than in action potentials recorded from ventricular fibers (especially endocardial fibers), and the duration of the plateau (phase 2) is longer.

Many premature activations of the atria that are conducted through the AV junction are blocked by the long refractory period of the Purkinje fibers. Therefore they fail to evoke a premature contraction of the ventricles. This function of protecting the ventricles against the effects of premature atrial depolarizations is especially pronounced at slow heart rates, because the action potential duration, and hence the effective refractory period of the Purkinje fibers, varies inversely with the heart rate (see Figure 2-20). At slow heart rates, the effective refractory period of the Purkinje fibers is especially prolonged; as the heart rate increases, the refractory period diminishes. Similar rate-dependent changes in the refractory period also occur in most of the other cells in the heart. However, in the AV node, the effective refractory period does not change appreciably over the normal range of heart rates, and it actually increases at very rapid heart rates. Therefore *at high heart rates, it is the AV node that protects the ventricles when atrial impulses arrive at excessive repetition rates.*

The first portions of the ventricles to be excited are the interventricular septum (except its basal portion) and the papillary muscles. The wave of activation spreads into the septum from both its left and its right endocardial surfaces. Early contraction of the septum tends to make it more rigid and allows it to serve as an anchor point for the contraction of the remaining ventricular myocardium. Also, early contraction of the papillary muscles prevents eversion of the AV valves during ventricular systole.

The endocardial surfaces of both ventricles are activated rapidly, but the wave of excitation spreads from endocardium to epicardium at a slower velocity (about

0.3 to 0.4 m/s). Because the right ventricular wall is appreciably thinner than the left, the epicardial surface of the right ventricle is activated earlier than the epicardial surface of the left ventricle. Also, apical and central epicardial regions of both ventricles are activated somewhat earlier than are their respective basal regions. The last portions of the ventricles to be excited are the posterior basal epicardial regions and a small zone in the basal portion of the interventricular septum.

AN IMPULSE CAN TRAVEL AROUND A REENTRY LOOP

Under certain conditions, a cardiac impulse may reexcite some region through which it had passed previously. This phenomenon, known as **reentry**, underlies many clinical disturbances of cardiac rhythm. Reentry may be **ordered** or **random**. In the ordered variety, the impulse traverses a fixed anatomical path, whereas in the random type, the path continues to change. The principal example of random reentry is **fibrillation**.

The conditions necessary for reentry are illustrated in Figure 3-12. In each of the four panels, a single bundle (S) of cardiac fibers splits into a left (L) and a right (R) branch with a connecting bundle (C) between the two branches. Normally, the impulse coming down bundle S is conducted along the L and R branches (panel A). As the impulse reaches connecting link C, it enters link C from both sides and becomes extinguished at the point of collision. The impulse from the left side cannot proceed further because the tissue beyond has just been depolarized from the other direction, and therefore it is absolutely refractory. The impulse cannot pass through bundle C from the right either, for the same reason.

Panel B of Figure 3-12 shows that the impulse cannot make a complete circuit if antegrade block exists in the two branches (L and R) of the fiber bundle. Furthermore, if **bidirectional** block exists at any point in the loop (e.g., branch R in panel C), the impulse will not be able to reenter.

A necessary condition for reentry is that at some point in the loop the impulse can pass in one direction but not in the other. This phenomenon is called **unidirectional block**. As shown in panel D, the impulse may travel down branch L normally and may be blocked in the antegrade direction in branch R. The impulse that was conducted down branch L and through the connecting

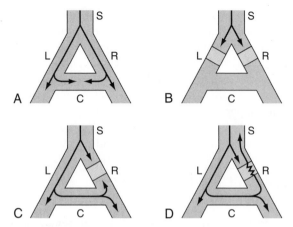

FIGURE 3-12 ■ The role of unidirectional block in reentry. **A,** An excitation wave traveling down a single bundle (S) of fibers continues down the left (L) and right (R) branches. The depolarization wave enters the connecting branch (C) from both ends and is extinguished at the zone of collision. **B,** The wave is blocked (*blue squares*) in the L and R branches **C,** Bidirectional block exists in branch R. **D,** Unidirectional block exists in branch R. The antegrade impulse is blocked (*blue square*), but the retrograde impulse is conducted through (*jagged line*) and reenters bundle S.

branch C may be able to penetrate the depressed region in branch R from the retrograde direction, even though the antegrade impulse was blocked previously at this same site. The antegrade impulse arrives at the depressed region in branch R earlier than the impulse that traverses a longer path and enters branch R from the opposite direction. The antegrade impulse may be blocked simply because it arrives at the depressed region during its effective refractory period. If the retrograde impulse is delayed sufficiently, the refractory period may have ended, and the impulse is conducted back into bundle S.

Unidirectional block is a necessary condition for reentry, but not a sufficient one. *The effective refractory period of the reentered region must also be less than the propagation time around the loop.* In panel D, if the retrograde impulse is conducted through the depressed zone in branch R and if the tissue just beyond is still refractory from the antegrade depolarization, branch S is not reexcited. Therefore the conditions that promote reentry are those that prolong conduction time or shorten the effective refractory period.

The functional components of reentry loops responsible for specific dysrhythmias in intact hearts are diverse. Some loops are very large and involve entire specialized conduction bundles; other loops are microscopic. The loop may include myocardial fibers, specialized conducting fibers, nodal cells, and junctional tissues, in almost any conceivable arrangement. Also, the cardiac cells in the loop may be normal or deranged.

CLINICAL BOX

Accessory AV pathways are present in some people. Such pathways often serve as a part of a reentry loop (see Figure 3-12), which could lead to serious cardiac rhythm disturbances in these patients. The **Wolff-Parkinson-White syndrome,** a congenital disturbance, is the most common clinical disorder in which a bypass tract of myocardial fibers serves as an accessory pathway between atria and ventricles. Ordinarily, the syndrome causes no functional abnormality. It is easily detected in the electrocardiographic reading, because a portion of the ventricular myocardium is preexcited via the bypass tract. Slightly later, the normal excitation of the remainder of the ventricular myocardium via the AV node and His-Purkinje system imparts a bizarre configuration to the ventricular (QRS) complex of the **electrocardiogram**. Occasionally, however, a reentry loop develops in which the atrial impulse travels to the ventricle via one of the two AV pathways (AV node or bypass tract), and then the impulse travels back to the atria through the other of the two pathways. Continuous circling around the loop leads to a very rapid rhythm (**supraventricular tachycardia**), which may be incapacitating because the rapid rate may not allow sufficient time for ventricular filling.

AFTERDEPOLARIZATIONS LEAD TO TRIGGERED ACTIVITY

Triggered activity is so named because it is always coupled to a preceding action potential. Consequently, dysrhythmias induced by triggered activity are difficult to distinguish from those induced by reentry, which is also always coupled to a previous action potential. Triggered activity is caused by **afterdepolarizations**. Two types of afterdepolarizations are recognized: **early afterdepolarizations (EADs)** and **delayed afterdepolarizations (DADs)**. EADs occur at the end of the plateau (phase 2) of an action potential or about

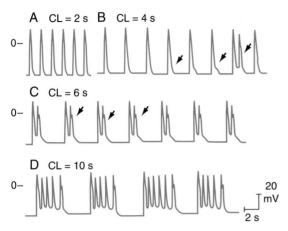

FIGURE 3-13 ■ Effect of pacing at different cycle lengths (CLs) on cesium-induced early afterdepolarizations (EADs) in a canine Purkinje fiber. **A,** EADs not evident. **B,** EADs first appear (*arrows*). The third EAD reaches threshold and triggers an action potential (*third arrow*). **C,** EADs that appear after each driven depolarization trigger an action potential. **D,** Triggered action potentials occur in salvos. (*Modified from Damiano BP, Rosen M: Effects of pacing on triggered activity induced by early afterdepolarizations.* Circulation *69:1013, 1984.*)

midway through repolarization (phase 3), whereas DADs occur near the very end of repolarization or just after full repolarization (phase 4).

Early Afterdepolarizations

EADs are more likely to occur when the prevailing heart rate is slow; rapid pacing suppresses EADs. In the experiment shown in Figure 3-13, EADs were induced by cesium in an isolated Purkinje fiber preparation. No afterdepolarizations were evident when the preparation was driven at a cycle length of 2 seconds (s). When the cycle length was increased to 4 s, EADs appeared; their incidence increased as cycle length increased to 6 and 10 s. Some EADs were subthreshold but eventually others reached threshold to trigger an action potential.

EADs may be produced experimentally by interventions that prolong the action potential. Because EADs may be initiated at either of two distinct levels of transmembrane potential, namely, at the end of the plateau and about midway through repolarization, two different mechanisms may be involved in generating them.

Considerable information has been obtained about the mechanism responsible for those EADs that appear at the end of the plateau. The more prolonged the action potential, the more likely are EADs to occur. For those action potentials that trigger EADs, the plateau appears to be prolonged enough so that those Ca^{++} channels that were activated at the beginning of the plateau and then inactivated would have sufficient time to be reactivated again before the plateau had expired. This secondary activation, which seems to depend on the activity of calcium/calmodulin-dependent protein kinase type II (CaMKII), can trigger an afterdepolarization. Less information is available about the cellular mechanisms responsible for those EADs that appear midway through repolarization.

CLINICAL BOX

The pathologic significance of EADs was recognized in connection with the congenital and drug-induced long QT syndrome (LQTS). As the action potential lengthens, EADs occur and caused triggered automaticity. In the electrocardiogram, this problem is manifested as polymorphic ventricular tachycardia, also called *torsades de pointes*. Episodes of torsades de pointes can be self-limited but may proceed to ventricular fibrillation and sudden death. Clinically, hypokalemia and bradycardia (see Figure 3-13) are hallmarks of its presentation. Restoring extracellular K^+ to normal levels and increasing heart rate are two approaches used to overcome the propensity for development of torsades de pointes.

Delayed Afterdepolarizations

In contrast to EADs, DADs tend to appear when the heart rate is high. The salient characteristics of DADs are shown in Figure 3-14. Transmembrane potentials were recorded from Purkinje fibers that were exposed to a high concentration of **acetylstrophanthidin,** a digitalis-like substance. In the absence of pacing stimuli, these fibers were quiescent. In each panel, a sequence of six driven action potentials was induced at various basic cycle lengths.

When the cycle length was 800 milliseconds (ms) (panel A), the last driven action potential was followed by a brief subthreshold DAD that did not reach

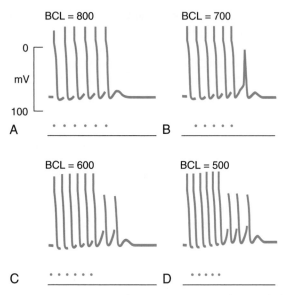

FIGURE 3-14 ■ Transmembrane action potentials recorded from isolated canine Purkinje fibers. Acetylstrophanthidin was added to the bath, and sequences of six driven beats (denoted by the *dots*) were produced at basic cycle lengths (BCL) of 800, 700, 600, and 500 ms. Note that delayed afterpotentials occurred after the driven beats and that these afterpotentials reached threshold after the last driven beat in panels **B** to **D** but not in panel **A**. *(From Ferrier GR, Saunders JH, Mendez C: A cellular mechanism for the generation of ventricular arrhythmias by acetylstrophanthidin.* Circ Res 32:600, 1973.)

threshold and, after the DAD had subsided, the transmembrane potential remained constant. When the basic cycle length was diminished to 700 ms (panel B), the DAD that followed the last paced beat reached threshold, and a triggered depolarization (or **extrasystole**) ensued. This extrasystole was itself followed by a subthreshold afterpotential. Diminution of the basic cycle length to 600 ms (panel C) evoked two extrasystoles after the last driven action potential. A sequence of three extrasystoles followed the six driven depolarizations that were separated by intervals of 500 ms (panel D). Slightly shorter basic cycle lengths or slightly greater concentrations of acetylstrophanthidin evoked a continuous sequence of nondriven beats, resembling a paroxysmal tachycardia (described later in this chapter).

DADs are associated with elevated intracellular Ca^{++} concentrations. The amplitudes of the DADs are increased by interventions that raise intracellular Ca^{++} concentrations, such as elevated extracellular Ca^{++} concentrations and toxic levels of digitalis glycosides. Elevations of intracellular Ca^{++} provoke the oscillatory release of Ca^{++} from the SR. Hence in myocardial cells, the DADs are accompanied by small changes in developed force. The high intracellular Ca^{++} concentrations also activate certain membrane channels that permit the passage of Na^+ and K^+. The net flux of these cations constitutes a **transient inward current**, I_{ti}, that is at least partly responsible for the afterdepolarization of the cell membrane.

ELECTROCARDIOGRAPHY DISPLAYS THE SPREAD OF CARDIAC EXCITATION

The electrocardiograph enables the physician to infer the rate, rhythm, and course of the cardiac impulse simply by recording the variations in electrical potential at various loci on the body surface. By analyzing the details of these potential fluctuations, the physician gains valuable insight concerning (1) the anatomical orientation of the heart; (2) the relative sizes of its chambers; (3) a variety of disturbances of rhythm and conduction; (4) the extent, location, and progress of ischemic damage to the myocardium; (5) the effects of altered electrolyte concentrations; and (6) the influence of certain drugs (notably digitalis derivatives and antidysrhythmic agents). The science of electrocardiography is extensive and complex; only its elementary basis is considered here.

Scalar Electrocardiography

The systems of leads used to record routine electrocardiograms are oriented in certain planes of the body. The diverse electromotive forces that exist in the heart at any moment can be represented by a three-dimensional vector. A system of recording leads oriented in a given plane detects the projection of the three-dimensional vector on that plane. Furthermore, the potential difference between two recording electrodes represents the projection of the vector on the line between the two leads. Components of vectors projected on such lines are not vectors but **scalar quantities** (having magnitude but not direction). Hence, a recording of the changes with time of the differences of potential between two points on the surface of the skin is called a **scalar electrocardiogram.**

Configuration of the Scalar Electrocardiogram

The scalar electrocardiogram detects the changes with time of the electrical potential between some point on the skin surface and an indifferent electrode or between pairs of points on the skin surface. The cardiac impulse progresses through the heart in a complex three-dimensional pattern. Hence, the configuration of the electrocardiogram varies from individual to individual, and in any given individual the pattern varies with the anatomical location of the leads.

In general, the pattern consists of P, QRS, and T waves (see Figure 3-7). The P-R interval (or more precisely, the P-Q interval) is a measure of the time from the onset of atrial activation to the onset of ventricular activation; it normally ranges from 0.12 to 0.20 s. A considerable fraction of this time involves passage of the impulse through the AV conduction system. Pathological prolongations of this interval are associated with disturbances of AV conduction produced by inflammatory, circulatory, pharmacological, or nervous mechanisms.

The configuration and amplitude of the QRS complex vary considerably among individuals. The duration is usually between 0.06 and 0.10 s. Abnormal prolongation may indicate a block in the normal conduction pathways through the ventricles (such as a block of the left or right bundle branch). During the ST interval the entire ventricular myocardium is depolarized and there is negligible potential difference in the ventricle. Therefore the ST segment lies on the **isoelectric line**, under normal conditions. Any appreciable deviation from the isoelectric line is noteworthy and may indicate ischemic damage of the myocardium. The Q-T interval is sometimes referred to as the period of "electrical systole" of the ventricles. Its duration is about 0.4 s, but it varies inversely with the heart rate, mainly because the myocardial cell action potential duration varies inversely with the heart rate (see Figure 2-20).

In most leads the T wave is deflected in the same direction from the isoelectric line as the major component of the QRS complex, although biphasic or oppositely directed T waves are perfectly normal in certain

leads. Deviation of the T wave and QRS complex in the same direction from the isoelectric line indicates that the repolarization process proceeds in a direction counter to the depolarization process. T waves that are abnormal in either direction or amplitude may indicate myocardial damage, electrolyte disturbances, or cardiac hypertrophy.

Standard Limb Leads

Einthoven devised the original electrocardiographic lead system. In his lead system the **resultant cardiac vector** (the vector sum of all electrical activity occurring in the heart at any given moment) was considered to lie in the center of a triangle (assumed to be equilateral) formed by the left and right shoulders and the pubic region (Figure 3-15). This so-called **Einthoven triangle** is oriented in the frontal plane of the body. Hence only the projection of the resultant cardiac vector on the frontal plane is detected by this system of leads. For convenience, the electrodes are connected to the right and left forearms rather than to the corresponding shoulders, because the arms represent simple extensions of the leads from the shoulders. Similarly, the leg is taken as an extension of the lead system from the pubis, and the third electrode is connected to the left leg (by convention).

Certain conventions dictate the manner in which these **standard limb leads** are connected to the galvanometer. Lead I records the potential difference between the left arm (LA) and right arm (RA). The galvanometer connections are such that when the potential at LA (V_{LA}) exceeds the potential at RA (V_{RA}), the galvanometer is deflected upward from the isoelectric line. In Figures 3-15 and 3-16 this arrangement of the galvanometer connections for lead I is designated by a + at LA and by a − at RA. Lead II records the potential difference between RA and LL (left leg) and yields an upward deflection when the potential at LL (V_{LL}) exceeds V_{RA}. Finally, lead III registers the potential difference between LA and LL and yields an upward deflection when V_{LL} exceeds V_{LA}. These galvanometer connections were arbitrarily chosen so that the QRS complexes will be upright in all three standard limb leads in most normal individuals.

Let the frontal projection of the resultant cardiac vector at some moment be represented by an arrow (tail negative, head positive), as in Figure 3-15. Then, the potential difference, $V_{LA} - V_{RA}$, recorded in lead I will be represented by the component of the vector projected along the horizontal line between LA and RA, as shown in Figure 3-16. If the cardiac vector makes an angle, θ, of 60 degrees with the horizontal (as in panel A of Figure 3-16), the magnitude of the potential recorded be lead I will equal the vector magnitude times cosine 60 degrees. The deflection recorded in lead I will be upward, because the positive arrowhead lies closer to LA than to RA. The deflection in lead II will also be upright, because the arrowhead lies closer to LL than to RA. The magnitude of the lead II

deflection will be greater than that in lead I because in this example the direction of the vector parallels that of lead II; therefore the magnitude of the projection on lead II exceeds that on lead I. Similarly, in lead III the deflection will be upright, and in this example, where θ = 60 degrees, its magnitude will equal that in lead I.

If the vector in panel A of Figure 3-16 is the result of the electrical events occurring during the peak of the QRS complex, the orientation of this vector is said to represent the **mean electrical axis** of the heart in the frontal plane. The positive direction of this axis is taken in the clockwise direction from the horizontal plane (contrary to the usual mathematical convention). For normal individuals, the average mean electrical axis is

FIGURE 3-15 ▪ Einthoven triangle, illustrating the galvanometer connections for standard limb leads I, II, and III. LA, left arm connection; LL, left leg connection; RA, right arm connection. The *arrow* shows the sum of electrical forces as the cardiac vector obtained from the limb leads.

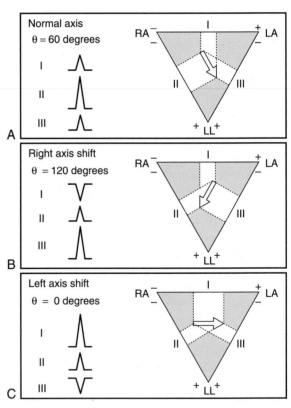

FIGURE 3-16 ▪ Magnitude and direction of the QRS complexes in limb leads I, II, and III, when the mean electrical axis (θ) is 60 degrees (**A**), 120 degrees (**B**), and 0 degrees (**C**). LA, left arm connection; LL, left leg connection; RA, right arm connection. The *white areas* indicate the projection on the frontal plane of QRS waves in each limb lead, and the *large white arrow* shows the resultant electrical axis of the cardiac vector.

approximately +60 degrees (as in panel A of Figure 3-16). Therefore the QRS complexes are usually upright in all three leads and largest in lead II.

With appreciable shift of the mean electrical axis to the right (panel B of Figure 3-16, in which θ = 120 degrees), the displacements of the QRS complexes in the standard leads change considerably. In this case the largest upright deflection is in lead III and the deflection in lead I is inverted, because the arrowhead is closer to RA than to LA. With left axis shift (panel C of Figure 3-16, where θ = 0 degrees), the largest upright deflection is in lead I, and the QRS complex in lead III is inverted.

As is evident from this discussion, the standard limb leads I, II, and III are oriented in the frontal plane at 0, 60, and 120 degrees, respectively, from the horizontal plane. Other limb leads, which are also oriented in the frontal plane, are usually recorded in addition to the standard leads. These "unipolar limb leads" lie along axes at angles of +90, −30, and −150 degrees from the horizontal plane. Such augmented lead systems are described in textbooks on electrocardiography and are not considered further here.

To obtain information concerning the projections of the cardiac vector on the sagittal and transverse planes of the body in scalar electrocardiography, the **precordial leads** are usually recorded. Most commonly, each of six selected points on the anterior and lateral surfaces of the chest in the vicinity of the heart is connected in turn to the galvanometer. The other galvanometer terminal is usually connected to a **central terminal,** which is composed of a junction of three leads from LA, RA, and LL, each in series with a 5000-ohm resistor. The voltage of this central terminal remains at a theoretical zero potential throughout the cardiac cycle.

Changes in the mean electrical axis may occur with alterations in the anatomical position of the heart or with changes in the relative preponderance of the right and left ventricles. For example, the axis tends to shift toward the left (more horizontal) in short, stocky individuals and toward the right (more vertical) in tall, thin persons. Also, with left or right **ventricular hypertrophy** (increased myocardial mass), the axis shifts toward the hypertrophied side.

DYSRHYTHMIAS OCCUR FREQUENTLY AND CONSTITUTE IMPORTANT CLINICAL PROBLEMS

Cardiac dysrhythmias reflect disturbances of either **impulse propagation** or **impulse initiation**. The principal disturbances of impulse propagation are conduction blocks and reentrant rhythms. Disturbances of impulse initiation include those that arise from the SA node and those that originate from various ectopic foci.

Altered Sinoatrial Rhythms

The frequency of pacemaker discharge varies by the mechanisms described earlier in this chapter (see Figure 3-3). Changes in SA nodal discharge frequency are usually produced by cardiac autonomic nerves. Examples of electrocardiograms of sinus tachycardia and sinus bradycardia are shown in Figure 3-17. The P, QRS, and T deflections are all normal, but the duration of the cardiac cycle (the **P-P interval**) is altered. Characteristically, when sinus bradycardia or tachycardia develops, the cardiac frequency changes gradually and requires

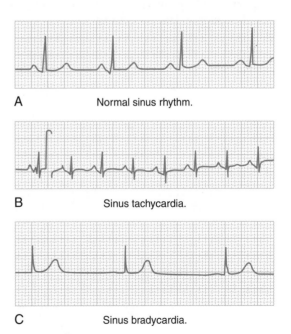

A   Normal sinus rhythm.

B   Sinus tachycardia.

C   Sinus bradycardia.

FIGURE 3-17 ■ Sinoatrial rhythms. **A,** Normal sinus rhythm. **B,** Sinus tachycardia. **C,** Sinus bradycardia.

several beats to attain its new steady-state value. Electrocardiographic evidence of respiratory cardiac dysrhythmia is common and is manifested as a rhythmic variation in the P-P interval at the respiratory frequency (see Figure 5-13).

Atrioventricular Transmission Blocks

Various physiological, pharmacological, and pathological processes can impede impulse transmission through the AV conduction tissue. The site of block can be localized more precisely by recording the **His bundle electrogram** (Figure 3-18). To obtain such tracings, an electrode catheter is introduced into a peripheral vein and threaded centrally until the tip containing the electrodes lies in the AV junctional region between the right atrium and ventricle. When the electrodes are properly positioned, a distinct deflection (Figure 3-18,H) is registered that represents the passage of the cardiac impulse down the bundle of His. The time intervals required for propagation from the atrium to the bundle of His (**A-H interval**) and from the bundle of His to the ventricles (**H-V interval**) may be measured accurately. Abnormal prolongation of the former or latter interval indicates block above or below the bundle of His, respectively.

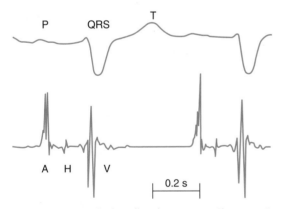

FIGURE 3-18 ■ His bundle electrogram (*lower tracing, retouched*) and lead II of the scalar electrocardiogram (*upper tracing*). The deflection, H, which represents the impulse conduction over the bundle of His, is clearly visible between the atrial, A, and ventricular, V, deflections. The conduction time from the atria to the bundle of His is denoted by the A-H interval; that from the bundle of His to the ventricles, by the H-V interval.

Premature Depolarizations

Premature depolarizations occur at times in most normal individuals but are more common under certain abnormal conditions. They may originate in the atria, AV junction, or ventricles. One type of premature depolarization is coupled to a normally conducted depolarization by a constant **coupling interval**. If the normal depolarization is suppressed temporarily (e.g., by vagal stimulation), the premature depolarization is also suppressed. Such premature depolarizations are called **coupled extrasystoles**, or simply extrasystoles, and they probably reflect a reentry phenomenon (see Figure 3-12). A second type of premature depolarization occurs as the result of enhanced automaticity in some ectopic focus. This ectopic center may fire regularly and may be protected from depolarization by the normal cardiac impulse. If this premature depolarization occurs at a regular interval or at a simple multiple of that interval, the disturbance is called **parasystole**.

A **premature atrial depolarization** is shown in the electrocardiogram in Figure 3-19A. The normal interval between beats was 0.89 s (heart rate, 68 beats/min). The premature atrial depolarization (second P wave in the figure) followed the preceding P wave by only 0.56 s. The configuration of the premature P wave differs from the configuration of the other, normal P waves because the path of atrial excitation, originating at some ectopic focus in the atrium, is different from the normal spread of excitation that originates in the SA node. The QRS complex of the premature depolarization is usually normal in configuration because the spread of ventricular excitation occurs over the usual pathways.

A **premature ventricular depolarization** appears in Figure 13-19B. Because the premature excitation originated at some ectopic focus in the ventricles, the impulse spread was aberrant, and the configurations of the QRS and T waves are entirely different from the normal deflections. The premature QRS complex followed the preceding normal QRS complex by only 0.47 s. The interval after the premature excitation is 1.28 s, considerably longer than the normal interval between beats (0.89 s). The interval (1.75 s), from the QRS complex just before the premature excitation to the QRS complex just after it, is virtually equal to the duration of two normal cardiac cycles (1.78 s).

The prolonged interval that usually follows a premature ventricular depolarization is called a **compensatory pause.** The reason for the compensatory pause after a premature ventricular depolarization is that the ectopic ventricular impulse does not disturb the natural rhythm of the SA node. Either the ectopic ventricular impulse is not conducted retrogradely through the AV conduction system or, if it is, the time required is such that the SA node has already fired at its natural interval before the ectopic impulse could have reached it. Likewise, the SA nodal impulse that was generated between the second and third QRS complexes in Figure 3-19B did not affect the ventricle because the AV junction and perhaps also the ventricles were still refractory from the premature excitation. In Figure 3-19B, the P wave that originated in the SA node at the time of the premature depolarization occurred at the same time as the T wave of the premature cycle and therefore cannot easily be identified in the tracing.

Ectopic Tachycardias

When a tachycardia originates from some ectopic site in the heart, the onset and termination are typically abrupt, in contrast to the more gradual changes in heart rate in sinus tachycardia. Such ectopic tachycardias are usually called **paroxysmal tachycardias** because of their sudden appearance and abrupt cessation. Such tachycardias may cause light-headedness or even transient loss of consciousness (syncope), because the very rapid contraction frequency does not permit adequate time for ventricular filling between heartbeats.

Paroxysmal tachycardias that originate in the atria or in the AV junctional tissues (Figure 3-20A) are usually indistinguishable, and therefore both are included in the term **paroxysmal supraventricular tachycardia.** The tachycardia often results from an impulse repetitively circling a reentry loop that includes atrial tissue, the AV junction, or both. The QRS complexes are often normal because ventricular activation proceeds over the normal pathways.

Paroxysmal ventricular tachycardia originates from an ectopic focus in the ventricles. The electrocardiogram is characterized by repeated, bizarre QRS complexes that reflect the aberrant intraventricular impulse conduction (Figure 3-20B). Paroxysmal ventricular tachycardia is much more ominous than supraventricular tachycardia because it is frequently a precursor of ventricular fibrillation, a lethal dysrhythmia described in the next section.

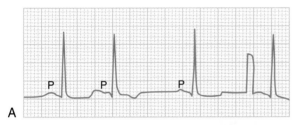

A

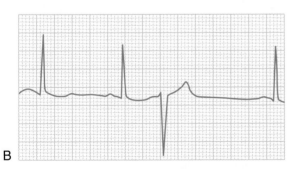

B

FIGURE 3-19 ■ A premature atrial depolarization (**A**) and a premature ventricular depolarization (**B**). Atrial depolarization indicated by P; the premature atrial depolarization (second beat in the top tracing) is followed by normal QRS and T waves. The interval after the premature depolarization is not much longer than the usual interval between beats. The brief rectangular deflection just before the last depolarization is a standardization signal. The premature ventricular depolarization (**B**) is characterized by bizarre QRS and T waves and is followed by a compensatory pause.

Episodes of ectopic tachycardia may persist for only a few beats or for many hours or days, and the episodes often recur. Paroxysmal tachycardias may occur as the result of (1) the rapid firing of an ectopic pacemaker; (2) triggered activity secondary to afterpotentials that reach threshold; or (3) an impulse circling a reentry loop repetitively.

Fibrillation

Under certain conditions, cardiac muscle undergoes an irregular type of contraction that is entirely ineffectual

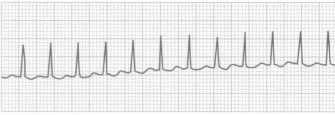

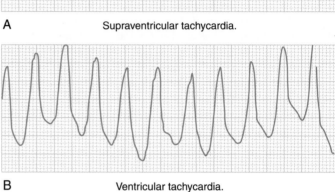

A   Supraventricular tachycardia.

FIGURE 3-20 ■ Paroxysmal tachycardias. **A,** Supraventricular tachycardia. **B,** Ventricular tachycardia.

B   Ventricular tachycardia.

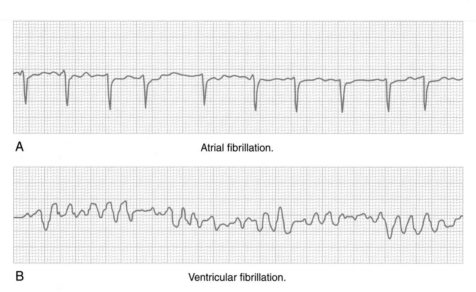

A   Atrial fibrillation.

B   Ventricular fibrillation.

FIGURE 3-21 ■ Atrial and ventricular fibrillation. **A,** Atrial fibrillation. **B,** Ventricular fibrillation.

in propelling blood. Such a dysrhythmia is termed **fibrillation** and may involve either the atria or the ventricles. Fibrillation probably represents a reentry phenomenon in which the reentry loop fragments into multiple, irregular circuits.

The tracing in Figure 3-21A illustrates the electrocardiographic changes in **atrial fibrillation** as seen in various types of chronic heart disease. The atria do not

contract and relax sequentially during each cardiac cycle and hence do not contribute to ventricular filling. Instead, the atria undergo a continuous, uncoordinated, rippling type of activity. In the electrocardiogram there are no P waves; they are replaced by continuous irregular fluctuations of potential, called **f waves**.

Although atrial fibrillation and flutter are compatible with life and even with full physical activity, the onset of **ventricular fibrillation** leads to loss of consciousness within a few seconds. The irregular, continuous, uncoordinated twitchings of the ventricular muscle fibers pump no blood. In the electrocardiogram in Figure 3-21B, irregular fluctuations of potential are manifest.

> In atrial fibrillation, the AV node is activated at intervals that may vary considerably from cycle to cycle. Hence there is no constant interval between QRS complexes and therefore between ventricular contractions. Because the strength of ventricular contraction depends on the interval between beats (see Figure 5-24), the volume and rhythm of the pulse are very irregular. In many patients the atrial reentry loop and the pattern of AV conduction are more regular. The rhythm is then referred to as **atrial flutter**.

Fibrillation is often initiated when a premature impulse arrives during the **vulnerable period**. In the ventricles, this period coincides with the downslope of the T wave. During this period, the excitability of the cardiac cells varies. Some fibers are still in their effective refractory periods, others have almost fully recovered their excitability, and still others are able to conduct impulses, but only at very slow conduction velocities. As a consequence, the action potentials are propagated over the chambers in multiple wavelets that travel along circuitous paths and at various conduction velocities. As a region of cardiac cells becomes excitable again, it will ultimately be reentered by one of the wave fronts traveling about the chamber. The process is self-sustaining.

Electric shock is sometimes used to treat ventricular fibrillation, and sometimes also atrial fibrillation, especially when the disturbance does not respond optimally to drugs. The timing of the shock is coordinated with the absolute refractory period of the ventricles (i.e., during or shortly after the QRS deflection of the electrocardiogram), so that the shock does not affect ventricular excitation. However, the shock will render all the atrial myocytes temporarily refractory, and thereby interrupt the prevailing reentry circuits.

SUMMARY

- Automaticity is characteristic of certain cells in the heart, notably those in the SA and AV nodes and in the specialized conducting system. Automaticity is achieved by a slow spontaneous depolarization of the membrane during phase 4.
- The SA node initiates the impulse that induces cardiac contraction. This impulse is propagated from the SA node to the atria, and the wave of excitation ultimately reaches the AV node.
- The AV node cells are slow-response fibers, and the impulse travels very slowly through the AV node. The consequent delay between atrial and ventricular depolarizations provides adequate time for atrial contraction to help fill the ventricles.
- Impulses may be initiated abnormally (1) by slow diastolic depolarization of automatic cells in ectopic sites or (2) by afterdepolarizations that reach threshold:
  - Ectopic foci: Automatic cells in the atrium, AV node, or His-Purkinje system may initiate propagated cardiac impulses either because the ordinarily more rhythmic, normal pacemaker cells are suppressed or because the rhythmicity of the ectopic foci is abnormally enhanced.
  - Afterdepolarizations: Under abnormal conditions, afterdepolarizations may appear early in phase 3 of a normally initiated beat, or they may be delayed until near the end of phase 3 or the beginning of phase 4. Such afterdepolarizations may themselves trigger propagated impulses.
- Disturbances of impulse conduction consist mainly of simple conduction block and reentry:
  - Simple conduction block: Failure of propagation in a cardiac fiber as the result of a disease process (e.g., ischemia, inflammation) or a drug.
  - Reentry: A cardiac impulse may traverse a loop of cardiac fibers and reenter previously excited tissue when the impulse is conducted slowly around the loop and the impulse is blocked unidirectionally in some section of the loop.
- The electrocardiogram is recorded from the surface of the body and traces the conduction of the cardiac

impulse through the heart. The component waves of the electrocardiogram are:

- P wave: Spread of excitation over the atria.
- QRS interval: Spread of excitation over the ventricles.
- T wave: Spread of repolarization over the ventricles.

ADDITIONAL READING

Anderson RH, Ho SY: The morphology of the cardiac conduction system, *Novartis Found Symp* 250:6, 2003.

Antzelevitch C, Shimuzu W, Yan GX, et al: The M cell. Its contribution to the ECG and to normal and abnormal electrical function of the heart, *J Cardiovasc Electrophysiol* 10:1124, 1999.

Boyett MR, Honjo H, Kodama I: The sinoatrial node, a heterogeneous pacemaker structure, *Cardiovasc Res* 47:658, 2000.

Gima K, Rudy Y: Ionic current basis of electrocardiographic waveforms, *Circ Res* 90:889, 2003.

Kleber AG, Rudy Y: Basic mechanisms of cardiac impulse propagation and associated arrhythmias, *Physiol Rev* 84:431, 2004.

Lakatta EG, DiFrancesco D: What keeps us ticking: a funny current, a calcium clock, or both? *J Mol Cell Cardiol* 47:157, 2009.

Li J, Greener ID, Inada S, et al: Computer three-dimensional reconstruction of the atrioventricular node, *Circ Res* 102:975, 2008.

Noble D, Noble PJ, Fink M: Competing oscillators in cardiac pacemaking: Historical background, *Circ Res* 106:1791, 2010.

Rohr S: Role of gap junctions in the propagation of the cardiac action potential, *Cardiovasc Res* 62:309, 2004.

Vassalle M, Yu H, Cohen IS: The pacemaker current in cardiac Purkinje myocytes, *J Gen Physiol* 106:559, 1995.

CASE 3-3

HISTORY

An 18-year-old high school student has seen a cardiologist regularly since it was discovered that she had symptoms of the long QT (LQT) syndrome 3 years ago. At that time, she experienced several episodes of light-headedness during a soccer game. Her family physician performed an analysis of systems, which found everything normal except for some electrocardiographic abnormalities. She was referred to the cardiologist whose examination included an ECG. The cardiologist reported a patient in normal sinus rhythm with a heart rate of 71 beats/min. Other ECG data were a PR interval of 0.14 s, QRS duration of 0.10 s, and a QT interval of 475 ms. The QT interval, even when corrected for heart rate, is abnormally long. Analysis of DNA revealed that the patient had a mutation in a gene linked to a cardiac potassium channel. The mutation (loss of function) results in less outward repolarizing current and therefore, a longer ventricular action potential. The phenotype of her syndrome is designated LQT1. The cardiologist had the patient walk around the office for light exercise. Immediately after exercising, her heart rate was increased and her QT interval had decreased, as expected. The cardiologist advised her not to participate in competitive athletics and prescribed a β-adrenergic antagonist (atenolol) to be taken daily. She has followed this regimen and has remained symptom-free since first diagnosed.

QUESTIONS

1. The PR interval of 0.14 s indicates that:
   a. impulse initiation in the SA node is unusually rapid.
   b. conduction of the impulse through the bundle branches is slower than normal.
   c. conduction time of the impulse from atria through the AV node and ventricular conducting system to ventricles are normal.
   d. atrial action potentials are initiated within normal limits.
   e. the contractile state of the left ventricle is weaker than normal.

2. The QT interval measures the average:
   a. interval between successive SA node impulses.
   b. conduction velocity of atrial muscle.
   c. time for impulse conduction through the AV node.
   d. velocity of conduction in the ventricular conducting system.
   e. duration of the ventricular action potential.

3. When the patient exercised, heart rate increased, and this can be measured in:
   a. reduced R-R interval.
   b. lengthened PR interval.
   c. increased duration of the QRS complex.
   d. decreased amplitude of P waves.
   e. increased R wave amplitude.

4. The long QT syndrome is associated with early afterdepolarizations (EADs) and can eventually produce torsades de pointes (a form of

ventricular fibrillation). During exercise, the patient's QT interval:

a. increased because of greater closing of repolarizing K channels.

b. decreased because of greater opening of depolarizing Na channels.

c. increased because of greater inactivation of Na channels.

d. decreased because of greater activation of repolarizing K channels.

e. increased because of greater tendency for reentry.

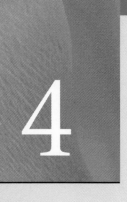

4

THE CARDIAC PUMP

OBJECTIVES

1. Learn how the microscopic and gross anatomy of the heart enables it to pump blood through the systemic and pulmonary circulations.

2. Indicate how electrical excitation of the heart is coupled to its contractions.

3. Elucidate the main factors that determine cardiac contractile force.

4. Describe and explain the pressure changes in the heart chambers and great vessels during a complete cardiac cycle.

5. Relate ATP metabolism to oxidation of fatty acids and carbohydrates.

6. Learn how O_2 consumption links cardiac substrate metabolism with ventricular function.

The heart exhibits a wide range of activity and functional capacity, and performs a tremendous amount of work over the lifetime of an individual. The heart can function independently of extracardiac stimuli, but its performance is strongly influenced by humoral and neural factors. Because all myocardial muscle cells are activated to contract on each beat, the strength of the heart's contraction is determined ultimately by the strength of contraction of all the individual myocardial cells. The strength of contraction of each cell is determined in turn by excitation-contraction coupling processes within it and by its (sarcomere) length, which is determined by the physical forces acting on the cell, both prior to contraction (**preload**) and during contraction (**afterload**). In this chapter we consider some of the basic intrinsic mechanisms (*viz.* those in myocardial cells and arising in the heart itself) that affect cardiac activity; the effects of extracardiac factors are discussed in subsequent chapters.

THE GROSS AND MICROSCOPIC STRUCTURES OF THE HEART ARE UNIQUELY DESIGNED FOR OPTIMAL FUNCTION

The Myocardial Cell

Several important morphological and functional differences exist between myocardial cells (Figures 4-1 to 4-4) and skeletal muscle cells. However, the contractile elements within the two types of cells are quite similar; each skeletal and cardiac muscle cell is made up of sarcomeres (from Z line to Z line) that contain thick filaments composed of myosin (in the A band) and thin filaments containing actin. The thin filaments extend

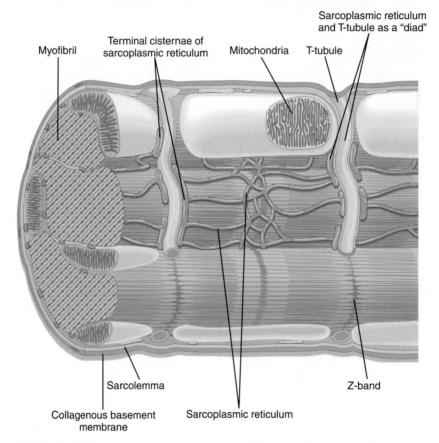

Myofibril

Terminal cisternae of sarcoplasmic reticulum

Mitochondria

T-tubule

Sarcoplasmic reticulum and T-tubule as a "diad"

Sarcolemma

Collagenous basement membrane

Sarcoplasmic reticulum

Z-band

FIGURE 4-1 ▪ Diagram of a cardiac sarcomere illustrating the relationships among components of the cardiac myocyte. *(Redrawn from Fawcett D, McNutt NS: The ultrastructure of the cat myocardium. I. Ventricular papillary muscle. J Cell Biol 42:1, 1969.)*

FIGURE 4-2 ▪ **A,** Low-magnification electron micrograph of a monkey heart (ventricle). Typical features of myocardial cells include the elongated nucleus (Nu), striated myofibrils (MF) with columns of mitochondria (Mit) between the myofibrils, and intercellular junctions (intercalated disks, ID). A blood vessel (BV) is located between two myocardial cells. **B,** Medium-magnification electron micrograph of monkey ventricular cells showing details of ultrastructure. The sarcolemma (SL) is the boundary of the muscle cells and is thrown into multiple folds where the cells meet at the ID region. The prominent MFs show distinct banding patterns, including the A band (A), dark Z lines (Z), I band regions (I), and M lines (M) at the center of each sarcomere unit. Mitochondria (Mit) occur either in rows between MFs or in masses just underneath the sarcolemma. Regularly spaced transverse tubules (TT) appear at the Z line levels of the myofibrils. **C,** High-magnification electron micrograph of a specialized intercellular junction between two myocardial cells of the mouse. Called a gap junction (GJ) or nexus, this attachment consists of very close apposition of the sarcolemmal membranes of the two cells and appears in thin section to consist of seven layers. **D,** Freeze-fracture replica of mouse myocardial gap junction, showing distinct arrays of characteristic intramembranous particles. Large particles (P) belong to the inner half of the sarcolemma of one myocardial cell, whereas the "pitted" membrane face (E) is formed by the outer half of the sarcolemma of the cell above.

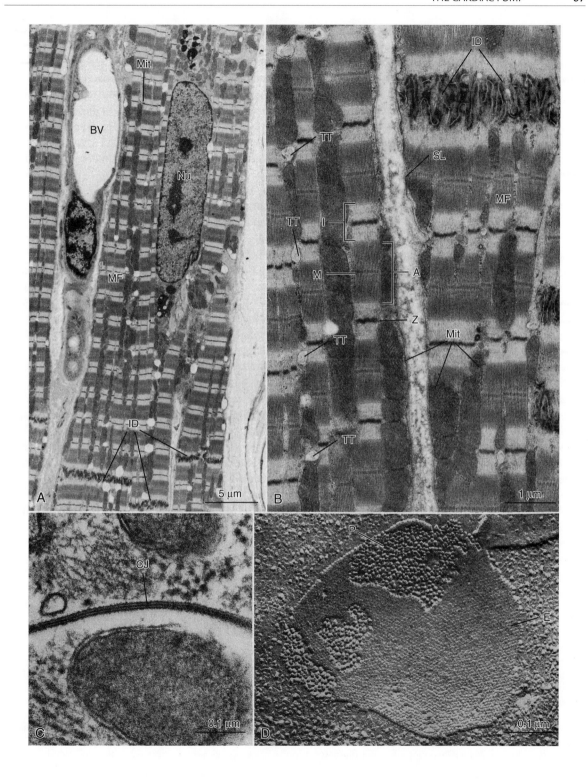

from the point where they are anchored to the Z line (through the I band) to interdigitate with the thick filaments. Shortening occurs by the sliding filament mechanism as in the case of skeletal muscle. Actin filaments slide along adjacent myosin filaments by cycling of the intervening cross-bridges, thereby bringing the Z lines closer together.

A striking difference between cardiac and skeletal muscle is the semblance of a syncytium in cardiac muscle with branching interconnecting fibers. The myocardium is not a true anatomic syncytium, because laterally the myocardial fibers are separated from adjacent fibers by their respective sarcolemmas, and the end of each fiber is separated from its neighbor by dense structures, called intercalated disks (IDs), that are continuous with the sarcolemma (see Figures 4-2 and 4-3). Nevertheless, cardiac muscle functions as a syncytium, because a wave of depolarization followed by contraction of the entire myocardium (an all-or-none response) occurs when a suprathreshold stimulus is applied to any one site.

As the wave of excitation approaches the end of a cardiac cell, the spread of excitation to the next cell depends on the electrical conductance of the boundary between the two cells. Gap junctions (nexi) with high conductances are present in the intercalated disks between adjacent cells (Figure 4-2C and D). These gap junctions, which mediate conduction of the cardiac impulse from one cell to the next, are made up of connexons, hexagonal structures that connect the cytosol of adjacent cells. Each connexon consists of six polypeptides surrounding a core channel approximately 1.6 to 2.0 nm wide, which serves as a low-resistance pathway for cell-to-cell conduction.

Cardiac impulses progress more rapidly in a direction parallel to (isotropic) the long axes of the constituent fibers than in a direction perpendicular to (anisotropic) the long axes of those fibers. Gap junctions exist in the borders between myocardial fibers that are in contact with each other longitudinally; they are very sparse in the lateral borders between myocardial fibers.

Cardiac and fast skeletal muscle fibers differ in the number of mitochondria in the two tissues. Fast skeletal muscle, which is called on for relatively short periods of repetitive or sustained contractions and which can metabolize anaerobically and build up a substantial O_2 debt, has relatively few mitochondria in its fibers. In contrast, cardiac muscle, which contracts repetitively for a lifetime and requires a continuous supply of O_2, is very rich in mitochondria (see Figures 4-1 to 4-3). Rapid oxidation of substrates with the synthesis of adenosine triphosphate (ATP) can keep pace with the myocardial energy requirements because of the large numbers of mitochondria containing the respiratory enzymes necessary for oxidative phosphorylation (see later in this chapter).

To provide adequate O_2 and substrate for its metabolism, the myocardium is endowed with a rich capillary supply, about one capillary per fiber. Thus, diffusion distances are short, and O_2, CO_2, substrates, and waste material can move rapidly between the myocardial cell and capillary. With respect to exchange of substances between the capillary blood and the myocardial cells, electron micrographs of myocardium show deep invaginations of the sarcolemma into the fiber at the Z lines (see Figure 4-3). These sarcolemmal invaginations constitute the transverse-tubular, or

---

FIGURE 4-3 ▣ **A,** Low-magnification electron micrograph of the right ventricular wall of a mouse heart. Tissue was fixed in a phosphate-buffered glutaraldehyde solution and postfixed in ferrocyanide-reduced osmium tetroxide. This procedure has resulted in the deposition of electron-opaque precipitate in the extracellular space, thus outlining the sarcolemmal borders (SL) of the muscle cells and delineating the intercalated disks (ID) and transverse tubules (TT). Nu, Nucleus of the myocardial cell. **B,** Mouse cardiac muscle in longitudinal section, treated as in **A**. The path of the extracellular space is traced through the ID region, and sarcolemmal invaginations that are oriented transverse to the cell axis (TT) or parallel to it (axial tubules, AT) are clearly identified. Gap junctions (GJ) are associated with the ID. Mitochondria are large and elongated and lie between the myofibrils. **C,** Mouse cardiac muscle. Tissue treated with ferrocyanide-reduced osmium tetroxide to identify the internal membrane system (sarcoplasmic reticulum, SR). Specific staining of the SR reveals its architecture as a complex network of small-diameter tubules that are closely associated with the myofibrils and mitochondria.

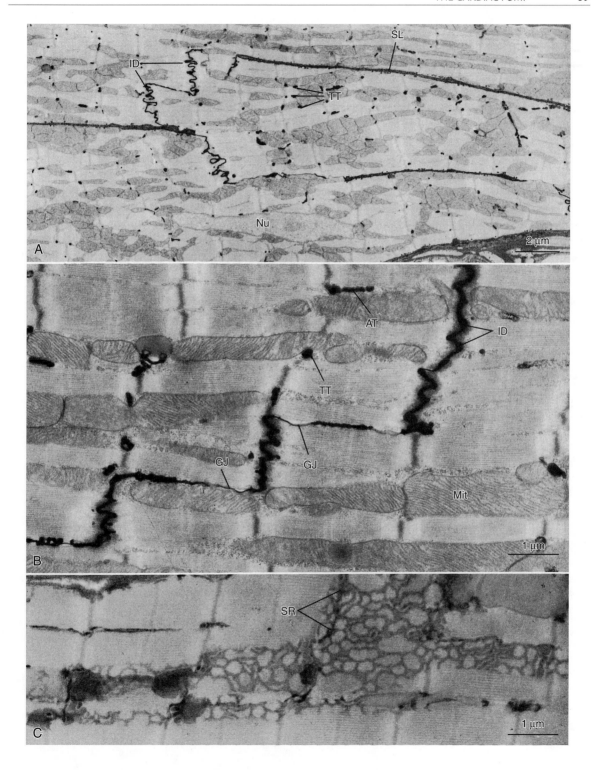

T-tubular, system. The T-tubule lumina are continuous with the bulk interstitial fluid; T-tubules play a key role in excitation-contraction coupling.

In mammalian ventricular cells, adjacent T-tubules are interconnected by longitudinally running or axial tubules that form an extensively interconnected lattice of "intracellular" tubules (see Figure 4-3). This T-tubular system is open to the interstitial fluid, is lined with a basement membrane continuous with that of the surface sarcolemma, and contains micropinocytotic vesicles. Thus, in ventricular cells the myofibrils and mitochondria have ready access to a space continuous with the interstitial fluid. The T-tubular system is absent or poorly developed in atrial myocytes and Purkinje cells of mammalian hearts.

A network of sarcoplasmic reticulum (SR) (Figure 4-3C) consisting of small-diameter sarcotubules is also present surrounding myofibrils; these sarcotubules are believed to be "closed" because colloidal tracer particles (2 to 10 nm in diameter) do not enter them. They do not contain basement membrane. Flattened elements of the SR are often found in close proximity to the T-tubular system as well as to the surface sarcolemma, forming "dyads" (Figure 4-4).

Structure of the Heart: Atria, Ventricles, and Valves

The mammalian heart is a four-chambered structure, consisting of two pumps in series; a "right heart," consisting of right atrium and right ventricle, that pumps venous blood to the pulmonary circulation, and a "left heart," consisting of left atrium and left ventricle, that pumps oxygenated blood into the systemic circulation at relatively high pressure (Figures 4-5 and 4-6). The atria are thin-walled, low-pressure chambers that function more as large reservoir conduits of blood for their respective ventricles than as important pumps for the forward propulsion of blood. The ventricles are formed by a continuum of muscle fibers that originates from the fibrous skeleton at the base of the heart (chiefly around the aortic orifice). These fibers sweep toward the apex at the epicardial surface and also pass toward the endocardium as they gradually undergo a 180-degree change in direction (Figure 4-7) to lie parallel to the epicardial fibers and form the endocardium and papillary muscles (see Figure 4-5). At the apex of the heart the fibers twist and turn inward to form papillary muscles. At the base and around the valve orifices (see Figure 4-6), the fibers form a thick, powerful muscle

FIGURE 4-4 ■ An electron micrograph of mammalian myocardium that shows a cross-section of a transverse tubule (TT) adjacent to junctional sarcoplasmic reticulum (JSR). Junctional processes (JP) extend from the JSR into the cell cytoplasm. The JPs are proteins that make up the calcium release channels from the SR and are also called ryanodine receptors because they bind the insecticide ryanodine. MIT, Mitochondrion; JG, junctional gap. (Courtesy Joachim R. Sommer.)

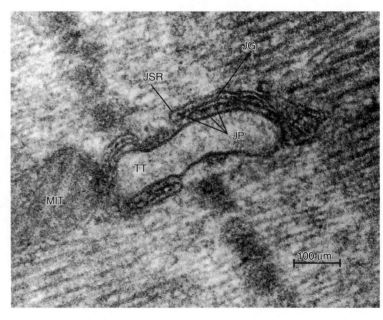

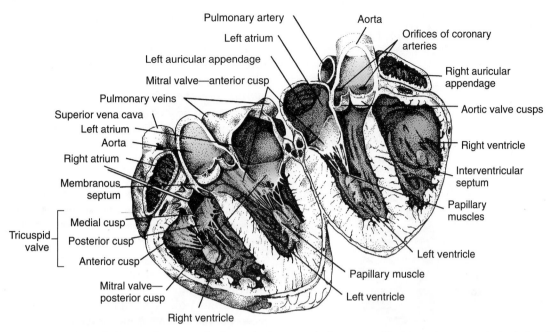

FIGURE 4-5 ■ Drawing of a heart split perpendicular to the interventricular septum illustrates the anatomical relationships of the leaflets of the atrioventricular and aortic valves.

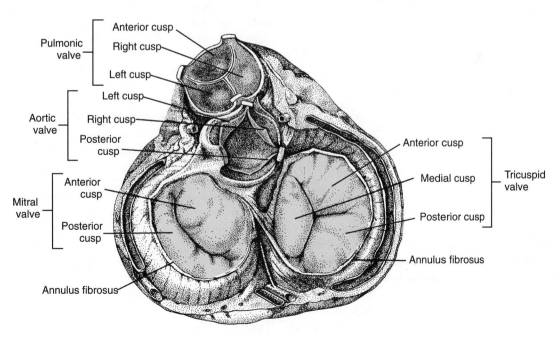

FIGURE 4-6 ■ Four cardiac valves as viewed from the base of the heart. Note how the leaflets overlap in the closed valves.

Endocardium

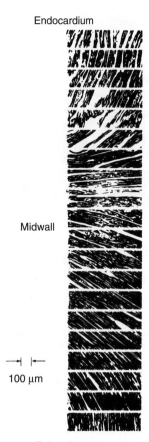

Midwall

—▸| |◂—
100 μm

Epicardium

FIGURE 4-7 ▪ Sequence of photomicrographs showing fiber angles in successive sections taken from the middle of the free wall of the left ventricle from a heart in systole. The sections are parallel to the epicardial plane. The fiber angle is 90 degrees at the endocardium, running through 0 degrees at the midwall to −90 degrees at the epicardium. *(From Streeter DD Jr, Spotnitz HM, Patel DP, et al: Fiber orientation in the canine left ventricle during diastole and systole.* Circ Res *24:339, 1969.)*

that not only decreases ventricular circumference for ejection of blood but also narrows the atrioventricular (AV) valve orifices as an aid to valve closure.

Ventricular ejection is accomplished by a reduction in circumference and by a decrease in the longitudinal axis with descent of the base of the heart. The earlier contraction of the apical part of the ventricles, coupled with approximation of the ventricular walls, propels the blood toward the outflow tracts. The right ventricle, which develops a mean pressure about one seventh of

that developed by the left ventricle, is considerably thinner than the left. The cardiac valves consist of thin flaps of flexible, tough, endothelium-covered fibrous tissue firmly attached at the bases to the fibrous valve rings. Movements of the valve leaflets are essentially passive, and the orientation of the cardiac valve is responsible for unidirectional flow of blood through the heart. There are two types of valves in the heart—the AV valves and the semilunar valves (see Figures 4-5 and 4-6).

Atrioventricular Valves
The valve between the right atrium and right ventricle is made up of three cusps (tricuspid valve), whereas the valve between the left atrium and left ventricle has two cusps (mitral valve). The total area of the cusps of each AV valve is approximately twice that of their respective AV orifices, so that there is considerable overlap of the leaflets in the closed position (see Figures 4-5 and 4-6). Attached to the free edges of these valves are fine, strong ligaments (chordae tendineae), which arise from the powerful papillary muscles of the respective ventricles and prevent eversion of the valves during ventricular systole.

Semilunar Valves
The valves between the right ventricle and the pulmonary artery and between the left ventricle and the aorta consist of three cuplike cusps attached to the valve rings (see Figures 4-5 and 4-6). At the end of the reduced ejection phase of ventricular systole, there is a brief reversal of blood flow toward the ventricles (shown as a negative flow in the phasic aortic flow curve in Figure 4-13) that snaps the cusps together and prevents regurgitation of blood into the ventricles. During ventricular systole the cusps do not lie back against the walls of the pulmonary artery and aorta but float in the bloodstream approximately midway between the vessel walls and their closed position. Behind the semilunar valves are small outpocketings of the pulmonary artery and aorta (sinuses of Valsalva), where eddy currents develop that tend to keep the valve cusps away from the vessel walls. The orifices of the right and left coronary arteries are behind the right and left cusps, respectively, of the aortic valve. Were it not for the presence of the sinuses of Valsalva and the eddy currents developed therein, the coronary ostia could be blocked by the valve cusps.

*The Pericardium Is an Epithelized Fibrous Sac
That Invests the Heart*

The pericardium consists of a visceral layer that adheres to the epicardium and a parietal layer that is separated from the visceral layer by a thin layer of fluid. This fluid provides lubrication for the continuous movement of the enclosed heart. The pericardium strongly resists a large, rapid increase in cardiac size because its distensibility is small. The pericardium plays a role in preventing sudden overdistention of the chambers of the heart because of this characteristic. However, with congenital absence of the pericardium or after its surgical removal, cardiac function is within physiological limits. Nevertheless, with the pericardium intact, an increase in diastolic pressure in one ventricle increases the pressure and decreases the compliance of the other ventricle.

CLINICAL BOX

If the heart becomes greatly distended with blood during diastole and becomes spherical, as may occur in cardiac failure, it is less efficient; more energy is required (greater wall tension) for the distended heart to eject the same volume of blood per beat than for the normal undilated heart. This is an example of Laplace's law (Chapter 8), which states that the tension (*T*, force/unit length) in the wall of a vessel equals the transmural pressure difference (pressure across the wall, or distending pressure, ΔP) times the radius (*r*) of the vessel. The Laplace relationship can be applied to the distended and spherical heart if correction is made for wall thickness. The equation is

$$T = \Delta Pr / 2w$$

where *T* is wall stress (force/area), ΔP is transmural pressure difference, *r* is radius, and *w* is wall thickness.

THE FORCE OF CARDIAC CONTRACTION IS DETERMINED BY EXCITATION-CONTRACTION COUPLING AND THE INITIAL SARCOMERE LENGTH OF THE MYOCARDIAL CELLS

Excitation-Contraction Coupling Is Mediated by Calcium

Contraction of the heart is triggered by the spread of electrical excitation throughout the syncytium of muscle cells. Ultimately, the strength of contraction of each cardiac cell is determined by the chemical processes linking or "coupling" this excitation to actomyosin cross-bridge cycling, a process known as "excitation-contraction coupling" (Figure 4-8). The excitation-contraction coupling processes are major determinants of the ability of the heart to contract, and thus of its contractility. For normal excitation-contraction coupling, the heart requires optimal concentrations of Na^+, K^+, and Ca^{++}. In the absence of Na^+, the heart is not excitable and will not beat because the action potential depends on extracellular Na^+. In contrast, the resting membrane potential is independent of the Na^+ gradient across the membrane (see Figure 2-7). Under normal conditions, the extracellular K^+ concentration is about 4 mM. A moderate reduction in extracellular K^+ has little effect on myocardial excitation and contraction, but it flattens the T wave of the electrocardiogram. A severe reduction in extracellular K^+ produces weakness, paralysis, and cardiac arrest. Large increases in extracellular K^+ produce dysrhythmias, depolarization, loss of excitability of the myocardial cells, and cardiac arrest in diastole. Ca^{++} is essential for cardiac contraction; removal of Ca^{++} from the extracellular fluid results in decreased contractile force and eventual arrest in diastole. Conversely, an increase in extracellular Ca^{++} enhances contractile force, and very high Ca^{++} concentrations induce cardiac arrest in systole (rigor). The free intracellular Ca^{++} concentration is responsible for the contractile state of the myocardium.

Initially, a wave of excitation spreads rapidly along the myocardial sarcolemma from cell to cell via gap junctions. Excitation also spreads to the cell interior via the T-tubules, which invaginate the cardiac fibers at the Z lines. Electrical stimulation at the Z line or the application of Ca^{++} to the Z lines in the skinned (sarcolemma removed) cardiac fiber elicits a localized contraction of adjacent myofibrils. During the plateau (phase 2) of the action potential, Ca^{++} permeability of the sarcolemma increases. Ca^{++} enters the cell through voltage-dependent L-type Ca^{++} channels in the sarcolemma and in the T-tubules (see Figure 4-8). The Ca^{++} channel protein is called the dihydropyridine receptor because it has high affinity for this group of Ca^{++} channel antagonists. Opening of the Ca^{++} channels is facilitated by phosphorylation of the channel proteins by a

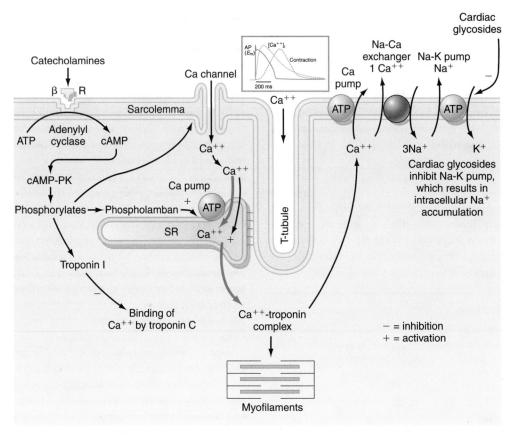

FIGURE 4-8 ■ Schematic diagram of the movement of calcium in excitation-contraction coupling in cardiac muscle. The influx of Ca^{++} from the interstitial fluid during excitation triggers the release of Ca^{++} from the sarcoplasmic reticulum (SR). The free cytosolic Ca^{++} activates contraction of the myofilaments (systole). Relaxation (diastole) occurs as a result of uptake of Ca^{++} by the SR, by extrusion of intracellular Ca^{++} by Na^+-Ca^{++} exchange, and to a limited degree by the Ca pump. ATP, adenosine triphosphate; βR, β-adrenergic receptor; cAMP, cyclic adenosine monophosphate; cAMP-PK, cAMP-dependent protein kinase; DHPR, dihydropyridine receptor; RyR, ryanodine receptor. *(Redrawn from Bers DM: Cardiac excitation-contraction coupling.* Nature *415:198, 2002.)*

cyclic adenosine monophosphate (cAMP)–dependent protein kinase. The primary source of extracellular Ca^{++} is the interstitial fluid (1 mM Ca^{++}). Some Ca^{++} also may be bound to the sarcolemma and to the **glycocalyx,** a mucopolysaccharide that covers the sarcolemma. The amount of Ca^{++} that enters the cell from the extracellular space is not sufficient to induce contraction of the myofibrils, but it serves as a trigger (trigger Ca^{++}) to release Ca^{++} from the intracellular Ca^{++} stores in the SR (see Figure 4-3). The Ca^{++} leaves the SR through calcium release channels, which are called **ryanodine receptors** because the channel protein, also

called **foot protein** or **junctional processes** of the SR, binds ryanodine avidly. During this process, called Ca^{++}-induced Ca^{++} release, the cytosolic free Ca^{++} increases from a resting level of about 0.1 μM to levels of 1 μM to 10 μM, and the Ca^{++} binds to the protein troponin C. The Ca^{++}-troponin complex interacts with tropomyosin to unblock active sites between the actin and myosin filaments, allowing cross-bridge cycling and hence contraction of the myofibrils (systole).

Mechanisms that raise systolic Ca^{++} increase the developed force, and those that lower Ca^{++} decrease the developed force. For example, catecholamines increase Ca^{++} entry into the cell by phosphorylation of the Ca^{++} channels via a cAMP-dependent protein kinase. Interestingly, when catecholamines enhance myocardial contractile force, they also elicit a limiting action by decreasing the sensitivity of the contractile machinery to Ca^{++} by phosphorylation of troponin I (see Figure 4-8). An increase in systolic Ca^{++} is also achieved by increasing extracellular Ca^{++} or decreasing the Na$^+$ gradient across the sarcolemma.

The sodium gradient can be reduced by increasing intracellular Na$^+$ or decreasing extracellular Na$^+$. Cardiac glycosides increase intracellular Na$^+$ by inhibiting the Na-K pump, which results in an accumulation of Na$^+$ in the cells. The elevated cytosolic Na$^+$ reverses the Na$^+$-Ca^{++} exchanger so that less Ca^{++} is removed from the cell. This Ca^{++} is stored in the SR. A lowered extracellular Na$^+$ results in a reduction in Na$^+$ entry into the cell and hence less exchange of Na$^+$ for Ca^{++} (see Figure 4-8).

Developed tension is diminished by a reduction in extracellular Ca^{++}, by an increase in the Na$^+$ gradient across the sarcolemma, or by administration of Ca^{++} blockers that prevent Ca^{++} from entering the myocardial cell (see Figure 2-15).

CLINICAL BOX

A patient in heart failure with a dilated heart, low cardiac output, fluid retention, high venous pressure, an enlarged liver, and peripheral edema may be treated with a diuretic and drugs that block the neurohumoral axis (sympathetic nervous and renin-angiotensin systems). The diuretic decreases extracellular fluid volume, thereby lessening the volume load (preload) on the heart and reducing venous pressure, liver congestion, and edema. Drugs that block the production (angiotensin-converting enzyme inhibitors) or action (angiotensin receptor antagonists) of angiotensin II reduce afterload, and drugs that block β-adrenergic receptors reduce heart rate and energy expenditure. Drugs that block angiotensin II or β-adrenergic receptors also interfere with the structural remodeling (hypertrophy) of the heart that occurs in patients with heart failure. In some instances, digoxin, a digitalis glycoside that inhibits the Na-K pump, is used. Indirectly, digoxin increases cardiomyocyte intracellular calcium stores via Na$^+$-Ca^{++} exchange, thereby enhancing contractile force.

At the end of systole, the Ca^{++} influx ceases and the sarcoplasmic reticulum is no longer stimulated to release Ca^{++}. In fact, the SR avidly takes up Ca^{++} by means of an ATP-energized Ca^{++} pump that is regulated by **phospholamban**. When phospholamban is phosphorylated by cAMP-dependent protein kinase (see Figure 4-8), its inhibition of the Ca^{++} pump is relieved. Phosphorylation of troponin I inhibits the Ca^{++} binding of troponin C, permitting tropomyosin to again block the sites for interaction between the actin and myosin filaments, and relaxation (diastole) occurs (see Figure 4-8).

Cardiac contraction and relaxation are both accelerated by catecholamines and adenylyl cyclase activation. The resulting increase in cAMP activates cAMP-dependent protein kinase, which phosphorylates the Ca^{++} channel in the sarcolemma. This allows a greater influx of Ca^{++} into the cell and thereby increases contraction. However, it also accelerates relaxation by phosphorylating phospholamban, which enhances Ca^{++} uptake by the SR and by phosphorylating troponin I, which inhibits the Ca^{++} binding of troponin C. Thus the phosphorylations by cAMP-dependent protein kinase serve to increase both the speed of contraction and the speed of relaxation.

The Ca^{++} that enters the cell to initiate contraction must be removed during diastole. The removal is primarily accomplished by the exchange of 3 Na$^+$ for 1 Ca^{++} (see Figure 4-8). Ca^{++} is also removed from the cell by a pump that utilizes ATP to transport Ca^{++} across the sarcolemma (see Figure 4-8).

Mechanics of Cardiac Muscle

The strength of contraction of individual myocardial cells is determined not only by the state of the excitation-contraction coupling processes but also by the initial length of the sarcomeres (see Figure 4-1), which determines the extent that actin-myosin cross-bridges can form and cycle (thus generating force and/or shortening). This length dependence of contraction can be observed in individual cardiac cells, in bundles of cells (as in ventricular strips or papillary muscles), and in the intact ventricles of the whole heart in the living organism. In the whole heart, the length dependence of cardiac contraction is manifest as the Frank-Starling

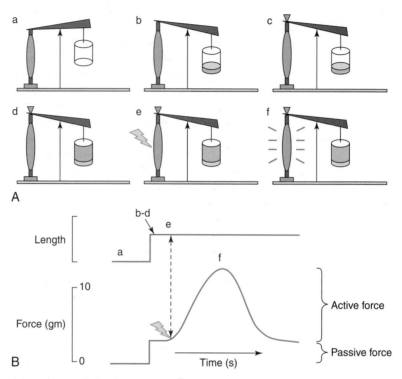

A

B

FIGURE 4-9 ▪ A simple experiment to determine the effect of preload on the strength of isometric cardiac muscle contraction. **A,** *a:* A strip of cardiac muscle, such as an isolated ventricular papillary muscle is attached to a lever and a fixed point. *b:* The other end of the lever is loaded, stretching the muscle. This load is the preload. *c:* A stop is placed against the lever, such that no further lengthening of the muscle can occur. *d:* Another weight is added (the afterload). Because of the stop, the muscle is not lengthened by this load. Only after it would begin to contract would this load exist on the muscle (hence the term afterload). In this case, the afterload is chosen to be so large that the muscle will not be able to lift it, and will therefore be forced to contract isometrically. *e:* The muscle is stimulated electrically to contract. *f:* The muscle contracts, generating force, but does not shorten. The contraction is isometric. **B,** The length of the muscle and the tension developed throughout the experiment in **A** are shown. The preload is a passive force that lengthens the muscle. When the muscle contracts, active tension is developed, but shortening cannot occur.

law of the heart, which is a major determinant of cardiac output. In the heart, the blood's pressure constitutes both a load on the heart that determines the length of the cardiac cells prior to each heart beat (the preload), and a load on the heart experienced as it ejects blood into its outflow tracts after it is electrically activated to contract (the afterload). The preload and afterload experienced by the heart in the intact circulation are determined by systemic factors, such as total peripheral resistance and blood volume, as explained further in this chapter and in Chapter 10.

Preload Determines the Strength of Cardiac Contraction

For an isolated strip of ventricular cardiac muscle or an isolated papillary muscle in an experimental situation (Figure 4-9), preload is the force (load) on the muscle prior (or pre-) to its being activated to

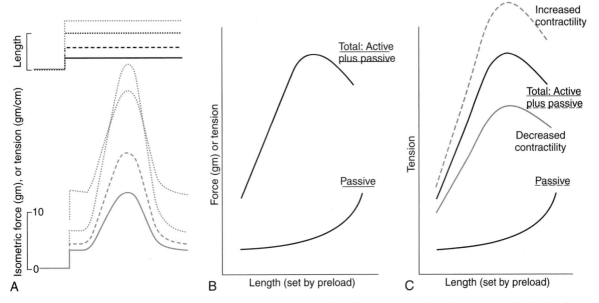

FIGURE 4-10 ■ The effect of preload on passive tension in a strip of cardiac muscle and on the active tension it develops. **A,** Recordings of muscle length and isometric tension, from experiments like those shown in Figure 4-9. *Dashed* and *dotted lines* show the response of the muscle to different preloads; increasing preload results in greater passive tension and greater active tension, until very high preloads, at which point peak active tension begins to decrease from that elicited by smaller preloads. **B,** Graph of results from experiments like those shown in **A**. The curve labeled "Passive" represents the passive force in the muscle produced by the preload, and the passive force is plotted as a function of the length of the muscle. Preload sets the initial muscle length, before it is stimulated to contract and produce active tension. The curve labeled "Total: Active plus Passive" represents the peak tension in the muscle during active contraction, as a function of its initial length. **C,** Increasing contractility, as produced by norepinephrine, causes increased active and total tension at any given initial muscle length. Decreased contractility, as might be caused by pharmacologic block of cardiac voltage–dependent Ca^{++} channels (see Figure 4-8) causes reduced active and total tension. Passive tension is largely unaffected.

contract. The preload applies tension to the muscle and stretches it *passively* to a new length. In the heart, preload is the stress exerted on the ventricle during diastole and can be represented by the Laplace equation for a thick-walled sphere. Thus muscle can be characterized by a *passive* length-tension relationship, obtained by measuring length at different preloads. Preload also determines the strength of an *active,* isometric contraction that begins from a particular length. The muscle may be forced to contract isometrically by the addition of a very large afterload that the muscle will not be able to lift (Figure 4-9). (The further lengthening of the muscle that would be caused by the afterload is prevented with a physical stop.) Then, upon electrical stimulation, the muscle contracts isometrically (i.e., without shortening) and develops the maximum *active* force of which it is capable, from that initial length. Increasing preload always stretches the

muscle further, causing both increased initial length (Figure 4-10A) and, up to a point, greater active force development. The total tension within the muscle at the peak of the contraction is the sum of the passive tension and active tension (Figure 4-10, B). When contractility is increased, as by norepinephrine (see Figure 4-8), the active tension and total tension are greatly increased (Figure 4-10C). The passive tension is largely unaffected when contractility increases, and thus the increase in total tension is due entirely to greater active tension. Conversely, a reduction in contractility, as might be caused by pharmacologic block of L-type Ca^{++} channels, results in reduced total tension, largely accounted for by decreased active tension development. The fact that active tension generated by cardiac muscle rises steeply with increasing initial muscle length is critical to the performance of the heart, allowing the heart to contract more strongly if it

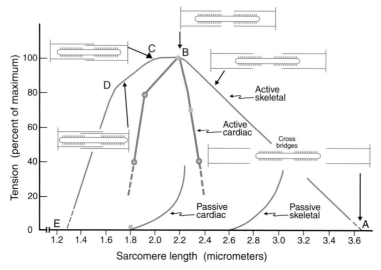

FIGURE 4-11 ■ Sarcomere length-tension relations for cardiac and skeletal muscle. Active tension (total tension − passive tension) is plotted as a function of initial sarcomere length. The diagrams of the myofilaments show the extent of overlap between thick and thin filaments at five specific sarcomere lengths in skeletal muscle. In skeletal muscle, maximum tension occurs at sarcomere lengths between 2.0 and 2.2 μm (between points B and C). Tension decreases between 2.2 and 3.65 μm of sarcomere length (between points A and B) because there is a decrease in the overlap between thick and thin filaments (between points C and D). In cardiac muscle, active tension falls steeply with sarcomere lengths greater or less than 2.2 μm. The increase in passive tension occurs at much shorter sarcomere lengths in cardiac muscle than in skeletal muscle. *(Redrawn from Gordon AM, Huxley AF, Julian FJ: Tension development in highly stretched vertebrate muscle fibres.* J Physiol 184:143, 1966; *and Braunwald E, Ross J Jr: Mechanisms of contraction of the normal and failing heart,* Boston, 1976, Little Brown.)

is stretched by a greater volume of blood prior to contraction.

The detailed relationship between sarcomere length and tension (passive and active) has also been examined (Figure 4-11). Cardiac sarcomere length has been determined with electron microscopy in papillary muscles and intact ventricles rapidly fixed during systole (contracted) or diastole (relaxed). The developed force is maximal when cardiac muscle begins its contractions at initial sarcomere length of 2.2 μm. At this length, there is optimal overlap of thick and thin filaments, and a maximal number of possible cross-bridge attachments. Although skeletal and cardiac muscles show somewhat similar length-tension relationships (see Figure 4-11), the two types of muscle are distinctly different with respect to the

normal operating range of sarcomere lengths. Cardiac muscle does not normally operate at very short (<1.8 μm) or very long (>2.2 μm) sarcomere lengths. Furthermore, the ascending limb of the cardiac muscle length-tension relation is very steep over the range of 1.8 μm to 2.0 μm, and this steepness cannot be accounted for entirely by more effective myofilament overlap, as it is in skeletal muscle. The active length-tension relation of skeletal muscle (see Figure 4-11) is obtained with constant levels of contractile activation, produced by tetanic stimulation, over the whole range of sarcomere lengths. Cardiac muscle, however, cannot be tetanized, and in cardiac muscle the level of contractile activation increases significantly over the range of 1.8 μm to 2.0 μm sarcomere length, thus accounting for the steep rise in active force. One mechanism, not present to the same extent in skeletal muscle, is that stretch of cardiac cells enhances the affinity of troponin C for Ca^{++}, thus resulting in the binding of a greater amount of Ca^{++} to troponin C and the formation of a greater number of cross-bridges. The mechanism responsible for this greater affinity of troponin C for Ca^{++} remains to be determined. One concept is that the thick and thin filaments are brought closer to each other as the diameter of the muscle fiber narrows during stretch, because the cell maintains constant volume. The protein, **titin**, may help in this process, in that it forms a scaffold to which actin and myosin filaments bind. Finally—another feature different from that of skeletal muscle—the amount of Ca^{++} released from the SR in cardiac muscle increases with increasing sarcomere length. This is a time-dependent phenomenon, developing slowly over many beats, after the sarcomere length has been increased. Thus, three cellular mechanisms contribute to the length dependence of cardiac muscle contraction from 1.8 μm to 2.2 μm: (1) changes in myofilament overlap, similar to those in skeletal muscle; (2) increased activation as a result of greater chemical affinity of troponin C for Ca^{++}; and (3) increased activation as a result of greater release of Ca^{++} from the sarcoplasmic reticulum.

Developed force of cardiac muscle is less than the maximal value when the sarcomeres are stretched beyond the optimal length, because the myofilaments overlap less and hence reduce cross-bridge cycling. At very short sarcomere lengths, the thin filaments overlap each other in the central region of the sarcomere. This 'double overlap' of the thin filaments diminishes contractile force.

In summary, the passive and active length-tension relations of cardiac muscle (see Figure 4-10B) arise from the mechanisms discussed above and, in the whole heart, are reflected in the relationship between volume of the heart and its actively developed pressure, as discussed later.

Afterload Determines the Velocity of Cardiac Muscle Shortening

A strip of cardiac muscle, and the intact heart, also experiences an additional load (force) against which it must contract, after it is activated (Figure 4-12). This load, known as afterload, determines the velocity with which the muscle can shorten. In the intact heart, this situation represents left ventricular ejection into the aorta. During ejection, the afterload is represented by the impedance due to aortic and intraventricular pressures, which are virtually equal to each other. Thus, the afterload is the stress applied to the ventricle during ejection of blood.

Experimentally, the effects of afterload may be examined in experiments (see Figure 4-12) similar to those for preload. If the afterload is such that the muscle can generate enough force to lift the load, then the muscle contracts isometrically until it generates enough force to lift the afterload, after which it can begin to shorten. The velocity of shortening is maximal (V_0) for no afterload and decreases monotonically to zero when the force (load) is too great for the muscle to lift at all (i.e., an isometric contraction). Norepinephrine increases the velocity of shortening at every level of afterload.

THE SEQUENTIAL CONTRACTION AND RELAXATION OF THE ATRIA AND VENTRICLES CONSTITUTE THE CARDIAC CYCLE

The sequence of electrical changes, pressures, and mechanical events within the heart and great vessels leading to and away from the heart during each beat is known as the cardiac cycle. Knowledge of the cardiac cycle is critical to understanding the physiologic regulation of cardiac output and for the clinician, for whom it is necessary in assessing cardiac function. During unchanging physiologic conditions, the events of the cardiac cycle are the same on each beat, but the cycle is often represented as beginning midway through diastole, as in Figure 4-13. In general, the cardiac cycle consists of a period of cardiac muscle relaxation, known as **diastole**, and a period of contraction, known as **systole**. Contraction of the ventricles is referred to as **ventricular systole**. The cardiac output (CO) is equal to the product of heart rate (HR) and stroke volume (SV), which is the output of the left ventricle on each stroke, or cycle. The SV of the left ventricle, which is ejected into the aorta during the ejection phase of the cardiac cycle, is simply the difference between the end-diastolic volume (EDV) and the end-systolic volume (ESV). Stroke volume into the

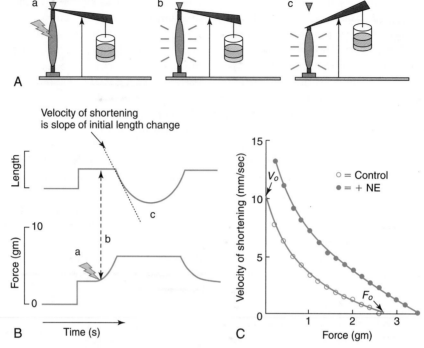

FIGURE 4-12 ■ The velocity of shortening of cardiac muscle depends on the afterload. Velocity of shortening is increased by norepinephrine (NE). **A** and **B,** Experiment to measure the effect of afterload on shortening velocity. *a:* A preload, stop, and small afterload are added. *b:* The muscle is stimulated to contract. It contracts isometrically at first, until it generates enough force to lift the afterload. *c:* When the muscle generates sufficient force to lift the afterload, muscle shortening can occur. The velocity of shortening is the slope of the initial length change. **C,** Force-velocity (F/V) curve. Velocity of shortening decreases monotonically as the afterload is increased, up to a level, F0, that the muscle cannot lift. The velocity of shortening is increased at all forces by increasing contractility, as through the action of norepinephrine (NE).

aorta is determined by strength and velocity of the left ventricular contraction. Thus, myocardial contractility (i.e., excitation-contraction coupling processes), preload (sarcomere length), and afterload are important determinants of stroke volume, because these factors determine the strength and velocity of the myocardial contraction.

Ventricular Systole

Isovolumic Contraction

The onset of ventricular contraction coincides with the peak of the R wave of the electrocardiogram and the initial vibration of the first heart sound. It is indicated

on the ventricular pressure curve as the earliest rise in ventricular pressure after atrial contraction. The phase between the start of ventricular systole and the opening of the semilunar valves (when ventricular pressure rises abruptly) is termed **isovolumic contraction** because ventricular volume is constant during this brief period (see Figure 4-13).

The increment in ventricular pressure during isovolumic contraction is transmitted across the closed valves. Isovolumic contraction has also been referred to as "isometric contraction." However, some fibers shorten and others lengthen, as evidenced by changes in ventricular shape; it is, therefore, not a true isometric contraction.

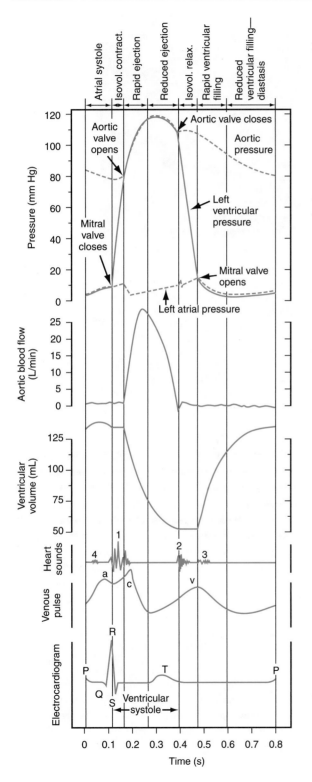

FIGURE 4-13 ■ Left atrial, aortic, and left ventricular pressure pulses correlated in time with aortic flow, ventricular volume, heart sounds, venous pulse, and the electrocardiogram for a complete cardiac cycle in a human subject. Isovol., isovolemic; relax., relaxation.

Ejection

Opening of the semilunar valves marks the onset of the ejection phase, which may be subdivided into an earlier, shorter phase (**rapid ejection**) and a later, longer phase (**reduced ejection**). The rapid ejection phase is distinguished from the reduced ejection phase by (1) the sharp rise in ventricular and aortic pressures that terminate at the peak ventricular and aortic pressures; (2) a more abrupt decrease in ventricular volume; and (3) a greater aortic blood flow (see Figure 4-13). The sharp decrease in the left atrial pressure curve at the onset of ejection results from the descent of the base of the heart and stretch of the atria. During the reduced ejection period, blood flow from the aorta to the periphery exceeds ventricular output, and therefore aortic pressure declines. Throughout ventricular systole, the blood returning to the atria produces a progressive increase in atrial pressure. Note that during approximately the first third of the ejection period, left ventricular pressure slightly exceeds aortic pressure and flow accelerates (continues to increase), whereas during the last two thirds of ventricular ejection, the reverse holds true. This reversal of the ventricular-aortic pressure gradient in the presence of continued flow of blood from the left ventricle to the aorta (caused by the momentum of the forward blood flow) is the result of the storage of potential energy in the stretched arterial walls, which produces a deceleration of blood flow into the aorta (see Chapter 7). The peak of the flow curve coincides in time with the point at which the left ventricular pressure curve intersects the aortic pressure curve during ejection. Thereafter, flow decelerates (continues to decrease) because the pressure gradient has been reversed.

With right ventricular ejection, there is shortening of the free wall of the right ventricle (descent of the

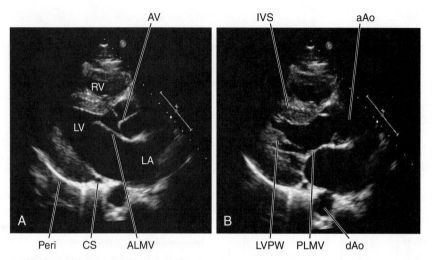

FIGURE 4-14 ■ Two-dimensional echocardiographic images of a normal human heart (young adult male) taken from the parasternal long-axis view. **A,** During diastole, the left atrium (LA) communicates freely with the cavity of the left ventricle (LV). The anterior leaflet (ALMV) and the posterior leaflet (PLMV, shown in **B**) of the mitral valve (MV) are open; the leaflets of the aortic valve (AV) are closed. **B,** During systole, the left ventricular (LV) interventricular septum (IVS), and posterolateral wall (LVPW) wall thicken; the LV cavity diminishes in volume. The LV cavity is open to the ascending aorta (aAo); the AV is open and the MV is closed. Also evident in the echocardiograms are the descending aorta (dAo), the coronary sinus (CS), the right ventricle cavity (RV), and the RV free wall. The pericardium (Peri) is evident as a very bright structure; a reverberation artifact is present. *(Courtesy of Dr. Peter Schulman.)*

tricuspid valve ring) and lateral compression of the chamber. However, with left ventricular ejection, there is very little shortening of the base-to-apex axis, and ejection is accomplished chiefly by compression of the left ventricular chamber.

The effect of ventricular systole on left ventricular diameter is shown in an echocardiogram in Figure 4-14. During ventricular systole, the septum and the free wall of the left ventricle become thicker and move closer to each other.

The venous pulse curve shown in Figure 4-13 has been taken from a jugular vein. The **a wave** is caused by atrial contraction, the **c wave** by the impact of the adjacent common carotid artery and to some extent by transmission of a pressure wave produced by the abrupt closure of the tricuspid valve in early ventricular systole, and the **v wave** by the pressure of blood returning from the peripheral vessels and the abrupt opening of the tricuspid valve. Note that except for the c wave, the venous pulse closely follows the atrial pressure curve.

At the end of ejection, a volume of blood approximately equal to that ejected during systole remains in the ventricular cavities. This **residual volume** (end-systolic volume) is fairly constant in normal hearts but is smaller with increased heart rate or reduced outflow resistance and larger when the opposite conditions prevail.

In addition to serving as a small adjustable blood reservoir, the residual volume to a limited degree can permit transient disparities between the outputs of the two ventricles.

CLINICAL BOX

In **heart failure,** the preload can be increased substantially because of the poor ventricular ejection and an increased blood volume caused by fluid retention. In **essential hypertension,** the high peripheral resistance augments the afterload by decreasing the peripheral runoff of the blood from the arterial system.

Ventricular Diastole

Isovolumic Relaxation Aortic valve closure produces the incisura on the descending limb of the aortic pressure curve and the second heart sound (with some vibrations evident on the atrial pressure curve) and marks the end of ventricular systole. The phase between the closure of the semilunar valves and the opening of the AV valves, termed **isovolumic relaxation,** is characterized by a precipitous fall in ventricular pressure without a change in ventricular volume.

Rapid Filling Phase The major part of the ventricular filling occurs immediately on opening of the AV valves, when the blood that had returned to the atria during the previous ventricular systole is abruptly released into the relaxing ventricles. This period of ventricular filling is called the **rapid filling phase**. In Figure 4-13 the onset of the rapid filling phase is indicated by the decrease in left ventricular pressure below left atrial pressure, resulting in the opening of the mitral valve. The rapid flow of blood from atria to relaxing ventricles produces a decrease in atrial and ventricular pressures and a sharp increase in ventricular volume.

Diastasis The rapid filling phase is followed by a phase of slow filling called **diastasis**. During diastasis, blood returning from the periphery flows into the right ventricle and blood from the lungs into the left ventricle. This small, slow addition to ventricular filling is indicated by a gradual rise in atrial, ventricular, and venous pressures and in ventricular volume (see Figure 4-13).

Atrial Systole The onset of atrial systole occurs soon after the beginning of the P wave of the electrocardiogram (atrial depolarization), and the transfer of blood from atrium to ventricle made by the peristalsis-like wave of atrial contraction completes the period of ventricular filling. Atrial systole is responsible for the small increases in atrial, ventricular, and venous (a wave) pressures as well as in ventricular volume shown in Figure 4-13. Throughout ventricular diastole, atrial pressure barely exceeds ventricular pressure, indicating a low-resistance pathway across the open AV valves during ventricular filling.

Atrial contraction can force blood in both directions because there are no valves at the junctions of the venae cavae and right atrium or at the junctions of the pulmonary veins and left atrium. Actually, little blood is pumped back into the venous tributaries during the brief atrial contraction, mainly because of the inertia of the inflowing blood.

Atrial contraction is not essential for ventricular filling, as can be observed in atrial fibrillation or complete heart block. However, its contribution is governed to a great extent by the heart rate and the structure of the AV valves. At slow heart rates, filling practically ceases toward the end of diastasis, and atrial contraction contributes little additional filling. During tachycardia, diastasis is abbreviated, and the atrial contribution can become substantial, especially if it occurs immediately after the rapid filling phase, when the AV pressure gradient is maximal. Should tachycardia become so great as to encroach on the rapid filling phase, atrial contraction becomes very important in rapidly propelling blood to fill the ventricle during this brief period of the cardiac cycle. Of course, if the period of ventricular relaxation is so brief that filling is seriously impaired, even atrial contraction cannot prevent inadequate ventricular filling. The consequent reduction in cardiac output may result in syncope. Obviously, if atrial contraction occurs simultaneously with ventricular contraction, no atrial contribution to ventricular filling can occur.

CLINICAL BOX

With slow, progressive, and sustained enlargement of the heart, as occurs in cardiac hypertrophy, or with a slow progressive increase in pericardial fluid, as occurs in pericarditis with pericardial effusion, the intact pericardium is gradually stretched.

Echocardiography Reveals Movement of the Ventricular Walls and of the Valves

Echocardiography consists of sending short pulses of high-frequency sound waves (ultrasound) through the chest tissues and the heart and recording the echoes reflected from the various structures. The timing and pattern of the reflected waves provide such information as the diameter of the heart, the ventricular wall thickness, and the magnitude and direction of the movements of various components of the heart. In Figure 4-14 the echocardiograph depicts the left heart in diastole (see Figure 4-14A) and in systole (see Figure 4-14B). During diastole, the mitral valve leaflets are open, allowing the cavity of the left atrium to be continuous with the cavity of the left ventricle. The anterior leaflet of the mitral valve is directed toward the interventricular septum, and the posterior leaflet is positioned along the inferolateral wall of the left ventricle. The open mitral valve is a funnel for the transfer of blood from atrium to ventricle. The aortic valve is closed. During systole, the aortic valve is open and the mitral valve is closed (see Figure 4-14B). The left ventricular wall and the interventricular septum are thickened as the ventricle contracts to eject blood into the aorta. The cavity of the left ventricle is diminished in volume.

The Two Major Heart Sounds Are Produced Mainly by Closure of the Cardiac Valves

Four sounds are usually produced by the heart, but only two are ordinarily audible through a stethoscope. With electronic amplification, the less intense sounds can be detected and recorded graphically as a **phonocardiogram**. This means of registering heart sounds that may be inaudible to the human ear helps to delineate the precise timing of the heart sounds relative to other events in the cardiac cycle.

A normal phonocardiogram taken simultaneously with an electrocardiogram is illustrated in Figure 4-15. The first heart sound is initiated at the onset of ventricular systole and consists of a series of vibrations of mixed, unrelated, low frequencies (a noise). It is the loudest and longest of the heart sounds, has a crescendo-decrescendo quality, and is heard best over the apical region of the heart. The tricuspid valve sounds are heard best in the fifth intercostal space just to the left of the sternum; the mitral sounds are heard best in the fifth intercostal space at the cardiac apex.

The first heart sound is chiefly caused by oscillation of blood in the ventricular chambers and vibration of the chamber walls. The vibrations are engendered in part by the abrupt rise of ventricular pressure with acceleration of blood back toward the atria, but primarily by sudden tension and recoil of the AV valves and adjacent structures with deceleration of the blood resulting from closure of the AV valves. The vibrations of the ventricles and the contained blood are transmitted through surrounding tissues and reach the chest wall, where they may be heard or recorded. The intensity of the first sound is a function of the force of

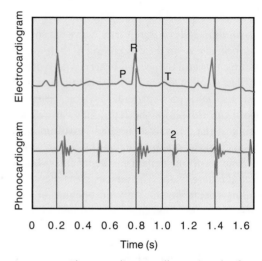

FIGURE 4-15 ■ Phonocardiogram illustrating the first (1) and second (2) heart sounds and their relationship to the P, R, and T waves of the electrocardiogram.

ventricular contraction and of the distance between the valve leaflets. The first sound is loudest when the leaflets are farthest apart, as occurs when the interval between atrial and ventricular systoles is prolonged (AV valve leaflets float apart) or when ventricular systole immediately follows atrial systole.

The second heart sound, which occurs with closure of the semilunar valves, is composed of higher-frequency vibrations (higher pitch), is of shorter duration and lower intensity, and has a more snapping quality than the first heart sound. The second sound is caused by abrupt closure of the semilunar valves, which initiates oscillations of the columns of blood and the tensed vessel walls by the stretch and recoil of the closed valve. The second sound caused by closure of the pulmonic valve is heard best in the second thoracic interspace just to the left of the sternum, whereas that caused by closure of the aortic valve is heard best in the same intercostal space but to the right of the sternum. Conditions that bring about a more rapid closure of the semilunar valves, such as rises in pulmonary artery or aortic pressure (e.g., pulmonary or systemic hypertension), increase the intensity of the second heart sound. In adults the aortic valve sound is usually louder than the pulmonic, but in cases of pulmonary hypertension the reverse is often true.

Note that the first sound, which starts just beyond the peak of the R wave, is composed of irregular waves and is of greater intensity and duration than the second sound, which appears at the end of the T wave. The third and fourth heart sounds do not appear on this record.

The third heart sound, which is sometimes heard in children with thin chest walls or in patients with left ventricular failure, consists of a few low-intensity, low-frequency vibrations heard best in the region of the apex. It occurs in early diastole and is believed to be the result of vibrations of the ventricular walls caused by abrupt cessation of ventricular distention and deceleration of blood entering the ventricles.

CLINICAL BOX

In overloaded hearts, as in congestive heart failure, when the ventricular volume is very large and the ventricular walls are stretched to the point at which distensibility abruptly decreases, a third heart sound may be heard. A third heart sound in patients with heart disease is usually a grave sign.

A fourth, or atrial, sound, consisting of a few low-frequency oscillations, is occasionally heard in normal individuals. It is caused by oscillation of blood and cardiac chambers created by atrial contraction.

Differences in the time of vibration of the two AV valves or two semilunar valves can sometimes be detected with the stethoscope because the onset and termination of right and left ventricular systoles are not precisely synchronous. Such asynchrony of valve vibrations, which may sometimes indicate abnormal cardiac function, is manifested as a **split sound** over the apex of the heart for the AV valves and over the base of the heart for the semilunar valves.

CLINICAL BOX

Mitral insufficiency and mitral stenosis produce, respectively, systolic and diastolic murmurs heard best at the cardiac apex, whereas aortic insufficiency and aortic stenosis produce, respectively, diastolic and systolic murmurs heard best in the second intercostal space just to the right of the sternum. The heart sounds may also be altered by deformities of the valves. Murmurs may be produced, and the character of a murmur

---

serves as an important guide in the diagnosis of valvular disease. When the third and fourth (atrial) sounds are accentuated, as occurs in certain abnormal conditions, triplets of sounds may occur, resembling the sound of a galloping horse. These gallop rhythms are essentially of two types: presystolic gallop caused by accentuation of the atrial sound, and protodiastolic gallop caused by accentuation of the third heart sound.

THE PRESSURE-VOLUME RELATIONSHIPS IN THE INTACT HEART

Examination of the relationship between pressure and volume in the heart during each cardiac cycle is useful, because this relationship reflects the properties and conditions of the myocardial cells, and also because this relationship provides a hemodynamic characterization of the heart. The effects of changes in preload, afterload, and cardiac contractility on stroke volume are readily revealed, in terms of the resulting changes in stroke volume. Pressure-volume relationships (Figures 4-16 and 4-17) can be recorded in humans and can be useful for evaluating cardiac function and other cardiovascular parameters. The relationship between left ventricular pressure and left ventricular volume throughout one entire cardiac cycle is known as the left ventricular pressure-volume loop (P-V loop; Figure 4-17), because the graph forms a complete loop, representing one complete cardiac cycle, which (typically) ends at the same pressures and volumes at which it began. Often, a theoretical passive pressure-volume relationship (labeled "Diastole" in Figure 4-16) and an active pressure-volume relationship (labeled "Systole" in Figure 4-16) are plotted on the same graph. These relationships reflect the passive and active length-tension relationships of strips of cardiac muscle (see Figure 4-10B), as they would be reflected in the whole heart. During each cardiac cycle, the heart operates within the limits imposed by these relationships

Passive or Diastolic Pressure-Volume Relationship

The passive length-tension relationship of isolated cardiac muscle determines the relationship between

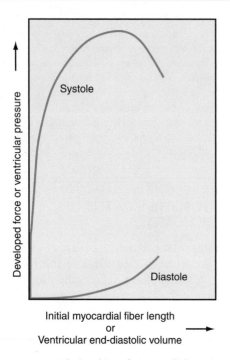

FIGURE 4-16 ■ Relationship of myocardial resting fiber length (sarcomere length) or end-diastolic volume to developed force or peak systolic ventricular pressure during ventricular contraction in the intact dog heart. *(Redrawn from Patterson SW, Piper H, Starling EH: The regulation of the heart beat.* J Physiol 48:465, 1914.)

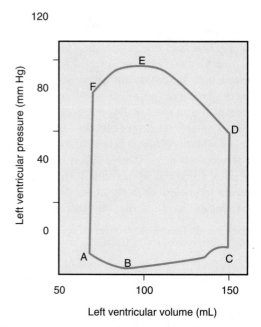

FIGURE 4-17 ■ Pressure-volume loop of the left ventricle for a single cardiac cycle (A through F). See text for explanation.

pressure and volume in the intact heart (see Figure 4-16) during diastole. For example, during diastole in the left ventricle, the pressure in the left ventricle increases, stretching the left ventricle (and thus increasing sarcomere length). The resulting relationship between pressure and volume reflects the length-tension relationship of the left ventricular cells. Thus, in general, the fiber length-force relationship for the papillary muscle also holds true for fibers in the intact heart. This relationship may be expressed graphically, as in Figure 4-16, by substitution of ventricular systolic pressure for force and of end-diastolic ventricular volume for myocardial resting fiber (and hence sarcomere) length. The lower curve in Figure 4-16 represents the pressure increment produced by each volume increment when the heart is in diastole.

Note that the pressure-volume curve in diastole is initially quite flat (compliant), indicating that large increases in volume can be accommodated with only small rises in pressure. Importantly, systolic pressure development is considerable at the lower filling pressures. However, the ventricle becomes much less distensible with greater filling, as evidenced by the sharp rise of the diastolic curve at large intraventricular volumes. In the normal intact heart, peak force may be attained at a filling pressure of 12 mm Hg. At this intraventricular diastolic pressure, which is about the upper limit observed in the normal heart, the sarcomere length is 2.2 μm. In the isolated heart, however, developed force peaks at filling pressures as high as 30 mm Hg; at even higher diastolic pressures (>50 mm Hg), the sarcomere length is no greater than 2.6 μm. This resistance to stretch of the myocardium at high filling pressures probably resides in the noncontractile constituents of the tissue (connective tissue) and serves as a safety factor protecting against overloading of the heart in diastole. Usually, ventricular diastolic pressure is about 0 to 7 mm Hg, and the average diastolic sarcomere length is about 2.2 μm. Thus the normal heart operates on the ascending portion of the Frank-Starling curve.

Active or End-Systolic Pressure-Volume Relationship

The upper curve in Figure 4-16 represents the theoretical peak pressure that could be developed by the ventricle during systole at each degree of filling. It arises from the Frank-Starling relationship of initial myocardial fiber length (or initial volume) to peak isovolumic force (or pressure) development by the ventricle, as illustrated previously in Figure 4-10. Experimentally, such a relationship could be obtained by closing off the aorta, and thereby forcing the left ventricle of an isolated heart to contract isovolumically. In this case, the ventricle would develop the maximum pressure of which it was capable, given its initial volume.

Pressure and Volume during the Cardiac Cycle: The P-V Loop

The changes in left ventricular pressure and volume throughout the cardiac cycle are shown in Figure 4-17 as a loop that lies between the passive or diastolic pressure-volume relationship and the theoretical end-systolic pressure-volume relationship. The element of time is not considered in this **pressure-volume loop**. Diastolic filling starts at A and terminates at C, when the mitral valve closes. With isovolumic contraction (C to D), there is a steep rise in pressure and no change in ventricular volume. At D, the aortic valve opens, and during the first phase of ejection (rapid ejection, D to E), the large reduction in volume is associated with a continued but less steep increase in ventricular pressure than the increase that occurred during isovolumic contraction. This volume reduction is followed by reduced ejection (E to F) and a small decrease in ventricular pressure. The aortic valve closes at F, and this event is followed by isovolumic relaxation (F to A),

characterized by a sharp drop in pressure and no change in volume. The mitral valve opens at A to complete one cardiac cycle.

Preload and Afterload during the Cardiac Cycle

For the intact left ventricle, the preload is experienced at the end of diastole, when ventricular filling is complete. Thus, preload and end-diastolic volume are closely related. To be specific, the left-ventricular end-diastolic pressure is considered the preload of the left ventricle (point C on the P-V loop, Figure 4-17).

At lower end-diastolic volumes, increments in filling pressure during diastole elicit a greater systolic pressure during the subsequent contraction. Systolic pressure increases until a maximal systolic pressure is reached at the optimal preload (see Figure 4-16). If diastolic filling continues beyond this point, no further rise in developed pressure occurs. At very high filling pressures, peak pressure development in systole is reduced. Afterload of the left ventricle is represented by the aortic pressure and left ventricular pressure during the ejection phase of the cardiac cycle. The afterload of the left ventricle is first experienced when the aortic valve opens. At this time, the left ventricle has generated enough pressure to force the aortic valve open and end the isovolumic contraction phase. The cardiac fibers may then shorten, and ejection begins. This is exactly analogous to the case with isolated strips of muscle, when the muscle generates enough force to lift the afterload, ending its isometric contraction phase and beginning to shorten. The load on the left ventricle during ejection is not constant however. The afterload of the left ventricle changes during ejection (D to F, Figure 4-17). Increased afterload will decrease the velocity with which the left ventricle can contract or shorten. In summary, preload of the left ventricle will affect the initial cardiac sarcomere length and thus the strength of the subsequent left ventricular contraction. Afterload will affect the velocity of the subsequent contraction. The amount of blood the left ventricle can eject, the stroke volume, will thus be affected by both preload and afterload.

Preload and afterload depend on certain characteristics of the vascular system and the behavior of the heart. With respect to the vasculature, the degree of venomotor tone and level of peripheral resistance influence preload and afterload. With respect to the heart, a change in rate or stroke volume can also alter preload and afterload. Hence cardiac and vascular factors interact to affect preload and afterload (see Chapter 10 for a full explanation).

Contractility

Contractility represents the performance of the heart at a given preload and afterload, and it depends on the state of the excitation-contraction coupling processes within the cells (see Figure 4-8). Contractility can be augmented by certain drugs, such as norepinephrine and digitalis, and by an increase in contraction frequency (**tachycardia**). The increase in contractility (**positive inotropic effect**) produced by any of these interventions is reflected by incremental increases in developed force and velocity of contraction. A reasonable index of myocardial contractility in the contracting heart can be obtained from the contour of ventricular pressure curves (Figure 4-18). These curves show the pressure in the left ventricle during one cardiac cycle.

CLINICAL BOX

In certain disease states, the AV valves may be markedly narrowed (stenotic). Under such conditions, atrial contraction plays a much more important role in ventricular filling than it does in the normal heart.

A hypodynamic heart is characterized by an elevated end-diastolic pressure, a slowly rising ventricular pressure, and a somewhat reduced ejection phase (curve C, Figure 4-18). A hyperdynamic heart (such as a heart stimulated by norepinephrine) shows reduced end-diastolic pressure, fast-rising ventricular pressure, and a brief ejection phase (curve B, Figure 4-18). The slope of the ascending limb of the ventricular pressure curve indicates the maximal rate of force development by the ventricle (maximal rate of pressure change with time, **maximal dP/dt**, as illustrated by the tangents to the steepest portion of the ascending limbs of the ventricular pressure curves in Figure 4-18). The slope is maximal during the isovolumic phase of systole. At any given degree of ventricular filling, the slope provides an index of the initial contraction velocity, and hence of contractility.

CLINICAL BOX

In the clinical determination of cardiac output, O_2 consumption is computed from measurements of the volume and O_2 content of expired air over a given interval of time. Because the O_2 concentration of peripheral arterial blood is essentially identical to that in the pulmonary veins, $[O_2]_{pv}$ is determined by measurement of a sample of peripheral arterial blood withdrawn by needle puncture. Pulmonary arterial blood actually represents mixed systemic venous blood. Samples for O_2 analysis are obtained from the pulmonary artery or right ventricle through a catheter.

Similarly, the contractile state of the myocardium can be obtained from the maximum velocity of blood flow in the ascending aorta during the cardiac cycle (i.e., the initial slope of the aortic flow curve; see Figure 4-13). Also, the **ejection fraction**, the ratio of the volume of blood ejected from the left ventricle per beat (stroke volume) to the volume of blood in the left ventricle at the end of diastole

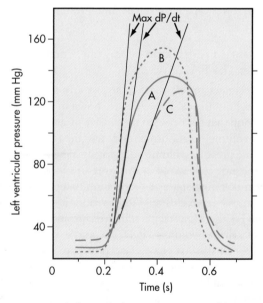

FIGURE 4-18 ■ Left ventricular pressure curves with tangents drawn to the steepest portions of the ascending limbs to indicate maximal (Max) dP/dt values. A, Control; B, hyperdynamic heart, as with norepinephrine administration; C, hypodynamic heart, as in cardiac failure.

(end-diastolic volume), is widely used clinically as an index of contractility. Other measurements (or combinations of measurements) that reflect the magnitude or velocity of the ventricular contraction have been used to assess the contractile state of the cardiac muscle.

THE FICK PRINCIPLE IS USED TO DETERMINE CARDIAC OUTPUT

In 1870 the German physiologist Adolph Fick contrived the first method for measuring cardiac output in intact animals and people. The basis for this method, called the **Fick principle,** is simply an application of the law of conservation of mass. It is derived from the fact that the quantity of O_2 delivered to the pulmonary capillaries via the pulmonary artery plus the quantity of O_2 that enters the pulmonary capillaries from the alveoli must equal the quantity of O_2 that is carried away by the pulmonary veins.

This principle is depicted schematically in Figure 4-19. The rate, q_1, of O_2 delivery to the lungs equals the O_2 concentration in the pulmonary arterial blood, $[O_2]_{pa}$, times the pulmonary arterial blood flow, Q, which equals the cardiac output; that is,

$$q_1 = Q[O_2]_{pa} \qquad (1)$$

Let q_2 be the net rate of O_2 uptake by the pulmonary capillaries from the alveoli. At equilibrium, q_2 equals the O_2 consumption of the body. The rate, q_3, at which O_2 is carried away by the pulmonary venous blood, $[O_2]_{pv}$, is multiplied by the total pulmonary venous

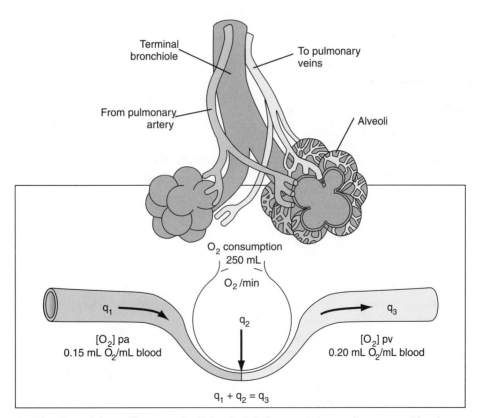

FIGURE 4-19 ▪ Schema illustrates the Fick principle for measuring cardiac output. The change in color from pulmonary artery (pa) to pulmonary vein (pv) represents the change in color of the blood as venous blood becomes fully oxygenated. q1, q2, q3, rates of O_2 delivery.

flow, which is virtually equal to the pulmonary arterial blood flow, Q; that is,

$$q_3 = Q[O_2]_{pv} \tag{2}$$

From conservation of mass,

$$q_1 + q_2 = q_3 \tag{3}$$

Therefore,

$$Q[O_2]_{pa} + q_2 = Q[O_2]_{pv} \tag{4}$$

Solving for cardiac output,

$$Q = q_2 / ([O_2]_{pv} - [O_2]_{pa}) \tag{5}$$

Equation 5 is the statement of Fick's principle.

An example of calculation of cardiac output in a normal, resting adult is illustrated in Figure 4-19. With an O_2 consumption of 250 mL/min, an arterial (pulmonary venous) O_2 content of 0.20 mL O_2/mL blood, and a mixed venous (pulmonary arterial) O_2 content of 0.15 mL O_2/mL blood, the cardiac output would equal $250 \div (0.20 - 0.15) = 5000$ mL/min.

The Fick principle is also used for estimating the O_2 consumption of organs in situ, when blood flow and the O_2 contents of the arterial and venous blood can be determined. Algebraic rearrangement reveals that O_2 consumption equals the blood flow times the arteriovenous O_2 concentration difference. For example, if the blood flow through one kidney is 700 mL/min, arterial O_2 content is 0.20 mL O_2/mL blood, and renal venous O_2 content is 0.18 mL O_2/mL blood, the rate of O_2 consumption by that kidney must be $700 (0.20 - 0.18) = 14$ mL O_2/min.

The Indicator Dilution Technique is a Useful Method for Measuring Cardiac Output

The indicator dilution technique for measuring cardiac output is also based on the law of conservation of mass and is illustrated by the model in Figure 4-20. Let a liquid flow through a tube at a rate of Q mL/s, and let q mg of dye be injected as a bolus into the stream at point A. Let mixing occur at some point downstream. If a small sample of liquid is continually withdrawn from point B farther downstream and passed through a densitometer, a curve of the dye concentration, c, may be recorded as a function of time, t, as shown in the lower half of Figure 4-20.

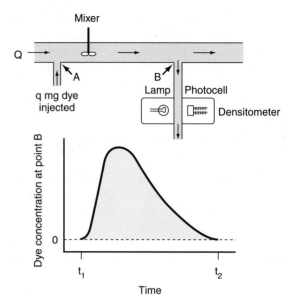

FIGURE 4-20 ■ Indicator dilution technique for measuring cardiac output. In this model (*upper section*), in which there is no recirculation, q mg of dye is injected instantaneously at point A into a stream flowing at Q mL/min. A mixed sample of the fluid flowing past point B is withdrawn at a constant rate through a densitometer. The resulting dye concentration curve at point B has the configuration shown in the *lower section* of the figure.

If no dye is lost between points A and B, the amount of dye, q, passing point B between times t_1 and t_2 will be

$$q = \bar{c} Q (t_2 - t_1) \tag{6}$$

where $\bar{c}$ is the mean concentration of dye. The value of $\bar{c}$ may be computed by dividing the area of the dye concentration by the duration $(t_2 - t_1)$ of that curve; that is

$$\bar{c} = \int_{t_1}^{t_2} cdt / (t_2 - t_1) \tag{7}$$

Substituting this value of $\bar{c}$ into equation 6 and solving for Q yields

$$Q = \frac{q}{\int_{t_1}^{t_2} cdt} \tag{8}$$

Thus flow may be measured by dividing the amount of indicator injected upstream by the area under the downstream concentration curve.

This technique had been widely used to estimate cardiac output in humans. A measured quantity of some indicator (a dye or isotope that remains within the circulation) is injected rapidly into a large central vein or into the right side of the heart through a catheter. Arterial blood is continuously drawn through a detector (densitometer or isotope rate counter), and a curve of indicator concentration is recorded as a function of time.

The most popular indicator dilution technique is **thermodilution**. The indicator is cold saline. The temperature and volume of the saline are measured accurately before injection. A flexible catheter is introduced into a peripheral vein and advanced so that the tip lies in the pulmonary artery. A small thermistor at the catheter tip records the changes in temperature. The opening in the catheter lies a few inches proximal to the tip. When the tip is in the pulmonary artery, the opening lies in or near the right atrium. The cold saline is injected rapidly into the right atrium through the catheter. The resultant change in temperature downstream is recorded by the thermistor in the pulmonary artery.

The thermodilution technique has the following advantages: (1) an arterial puncture is not necessary; (2) the small volumes of saline used in each determination are innocuous, allowing repeated determinations to be made; and (3) recirculation is negligible. Temperature equilibration takes place as the cooled blood flows through the pulmonary and systemic capillary beds, before it flows by the thermistor in the pulmonary artery the second time.

Metabolism of ATP and its Relation to Mechanical Function

The chemical energy that fuels cardiac contractile work and relaxation is derived from ATP hydrolysis (Figure 4-21). The healthy heart has a relatively constant level of ATP (~ 5 µmol/g wet weight) despite an extremely high rate of ATP hydrolysis (≈ 0.3 µmol g^{-1} second^{-1}). The tissue content of ATP is low relative to the rate of breakdown and production, with a complete turnover of the myocardial ATP content approximately every 12 seconds (s) in the heart at rest. The hydrolysis of ATP provides energy for contractile work (actin-myosin interaction and cell shortening), pumping Ca^{++} back into the sarcoplasmic reticulum at the end of systole, and maintaining normal ion gradients (low Na^+ and high K^+ in the cell).

Approximately two thirds of the ATP hydrolyzed by the heart is used to fuel contractile work, with the remaining third used for ion pumps and "housekeeping" functions like synthesis of proteins and nucleic acids. The sarcoplasmic reticulum Ca^{++}-ATPase is the primary ion pump consuming ATP. This process occurs during the end of systole, when cytosolic Ca^{++} is rapidly sequestered into the sarcoplasmic reticulum to initiate diastolic relaxation (see Figure 4-8). In the healthy heart the rate of ATP hydrolysis (breakdown) is exquisitely matched to the rate of ATP resynthesis. There is no significant change in the concentrations of ATP or ADP even with the onset of heavy exercise. The primary means for ATP resynthesis is via oxidative phosphorylation in mitochondria (>98%) with a small amount from glycolysis (<2%). Oxidative phosphorylation requires O_2 and dihydrogen (H_2). The O_2 is delivered to the myocardium and consumed in the mitochondria at complex IV to make H_2O, whereas the H_2 is from the metabolism of carbon fuels (mainly fatty acids, glucose, and lactate) and the generation of NADH (reduced form of nicotinamide adenine dinucleotide) and $FADH_2$ (reduced form of flavin adenine dinucleotide). ATP is formed from ADP and inorganic phosphate when H^+ is consumed by complex V (Figure 4-22). Importantly, the rates of ATP formation and breakdown depend on an adequate delivery of O_2 to the myocardium, which is a function of myocardial blood flow and oxygenation of arterial blood. An increase in ATP breakdown in the myocardium, such as occurs when heart rate, systolic blood pressure, and contractility are increased (as during exercise), requires an increase in O_2 delivery to the myocardium so that the mitochondria can generate sufficient ATP by oxidative phosphorylation to meet the demand for ATP. Thus, the rate of myocardial O_2 consumption is tightly linked to the work rate (or power) of the myocardium.

There is also ATP resynthesis from the breakdown of creatine phosphate by the creatine phosphokinase (CPK) reaction:

$$\text{Creatine phosphate} + \text{ADP} \rightarrow \text{ATP} + \text{Creatine}$$

This is a very fast reaction that acts to "buffer" the ATP concentration when the rate of ATP hydrolysis is suddenly increased, as with the onset of exercise, or

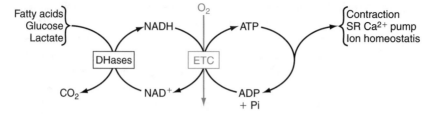

FIGURE 4-21 ■ Linkages between cardiac cell functions, adenosine triphosphate (ATP) hydrolysis, oxidative phosphorylation, and NADH (reduced form of nicotinamide adenosine dinucleotide) generation by dehydrogenases (DHases) in metabolism. ADP, adenosine diphosphate; ETC, electron transport chain; NAD$^+$, nicotinamide adenosine dinucleotide; SR, sarcoplasmic reticulum.

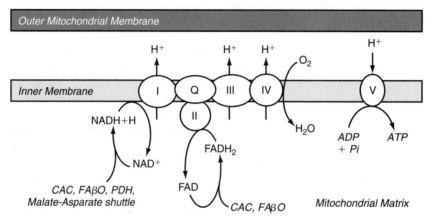

FIGURE 4-22 ■ The electron transport chain. ADP, adenosine diphosphate; ATP, adenosine triphosphate; CAC, citric acid cycle; FAβO, fatty acid β-oxidation; FAD, flavin adenine dinucleotide; FADH$_2$, reduced form of FAD; I through IV, Complexes I through IV; NAD$^+$, nicotinamide adenosine dinucleotide; NADH, reduced form of NAD; PDH, pyruvate dehydrogenase; Pi, inorganic phosphate; Q, ubiquinone; V, Complex V, or ATP Synthase.

when there is an abrupt decrease in oxidative phosphorylation, such as occurs with myocardial ischemia.

There is a stoichiometric link among the rate of oxidation of carbon fuels, NADH and FADH$_2$ reduction, flux through the electron transport chain, O$_2$ consumption, oxidative phosphorylation, ATP hydrolysis, actin-myosin interaction, and external contractile power produced by the heart (Figures 4-21 and 4-23). Thus an increase in contractile power results in a concomitant increase in all of the components in the system. The ATP concentration in the heart remains constant, even when the heart is stressed. Cardiac muscle has the highest mitochondrial content of any cell type (≈30% of cell volume is occupied by mitochondria). The citric acid or Krebs cycle provides

reducing equivalents (NADH and FADH$_2$) for oxidative phosphorylation, resulting in the condensation of ADP and inorganic phosphate to regenerate ATP. The citric acid cycle is fueled by acetyl–coenzyme A (CoA) formed primarily from oxidation of pyruvate and fatty acids. Cardiomyocytes oxidize fatty acids derived from both the plasma and the breakdown of intracellular triacylglycerol stores, whereas pyruvate is derived from either lactate dehydrogenase or glycolysis. The rates of these metabolic pathways are tightly coupled to the rate of contractile work, and conversely, contractile work is coupled to the supply of O$_2$ and the rate of oxidative phosphorylation. After an overnight fast, fatty acids are the major oxidative fuel for the heart (60%-100% of the O$_2$ consumption), with a lesser

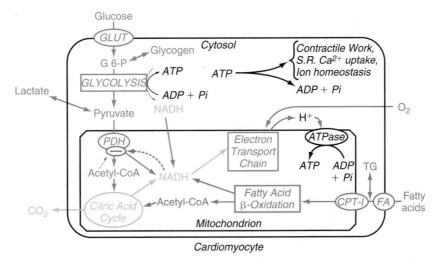

FIGURE 4-23 ■ Regulation of the oxidation of glucose and lactate by pyruvate dehydrogenase (PDH). The activity of PDH is inhibited by product inhibition from acetyl-CoA (coenzyme A) and NADH (reduced form of nicotinamide adenosine dinucleotide) (*dashed arrows*). Also, PDH activity is inhibited when phosphorylated by PDH kinase and activated when dephosphorylated by PDH phosphatase. ADP, adenosine diphosphate; ATP, adenosine triphosphate; CPT-I, carnitine palmitoyltransferase; G-6-P, glucose-6-phosphate; GLUT, glucose transporter; Pi, inorganic phosphate; S.R., sarcoplasmic reticulum.

contribution from lactate and glucose (0%-20% from each). The regulation of myocardial metabolism is complex in that it is linked to arterial substrate and hormone levels, coronary flow, inotropic state, and the nutritional status of the tissue.

Fatty Acid Metabolism

The heart readily extracts free fatty acids from the plasma and either oxidizes it or converts it to triglyceride stores. The rate of uptake of free fatty acids depends mainly on their concentration in the plasma and the concentration of the fatty acid transporter (FAT) in the plasma membrane. Thus fatty acid uptake is increased when fatty acid levels are increased, as with fasting or diabetes and decreased when they are low, such as following ingestion of a meal.

Esterified fatty acids are transferred across the mitochondrial membrane into the mitochondrial matrix by the carnitine–fatty acyl transport system (see Figure 4-24). The first one in the sequence, carnitine palmitoyltransferase I (CPT I), catalyzes the

formation of long-chain acylcarnitine from long-chain acyl-CoA in the compartment between the inner and outer mitochondrial membranes. The second enzyme, carnitine:acylcarnitine translocase, transports long-chain acylcarnitine across the inner mitochondrial membrane, whereas the last one in the sequence, CPT II, regenerates long-chain acyl-CoA in the mitochondrial matrix. Of the three enzymes involved in the transmitochondrial membrane transport, CPT I serves the key regulatory role. CPT I transfers the fatty acid moiety from acyl-CoA to carnitine to form long-chain acylcarnitine, which is then transported to the mitochondrion. CPT I activity is inhibited by malonyl-CoA. Once in the mitochondrial matrix, long-chain acyl-CoA passes through the β-oxidation to produce acetyl-CoA.

Acetyl-CoA can also be formed from the oxidation of ketone bodies (acetoacetate and β-hydroxybutyrate), which are taken up by the myocardium from the plasma (see Figure 4-24). Normally the heart does not use a significant number of ketone bodies as a fuel simply because their plasma concentration is very low. In

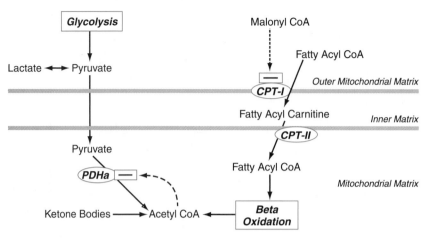

FIGURE 4-24 ■ The pathways and regulatory points of myocardial substrate metabolism. Regulation of fatty acid oxidation, and fatty acid inhibition of flux through PDHa. CoA, coenzyme A; CPT, carnitine palmitoyltransferase; PDH, pyruvate dehydrogenase; PDHa, active dephosphorylated PDH.

poorly controlled diabetes or during starvation, the concentration of ketone bodies increases dramatically and they become a significant source of fuel for the heart.

Carbohydrate Metabolism

Regulation of Glucose Uptake The three primary sources of carbohydrate substrate for the myocardium are extracellular glucose, glycogen stores, and extracellular lactate. The uptake of extracellular glucose is regulated by the transmembrane glucose gradient and the concentration and activity of glucose transporters in the plasma membrane. Two isoforms of the glucose transporter (GLUT) family have been identified in the myocardium, GLUT 1 and GLUT 4; the two are located both in the sarcolemmal membrane and in intracellular microsomal vesicles. GLUT 4 is the predominant isoform in the heart. Insulin and ischemia result in a translocation of GLUT 4 and GLUT 1 from the intracellular site into the plasma membrane, resulting in an increase in the membrane capacitance for glucose transport. The transmembrane glucose gradient is determined by the interstitial glucose and intracellular free glucose concentrations. The interstitial glucose level is a function of the arterial glucose concentration and blood flow; thus interstitial glucose levels and the transmembrane glucose gradient are decreased during ischemia and are increased by hyperglycemia. Upon entering the cell, free glucose is rapidly phosphorylated by hexokinase to form glucose-6-phosphate (G-6-P), which is impermeable to the cell membrane.

Regulation of Glycolysis Given a constant supply of G-6-P, the primary regulators of glycolytic rate are the activity of phosphofructokinase (PFK), and the ability to form NADH (Figure 4-25). Nicotinamide adenine dinucleotide (NAD+) is reduced to NADH by the conversion of glyceraldehyde 3-phosphate (GAP) to 3-phosphoglycerol phosphate by the enzyme GAP dehydrogenase (GAP-DH). Cytosolic NADH can be converted back to NAD+ through the conversion of pyruvate to lactate by lactate dehydrogenase (LDH), or the reducing equivalents can be shuttled into the mitochondria via the malate-aspartate shuttle. The rate of glycolysis in the myocardium is increased during exercise; however, the NADH and pyruvate are oxidized in mitochondria to CO_2, H_2O, and NAD+. Glycolysis is also increased when myocardial blood flow is below normal, a condition called myocardial ischemia. In this situation, mitochondrial oxidation of pyruvate and NADH is insufficient, and they are converted to lactate and NAD+ in the cytosol.

Regulation of Pyruvate and Lactate Oxidation Lactate is a major source of pyruvate formation under well-perfused conditions in vivo. Under

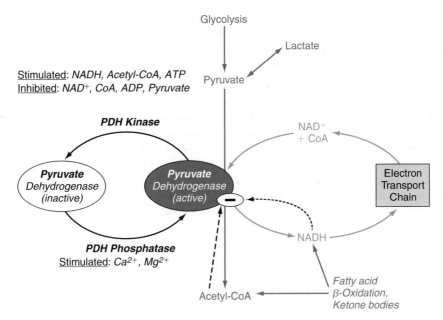

FIGURE 4-25 ■ Regulation of the oxidation of glucose and lactate by pyruvate dehydrogenase (PDH). The activity of PDH is inhibited by product inhibition from acetyl-CoA (coenzyme A) and NADH (reduced form of nicotinamide adenosine dinucleotide), and by phosphorylation by PDH kinase and dephosphorylation by PDH phosphatase. Inhibition of myocardial fatty acid oxidation reduces inhibition on PDH and thus increases pyruvate oxidation. ADP, adenosine diphosphate; ATP, adenosine triphosphate; NAD⁺, nicotinamide adenosine dinucleotide.

some conditions, lactate uptake can exceed glycolysis as a source of pyruvate. Lactate that is extracted by the heart is rapidly oxidized by lactate dehydrogenase, decarboxylated by pyruvate dehydrogenase (PDH) and oxidized to CO_2 in the citric acid cycle (see Figure 4-23).

Pyruvate decarboxylation is the key irreversible step in carbohydrate oxidation and is catalyzed by PDH (see Figure 4-25). PDH is a multienzyme complex located in the mitochondrial matrix. The activity of PDH is regulated by a variety of mechanisms; in particular, it is inactivated when phosphorylated by a specific PDH kinase and is activated when dephosphorylated by a specific PDH phosphatase (see Figure 4-25). The rate of pyruvate oxidation depends on the degree of phosphorylation of PDH and also on the mitochondrial concentrations of its substrates, and products as these control flux through the active dephosphorylated form of the enzyme. The activity of PDH phosphatase is increased by Ca^{++} and Mg^{++}, whereas PDH kinase is inhibited by pyruvate and ADP and activated by increases in acetyl-CoA/CoA and NADH/NAD⁺ (see Figure 4-25). Pyruvate oxidation and the activity of PDH in the heart are decreased by elevated rates of fatty acid oxidation caused by increased plasma levels of free fatty acid, and are enhanced by suppression of free fatty acid oxidation induced by a decrease in plasma free fatty acid levels or by inhibition of CPT I. Positive inotropic agents increase the amount of active enzyme by a Ca^{++}-dependent activation of PDH phosphatase, whereas PDH kinase activity is increased and the enzyme is more inactivated when carbohydrate reserves are low as in starvation or diabetes.

Interrelation Between Fatty Acid and Carbohydrate Metabolism

High rates of fatty acid oxidation feed back to inhibit uptake of glucose and lactate. In humans, there is a strong negative correlation between the concentration of free fatty acids in the arterial plasma and the extraction of glucose and lactate by the heart. Fatty acid oxidation inhibits the oxidation of lactate and glucose by a variety of mechanisms. The phenomenon of fatty acid inhibition of glucose uptake and oxidation is called the **glucose–fatty acid cycle**. First, high rates of fatty acid oxidation result in an increase in citrate content in the mitochondria, which then leads to an higher citrate content in the cytosol and inhibition of PFK activity and decreased rate of glycolysis. High rates of fatty acid oxidation also inhibit PDH activity. Raised mitochondrial levels of acetyl-CoA and NADH activate PDH kinase that then phosphorylates and inhibits PDH (see Figure 4-25). Also, it has been shown in isolated heart mitochondria that elevated rates of fatty acid oxidation inhibit flux through PDH for any given PDH phosphorylation state. Pharmacologic inhibition of CPT I inhibits fatty acyl-CoA transport into the mitochondria and its subsequent oxidation to acetyl-CoA and results in greater pyruvate oxidation by lowering acetyl-CoA levels and relieving tonic inhibition of PDH.

Effects of Plasma Substrate and Insulin Levels

Under most conditions, plasma free fatty acid levels are a primary regulator of myocardial glucose and lactate oxidation. High plasma free fatty acid levels (>0.8 mM) inhibit both the uptake and oxidation of glucose and lactate in human myocardium, whereas pharmacologic lowering of plasma free fatty acid levels (<0.3 mM) results in an increase in myocardial glucose and lactate uptake. This increase is primarily related to the release of product inhibition on PDH and glycolysis as free fatty acid concentration decreases in the perfusate. Arterial lactate concentration is not a key regulator of lactate uptake and oxidation under normal resting conditions in humans, when levels are rather constant at about 0.6 to 1.2 mM. However, during and after exercise, arterial lactate levels increase and arterial lactate concentration becomes the major regulator of lactate oxidation. Plasma glucose concentration is not a major regulator of glucose uptake and oxidation under well-perfused conditions, in which plasma insulin and free fatty acid are held constant.

Plasma insulin levels regulate directly myocardial carbohydrate metabolism by stimulating glucose transport into cardiomyocytes and indirectly by inhibiting lipolysis in adipocytes and thus lowering plasma free fatty acid levels. The direct action of insulin on glucose uptake occurs by increasing the incorporation of GLUT 4 and GLUT 1 into the sarcolemmal membrane. Insulin also results in stimulation of hexokinase and glycogen synthetase activities, resulting in increased glucose phosphorylation and glycogen synthesis; the mechanism for this effect in the heart is unclear but could be at least partially due to the increase in glucose and G-6-P that occurs secondary to insulin-stimulated glucose transport. In addition to these direct effects, insulin indirectly increases flux through glycolysis and PDH by decreasing plasma free fatty acid levels and thereby releasing fatty acid inhibition, causing an increase in glucose and lactate uptake and oxidation.

What is the significance of insulin in terms of substrate use in the human heart? With fasting, insulin levels are reduced, resulting in less insulin inhibition of fatty acid release from adipocytes, an increase in plasma free fatty acid concentration (>0.8 mM), a high rate of fatty acid oxidation by the heart, and inhibition of glucose and lactate uptake and oxidation by the heart. In contrast, after a meal, insulin levels increase dramatically and the free fatty acid levels fall, resulting in greater glucose and lactate uptake and oxidation by the heart. Diabetes is similar to fasting in that there are frequently periods of low insulin and high fatty acid concentrations in the plasma and low rates of glucose and lactate uptake and oxidation.

Cardiac O_2 Consumption and the Link between Ventricular Function and Cardiac Metabolism

The rates of ATP hydrolysis and synthesis under nonischemic conditions are coupled to the mechanical power output of the left ventricle (see Figure 4-21). The rate of citric acid cycle flux and O_2 consumption by the myocardium ($\dot{V}_{O_2}$) varies proportionately with ventricular power output because almost all of the ATP synthesis occurs by oxidative phosphorylation. The $\dot{V}_{O_2}$ is the amount of O_2 consumed by the myocardium each minute and is the difference between the amount of O_2 that flows into the myocardium and the amount that flows out.

Estimation of cardiac work is important in clinical practice because cardiac work determines the O_2 needs of the heart. Cardiac work has external and internal components. External mechanical work, **W**, (force times distance) is that done by the heart on moving the blood within it and can be written as

$$W = \int_{t_1}^{t_2} PdV + \rho v^2 / 2 \qquad (9)$$

The first term on the right side of Equation 9 is P-V work; that is, each small increment of volume that is pumped, **dV**, is multiplied by the associated pressure, **P**, and the products, **PdV**, are integrated over the duration of the stroke volume, **t₂ − t₁**. The second term is kinetic work due to the speed at which the blood moves, where ρ is the density of blood and **v** is its velocity. At resting levels of cardiac output, the kinetic energy component is less than 5% in the left ventricle. However, at high cardiac outputs, as in strenuous exercise, the kinetic energy component can account for up to 50% of total cardiac work in the right ventricle. This follows because work in the right ventricle is about 15% of that in the left ventricle inasmuch as the pulmonary vascular resistance is much less than systemic vascular resistance.

The internal work of the heart can be written as

$$W = \alpha \int T dt \qquad (10)$$

where α is proportionality constant that converts Tdt into units of work, that converts Tdt into units of energy. **T** is tension, and **dt** is time. Clinically, $\dot{V}_{O_2}$ and left ventricular power are difficult to measure; however, they are both closely related to the **rate-pressure product**, which is the heart rate times the systolic arterial blood pressure, **P_sys**. Such measurements are important because internal work is a large determinant of myocardial O_2 need.

The magnitude and duration of the left ventricular pressure and wall tension, as well as heart rate and contractility, are related to left ventricular O_2 consumption ($\dot{V}_{O_2}$). An alternative approach to evaluate cardiac work and its relation to has been developed. With this method, P-V loops (see Figure 4-17) are examined under conditions with varied preload and afterload; contractility is maintained constant. Integration of the area subtended by the end-systolic and end-diastolic P-V relations and by the systolic component of the P-V loop trajectory (Figure 4-26A, *shaded area*) yields a product, the P-V area (mm Hg × mL).

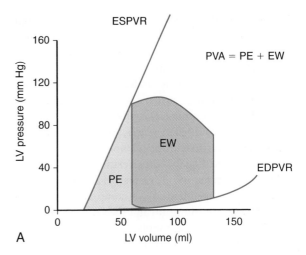

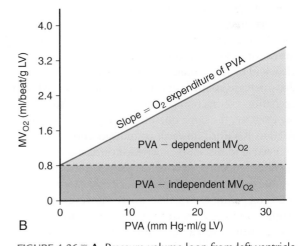

FIGURE 4-26 ■ **A,** Pressure-volume loop from left ventricle (LV) with areas corresponding to external work (EW) and mechanical potential energy (PE) integrated and summed to yield pressure-volume area (PVA). The end-systolic pressure-volume relation (ESPVR) is an index of contractility; EDPVR is the end-diastolic pressure-volume relation. **B,** Plot of myocardial O_2 consumption (MV_{O_2}; mL/beat per gram LV) as a function of the PVA (mm Hg · mL per gram LV). The linear regression slope gives the O_2 consumption dependent on PVA. The area below the intercept with the ordinate indicates the O_2 consumption that is independent of PVA. *(Redrawn from Suga H: Ventricular energetics. Physiol Rev 70:247, 1990).*

This includes the external work (EW) and potential energy (PE) underlying cardiac function and represents the total mechanical energy of the ventricle. The relation between O_2 consumption and the P-V area is measured experimentally under varied preload and afterload conditions. When O_2 consumption ($\dot{V}_{O2}$, mL O_2/beat/g left ventricle) is plotted against the P-V area (mm Hg × mL/g left ventricle), as shown in Figure 4-26B, a positive linear relation is obtained. The intercept of the $\dot{V}_{O2}$-P-V area relation is the $\dot{V}_{O2}$ for unloaded contractions. The area below the intercept (P-V area–independent $\dot{V}_{O2}$) comprises the basal metabolic O_2 consumption and the O_2 consumed for excitation-contraction coupling. The area above the intercept gives the P-V area–dependent $\dot{V}_{O2}$; this is the O_2 consumed by the contractile proteins during cross-bridge cycling. The inverse of the slope gives the thermodynamic efficiency of the utilization of O_2 for the total mechanical energy of contraction. In the human heart, this amounts to 0.35 or 35%. The efficiency of O_2 utilization does not change with agents that increase contractility, but the O_2 consumed for excitation-contraction coupling increases. Thus, during exercise, the slope does not change but the linear relation is shifted upward, an indication of the extra O_2 needed to sustain the increased cardiac output.

Simultaneously halving the aortic pressure and doubling the cardiac output, or vice versa, results in the same value for cardiac work. However, the O_2 requirements are greater for any given amount of cardiac work when a major proportion of the work is pressure work, as opposed to volume work. An increase in cardiac output at a constant aortic pressure (volume work) is accomplished with only a small increase in left ventricular $\dot{V}_{O2}$, whereas increased arterial pressure at constant cardiac output (pressure work) is accompanied by a large increase in $\dot{V}_{O2}$.

At rest, the $\dot{V}_{O2}$ of the two ventricles is about 9 mL O_2/100 g/min. The healthy human heart can increase the $\dot{V}_{O2}$, coronary blood flow, and left ventricular external power approximately fourfold to fivefold over resting conditions to maximal exercise (see also Chapter 13). In other words, in the absence of coronary artery disease, there is a "reserve" of approximately 400% in the capacity of the myocardium to increase its blood flow, rates of citric acid cycle flux, oxidative

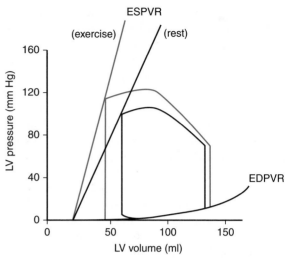

FIGURE 4-27 ▪ Pressure-volume loop indicating the pressure-volume area (PVA) of the left ventricle (LV) at rest (area bounded by *black lines*) and during exercise (area bounded by *blue lines*). The end-systolic pressure-volume relation (ESPVR) slope is increased because contractility is greater. The increased area during exercise shows the increased PVA or work done by the left ventricle; this necessitates an increased O_2 consumption. EDPVR, end-diastolic pressure-volume relation. *(Redrawn from Suga H: Ventricular energetics.* Physiol Rev *70:247, 1990).*

phosphorylation, $\dot{V}_{O2}$, and rate of external power generation. The power generation by the left ventricle is the product of the heart rate and the area contained within the PV loop. This "loop area" is the amount of external work generated by the left ventricle by a single heart beat.

Physical exercise requires a greater cardiac output to deliver O_2 to the working skeletal muscles. This is accomplished by increasing both heart rate and stroke volume (see Chapter 13; Figure 13-3). An increase in the amount of cardiac work is generated with each heartbeat, as illustrated in Figure 4-27. Physical exercise causes an increase in myocardial contractility, preload, and afterload; thus the LV P-V loop area increases because of a greater end-diastolic volume, a greater peak systolic pressure, and a decrease in end-systolic volume. The power generation (power = work/time) of the left ventricle increases because of the greater loop area and heart rate.

SUMMARY

- Although the myocardium is made up of individual cells with discrete membrane boundaries, the cardiac myocytes that constitute the ventricles contract almost in unison, as do those of the atria. The myocardium functions as a syncytium with an all-or-none response to excitation. Cell-to-cell conduction occurs through gap junctions that connect the cytoplasm of adjacent cells.

- An increase in myocardial fiber length, as occurs with an augmented ventricular filling during diastole (preload), produces a more forceful ventricular contraction. This relation between initial fiber length and strength of contraction is known as the Frank-Starling law of the heart.

- On excitation, voltage-gated Ca^{++} channels open to admit extracellular Ca^{++} into the cell. This Ca^{++} influx triggers the release of Ca^{++} from the sarcoplasmic reticulum. The elevated intracellular Ca^{++} promotes cross-bridge cycling between thick and thin filaments that causes contraction of the cell.

- Relaxation is accomplished via restoration of the resting cytosolic Ca^{++} level by pumping it back into the sarcoplasmic reticulum and by exchanging it for extracellular Na^+ across the sarcolemma.

- Velocity and force (afterload) of contraction are functions of the intracellular concentration of free Ca^{++}. Afterload and velocity are inversely related, so that with no load, velocity is maximal. In an isometric contraction, in which no external shortening occurs, total load is maximal and velocity is zero.

- In ventricular contraction, the preload is the stress (pressure) in the ventricle, prior to contraction, that stretches the myocardial cells. The afterload is the aortic pressure against which the left ventricle ejects the blood.

- Contractility is an expression of cardiac performance at a given preload and afterload. Contractility is increased mainly by interventions that raise intracellular Ca^{++} and is decreased by interventions that lower intracellular Ca^{++}.

- Simultaneous recording of left atrial, left ventricular, and aortic pressures, ventricular volume; heart sounds, and the electrocardiogram graphically portray the sequence of related electrical and cardiodynamic events throughout a cardiac cycle. The first heart sound is caused mainly by abrupt closure of the AV valves; the second heart sound is caused by abrupt closure of the semilunar valves.

- Cardiac output can be determined, according to the Fick principle, by measuring the O_2 consumption of the body, $\dot{V}_{O2}$, and the O_2 content of arterial, $[O_2]_a$, and mixed venous, $[O_2]_v$, blood. Cardiac output = $\dot{V}_{O2}/([O_2]_a - [O_2]_v)$. It can also be measured by dye dilution or thermodilution techniques. The greater the cardiac output, the greater is the dilution of the injected dye or cold saline by the arterial blood.

- The total mechanical energy of the left ventricle can be obtained from the sum of the area inscribed by the P-V loop and the potential energy derived from the systolic component of the P-V loop trajectory. When $\dot{V}_{O2}$ is plotted against the P-V area, a linear relation is obtained. The P-V area–independent $\dot{V}_{O2}$ is a measure of the O_2 used for excitation-contraction coupling and for basal metabolism. The P-V area–dependent $\dot{V}_{O2}$ is the O_2 consumed during cross-bridge cycling.

ADDITIONAL READING

Bers DM: *Excitation-Contraction Coupling and Cardiac Contractile Force*, ed 2, Boston, 2001, Kluwer Academic.

Blaustein MP, Lederer WJ: Sodium/calcium exchange: Its physiological implications, *Physiol Rev* 79:763, 1999.

de Tombe PP: Cardiac myofilaments: Mechanics and regulation, *J Biomech* 36:721, 2003.

Gibbs CL: Cardiac energetics: sense and nonsense, *Clin Exp Pharmacol Physiol* 30:598, 2003.

Gibbs CL, Loiselle DS: Cardiac basal metabolism, *Jap J Physiol* 51:399, 2001.

Katz AM: *Physiology of the Heart*, ed 5, Philadelphia, 2011, Wolters Kluwer/Lippincott Williams & Wilkins Health.

Lorenz JN, Kranias EG: Regulatory effects of phospholamban on cardiac function in intact mice, *Am J Physiol* 273:H2826, 1997.

Niggli E: Ca^{++} sparks in cardiac muscle: Is there life without them? *News Physiol Sci* 14:129, 1999.

Shannon TR, Bers DM: Integrated Ca^{2+} management in cardiac myocytes, *Ann N Y Acad Sci* 1015:28, 2004.

Soeller C, Cannell MB: Analysing cardiac excitation-contraction coupling with mathematical models of local control, *Prog Biophys Mol Biol* 85:141, 2004.

Suga H: Ventricular energetics, *Physiol Rev* 70:247, 1990.

Verdonck F, Mubagwa K, Sipido KR: [Na$^+$] in the subsarcolemmal "fuzzy" space and modulation of [Ca^{2+}]$_i$ and contraction in cardiac myocytes, *Cell Calcium* 35:603, 2004.

Wier WG, Balke CW: Ca^{++} release mechanisms, Ca^{++} sparks, and local control of excitation-contraction coupling in normal heart muscle, *Circ Res* 85:770, 1999.

CASE 4-1

HISTORY

A 60-year-old woman entered the hospital complaining of shortness of breath, fatigue, and swelling of her ankles and lower legs. She had had these symptoms for about 3 years but refused medical treatment until they became severe. As a child she had rheumatic fever and experienced a murmur, which was diagnosed as mitral stenosis. Physical examination revealed a dyspneic, slightly cyanotic woman with ankle and pretibial edema, distended neck veins, an enlarged tender liver, ascites, and rales at the lung bases. The electrocardiogram showed atrial fibrillation and right axis deviation. A chest x-ray showed an enlarged heart and shadows at the lung bases that were compatible with pulmonary edema. A cardiac workup showed a low cardiac output. After a week of treatment for the congestive heart failure, the patient's symptoms abated and she was sent home with medication therapy.

QUESTIONS

1. Auscultation of the heart revealed a:
   a. harsh systolic murmur heard best at the cardiac apex.
   b. harsh systolic murmur heard best in the second interspace to the left of the sternum.
   c. soft, high-pitched diastolic murmur heard best in the second interspace to the left of the sternum.
   d. rumbling, low-pitched diastolic murmur heard best at the cardiac apex.
   e. high-pitched systolic murmur heard best in the second interspace to the right of the sternum.

2. Which of the following is observed in atrial fibrillation?
   a. A regular heartbeat.
   b. The heart rate measured by auscultation over the precordium is less than that measured by palpation of the radial artery.
   c. A very rapid irregular rate.
   d. A constant strength of the heartbeats as palpated at the wrist.
   e. Regular P waves in the electrocardiogram.

3. Which of the following therapeutic measures would help this patient?
   a. Insertion of a pacemaker to correct the dysrhythmia.
   b. Administration of a diuretic such as furosemide to reduce preload.
   c. Saline infusion to increase preload and cardiac rhythm.
   d. Intravenous adenosine to restore normal cardiac output.
   e. Administration of a calcium entry blocker such as diltiazem.

4. Which of the following findings would be true for this patient?
   a. Increased serum albumin.
   b. Increased pulmonary wedge pressure (measured by threading a catheter via a peripheral vein as far as it will go into a branch of the pulmonary artery).
   c. Increased sodium excretion.
   d. Reduced peripheral resistance.
   e. Increased pulse pressure.

5. The patient's whole body oxygen consumption was 300 mL/min and the pulmonary artery and the brachial artery blood oxygen content were 8 mL/dL and 18 mL/dL, respectively. What was the patient's cardiac output?
   a. 2.0 L/min.
   b. 4.8 L/min.
   c. 3.0 L/min.
   d. 1.3 L/min.
   e. 1.2 L/min.

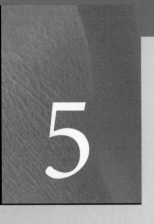

5 REGULATION OF THE HEARTBEAT

OBJECTIVES

1. Describe the neural control of heart rate.
2. Explain the role of preload in the regulation of myocardial contraction.
3. Describe the neural regulation of myocardial contraction.
4. Explain the effects of hormones on myocardial contraction.
5. Explain the effects of blood gases on myocardial contraction.

T he quantity of blood pumped by the heart each minute (i.e., **cardiac output, CO**) may be varied by changing the frequency of its beats (i.e., **heart rate, HR**) or the volume ejected per stroke (i.e., **stroke volume, SV**). Cardiac output is the product of heart rate and stroke volume; that is,

$$CO = HR \times SV$$

A discussion of the control of cardiac activity may therefore be subdivided into considerations of the regulation of pacemaker activity and the regulation of myocardial contraction. However, in the intact organism, a change in the function of one of these features of cardiac activity almost invariably alters the other.

Certain local factors, such as temperature changes and tissue stretch, can affect the discharge frequency of the sinoatrial (SA) node. However, the principal control of heart rate is relegated to the autonomic nervous system, and the discussion is restricted to this aspect of heart rate control. Also considered are the intrinsic and extrinsic factors that regulate myocardial performance.

HEART RATE IS CONTROLLED MAINLY BY THE AUTONOMIC NERVES

In normal adults the average heart rate at rest is approximately 70 beats per minute (beats/min); the rate is significantly higher in children. During sleep the heart rate decelerates by 10 to 20 beats/min, but during emotional excitement or muscular activity it may accelerate to rates considerably above 100 beats/min. In well-trained athletes at rest, the rate is usually only about 50 beats/min.

The SA node is usually under the tonic influence of both divisions of the autonomic nervous system. The sympathetic system enhances automaticity, whereas the parasympathetic system inhibits it. Changes in heart rate usually involve a reciprocal action of the two divisions of the autonomic nervous system. Thus, an

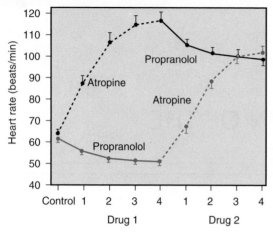

FIGURE 5-1 ■ Effects of four equal doses of atropine (0.04 mg/kg total) and of propranolol (0.2 mg/kg total) on the heart rate of 10 healthy young men (mean age, 21.9 years). In half of the trials, atropine was given first (*top curve*); in the other half, propranolol was given first (*bottom curve*). (*Redrawn from Katona PG, McLean M, Dighton DH, et al: Sympathetic and parasympathetic cardiac control in athletes and nonathletes at rest.* J Appl Physiol *52:1652, 1982.*)

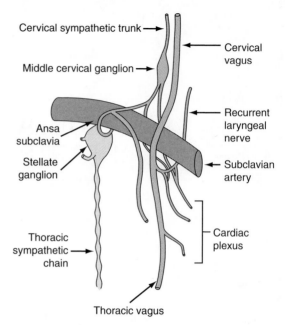

FIGURE 5-2 ■ The cardiac autonomic nerves on the right side of the human body.

increased heart rate is produced by a diminution of parasympathetic activity and a concomitant increase in sympathetic activity; deceleration is usually achieved by the opposite mechanisms. Under certain conditions, the heart rate may be changed by selective action of just one division of the autonomic nervous system rather than by reciprocal changes in both divisions.

Ordinarily, parasympathetic tone predominates in healthy, resting individuals. Blockade of parasympathetic effects by administration of **atropine** (a **muscarinic receptor antagonist**) usually increases heart rate substantially, whereas blockade of sympathetic effects by administration of **propranolol** (a **β-adrenergic receptor antagonist**) usually decreases heart rate only slightly (Figure 5-1). When both divisions of the autonomic nervous system are blocked, the heart rate of young adults averages about 100 beats/min. The rate that prevails after complete autonomic blockade is called the **intrinsic heart rate.**

Parasympathetic Pathways

Cardiac parasympathetic fibers originate in the medulla oblongata, in cells that lie in the **dorsal motor**

nucleus of the vagus or in the **nucleus ambiguus.** The precise location varies from species to species. Efferent vagal fibers pass inferiorly through the neck as the cervical vagus nerves (Figure 5-2), which lie close to the common carotid arteries. They then pass through the mediastinum to synapse with postganglionic cells on the epicardial surface or within the walls of the heart itself. Most of the cardiac ganglion cells are found in plexuses and are located near the SA node and atrioventricular (AV) conduction tissue.

The right and left vagi are distributed differentially to the various cardiac structures. The right vagus nerve affects the SA node predominantly; its stimulation slows SA nodal firing or may even stop it for several seconds. The left vagus nerve mainly inhibits AV conduction tissue to produce various degrees of AV block. However, the distributions of the efferent vagal fibers overlap, such that left vagal stimulation also depresses the SA node and right vagal stimulation impedes AV conduction.

The SA and AV nodes are rich in **cholinesterase.** Hence the effects of any given vagal impulse are brief because cholinesterase rapidly hydrolyzes the neurally released acetylcholine. The effects of vagal activity on

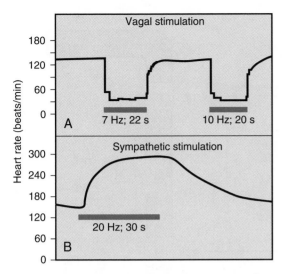

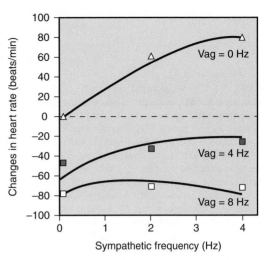

FIGURE 5-3 ■ Changes in heart rate evoked by stimulation (*horizontal bars*) of the vagus (**A**) and sympathetic (**B**) nerves in an anesthetized dog. *(Modified from Warner HR, Cox AJ: A mathematical model of heart rate control by sympathetic and vagus efferent information.* J Appl Physiol *17:349, 1962.)*

FIGURE 5-4 ■ Changes in heart rate in an anesthetized dog when the vagus and cardiac sympathetic nerves were stimulated simultaneously. The sympathetic nerves were stimulated at 0, 2, and 4 Hz; the vagus nerves at 0, 4, and 8 Hz. As the frequency of sympathetic stimulation increased from 0 to 4 Hz, the heart rate rose by about 80 beats/min in the absence of vagal stimulation (Vag = 0 Hz). However, when the vagi were stimulated at 8 Hz, increasing the sympathetic stimulation frequency from 0 Hz to 4 Hz had a negligible influence on heart rate. The *symbols* represent the observed changes in heart rate; the curves were derived from a computed regression equation. *(Modified from Levy MN, Zieske H: Autonomic control of cardiac pacemaker activity and atrioventricular transmission.* J Appl Physiol *27:465, 1969.)*

SA and AV nodal function also display a very short latency (about 50 to 100 milliseconds), because the released acetylcholine activates special K^+ channels ($I_{K,ACh}$, an inwardly rectifying potassium channel) in the cardiac cells. The opening of these channels is so prompt because it does not require the operation of a second messenger, such as **cyclic adenosine monophosphate** (**cAMP**).

When the vagus nerves are stimulated at a constant frequency for several seconds, the heart rate decreases abruptly and attains a steady-state value within one or two cardiac cycles (Figure 5-3A). Also, when stimulation is discontinued, the heart rate returns very quickly to its basal level. The combination of the brief latency and rapid decay of the response (because of the abundance of cholinesterase) allows the vagus nerves to exert a beat-by-beat control of SA and AV nodal function.

Parasympathetic influences predominate over sympathetic effects at the SA node, as shown in Figure 5-4. This vagal predominance in the regulation of heart rate is mediated mainly by suppression of the release of norepinephrine from the sympathetic nerve endings by the acetylcholine released from neighboring vagus nerve endings. This nerve-nerve interaction between the two divisions of the autonomic nervous system is discussed more fully in association with Figure 5-5.

Sympathetic Pathways

The cardiac sympathetic fibers originate in the intermediolateral columns of the upper five or six thoracic and lower one or two cervical segments of the spinal cord. They emerge from the spinal column through the white communicating branches and enter the paravertebral chains of ganglia. Preganglionic and postganglionic neurons synapse mainly in the stellate and middle cervical ganglia (see Figure 5-2). The middle cervical ganglia lie close to the vagus nerves in the superior portion of the mediastinum. Sympathetic and parasympathetic fibers then join to form a plexus of mixed efferent nerves to the heart (see Figure 5-2).

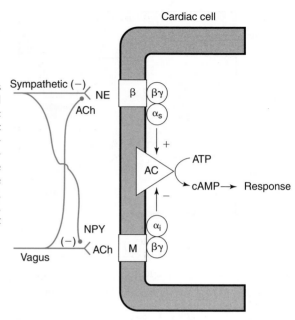

FIGURE 5-5 ■ Interneuronal and intracellular mechanisms responsible for the interactions between the sympathetic and parasympathetic systems in the neural control of cardiac function. Acetylcholine (ACh) and norepinephrine (NE) act on muscarinic (M) and β-adrenergic (β) receptors, respectively. Inhibitory (α_i) and stimulatory (α_s) components of guanine nucleotide–binding proteins transduce the neurotransmitter signals to adenylyl cyclase (AC) to regulate synthesis of cyclic adenosine monophosphate (cAMP). ATP, adenosine triphosphate; βγ, βγ subunit of G protein; NPY, neuropeptide Y. *(Modified from Levy MN: in Kulbertus HE, Franck G, editors:* Neurocardiology, *Mt Kisco, NY, 1988, Futura.)*

Postganglionic cardiac sympathetic fibers approach the base of the heart along the adventitial surface of the great vessels. On reaching the base of the heart, these fibers are distributed to the various chambers as an extensive epicardial plexus. They then penetrate the myocardium, usually along the coronary vessels. *The adrenergic receptors in the nodal regions and in the myocardium are predominantly of the β type;* that is, they are activated by β-adrenergic agonists, such as **isoproterenol,** and are inhibited by β-adrenergic blocking agents, such as **propranolol.**

Like the vagus nerves, the left and right sympathetic fibers are distributed differentially. In the dog, for example, fibers on the left side have more pronounced effects on myocardial contractility than do fibers on the right side, whereas the fibers on the left side have much less effect on heart rate than do the fibers on the right side (Figure 5-6). In some dogs, left cardiac sympathetic nerve stimulation may not affect the heart rate at all. This bilateral asymmetry probably also exists in humans. In one group of patients, block of the right stellate ganglion caused a mean reduction in heart rate of 14 beats/min, whereas left-sided blockade decreased heart rate by only 2 beats/min.

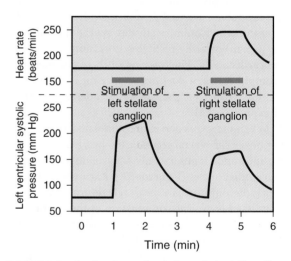

FIGURE 5-6 ■ In the dog, stimulation of the left stellate ganglion has a greater effect on ventricular contractility than does right-sided stimulation, but a lesser effect on heart rate. In this example, traced from an original record, left stellate ganglion stimulation had no detectable effect at all on heart rate but had a considerable effect on ventricular performance in an isovolumic left ventricle preparation. *(From Levy MN: Unpublished tracing.)*

Figures 5-3B and 5-6 show that the effects of sympathetic stimulation decay very gradually after the cessation of stimulation, in contrast to the abrupt termination of the response after vagal activity (see Figure 5-3A). Most of the norepinephrine released during sympathetic stimulation is taken up again by the nerve terminals, and much of the remainder is carried away by the bloodstream. These processes are relatively slow. Furthermore, at the beginning of sympathetic stimulation, the facilitatory effects on the heart attain steady-state values much more slowly than do the inhibitory effects of vagal stimulation (see Figure 5-3).

At least two factors are responsible for the more gradual onset of the heart rate response to sympathetic activity than to vagal activity. First, the response to sympathetic activity depends mainly on the intracellular production of second messengers, mainly cAMP, in the automatic cells in the SA node (see Figure 5-5). This is a slower process than the process that transduces the response to vagal activity. The **muscarinic receptors** that respond to the acetylcholine released from the vagal terminals are coupled directly to the acetylcholine-regulated K^+ channels by a G protein; this direct coupling allows a prompt response. Second, the postganglionic nerve endings of each of the two autonomic divisions release neurotransmitters at different rates. Intense vagal activity releases enough acetylcholine during a brief period (e.g., 1 s) to arrest the heartbeat. Conversely, even during intense sympathetic activity, enough **norepinephrine** is released during each cardiac cycle to change cardiac behavior by only a small increment. Thus the vagus nerves are able to exert beat-by-beat control of heart rate, whereas the sympathetic nerves are not able to alter cardiac function very much within one cardiac cycle.

The predominance of parasympathetic over sympathetic effects on SA and AV node activities depends on the nature of their interactions. There are prejunctional (nerve-nerve) and postjunctional (within the cardiac cell) interactions between vagal and sympathetic neurons (see Figure 5-5). Within the terminal autonomic innervation, parasympathetic and sympathetic fibers are interlaced within micrometer distances of each other.

The experiment illustrated in Figure 5-7 demonstrates that stimulation of the cardiac sympathetic

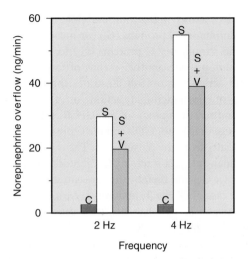

FIGURE 5-7 ■ Mean rates of overflow of norepinephrine into the coronary sinus blood in a group of seven dogs under control conditions (C), during cardiac sympathetic stimulation (S) at 2 or 4 Hz, and during combined sympathetic and vagal stimulation (S + V). The combined stimulus consisted of sympathetic stimulation at 2 or 4 Hz and vagal stimulation at 15 Hz. *(Redrawn from Levy MN, Blattberg B: Effect of vagal stimulation on the overflow of norepinephrine into the coronary sinus during cardiac sympathetic nerve stimulation in the dog.* Circ Res 38:81, 1976.)

nerves results in the overflow of substantial amounts of norepinephrine into the coronary sinus blood. The amount of norepinephrine that overflows into the coronary sinus blood parallels the amount of norepinephrine released at cardiac sympathetic terminals. Concomitant vagal stimulation reduces the overflow of norepinephrine by about 30%. The sympathetic adrenergic terminal membrane has muscarinic receptors activated by acetylcholine that causes inhibition of norepinephrine release. Thus, vagal activity decreases cardiac frequency (see Figure 5-4) and contractility (see Figure 5-31) partly by antagonizing the facilitatory effects of any concomitant sympathetic activity. Physiologically, **neuropeptide Y (NPY),** a cotransmitter with norepinephrine in sympathetic adrenergic nerves, can inhibit acetylcholine from neighboring vagal fibers (see Figure 5-5).

Postjunctional interaction of parasympathetic and sympathetic transmitter occurs largely, but not exclusively, through regulation of cAMP formation (see Figure 5-5). Postjunctional targeting of transmitter action begins at guanine nucleotide–coupled receptors

(GPCRs), namely muscarinic and β-adrenergic receptors. Inhibitory G proteins (G$_i$) for muscarinic receptor and stimulatory G proteins (G$_s$) for β-adrenergic receptors provide another means of targeting transmitter action. Figure 5-8 illustrates the general features of postjunctional action of a transmitter. Transmitter occupancy of its GPCR facilitates the exchange of GTP for GDP and the G protein α subunit dissociates from the βγ subunits. The α subunit regulates adenylyl cyclase activity (inhibition via G$_i$, stimulatory via G$_a$) and thereby the concentration of cAMP. In the case of G$_i$, the βγ subunits serve as a transducer to activate I$_{K,ACh}$ channels that cause membrane hyperpolarization in SA (see Figure 3-5) and AV (see Figure 3-10) nodes. Cyclic AMP is a water-soluble substance whose message is targeted by intracellular compartments of its synthetic enzyme, adenylyl cyclase, its hydrolytic enzymes, phosphodiesterases, and its anchoring peptides, cyclic AMP-dependent protein kinase anchoring proteins (AKAPs). Thus,

norepinephrine raises intracellular cAMP, which interacts with its cognate protein kinase to regulate cardiac function by phosphorylation of strategic proteins (troponin I, phospholamban, various ionic channels, glycolytic enzymes). Acetylcholine, by reducing cAMP formation, exerts opposite actions on these intracellular effectors. Thus, the postjunctional interaction between these autonomic transmitters adds another level of integration to their regulation of heart function (see Figure 5-8).

> There are many targets at which signals initiated at G protein-coupled receptors (GPCRs) can be modified (see Figure 5-8). Among these are regulators of G protein signaling (RGSs), proteins that inactivate G proteins by augmenting their intrinsic GTPase activity. Thus, the signal from GPCR is reduced when α-GTP is degraded to α-GDP. RGS6 is a protein found in heart muscle, where it interacts with the β subunit to limit

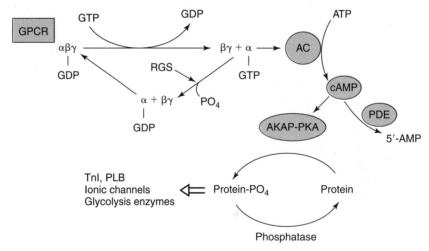

FIGURE 5-8 ▪ General reaction scheme for regulation of adenylyl cyclase (AC) by a G protein–coupled receptor (GPCR). Agonist occupancy of GPCR promotes exchange of guanosine triphosphate (GTP) for guanosine diphosphate (GDP) on the α subunit; this exchange stimulates (α$_s$-GTP) or inhibits (α$_i$-GTP) AC activity and synthesis of cyclic adenine monophosphate (cAMP). The βγ subunit of G$_i$ can activate muscarinic potassium (K$_{ACh}$) channels in heart. The deactivation of α subunits is effected by regulators of G proteins (RGSs). Phosphodiesterases (PDEs) regulate cAMP concentration by hydrolysis to 5′-AMP. cAMP activates cAMP-dependent protein kinase (PKA) to phosphorylate proteins in compartments determined by the presence of PKA-kinase-anchoring proteins (AKAPs). The state (phosphorylated/dephosphorylated) of various proteins—troponin I (TnI), phospholamban (PLB), ionic channels, enzymes—regulates their function.

signals through G_i. Knockout of RGS6 removes this restraint on inhibition by G_i-mediated signaling. Subsequently, mice displayed a resting bradycardia (reduced heart rate). In atrial cells from these animals, activation of K_{ACh} channels by agonist persisted for a longer time. Also, muscarinic agonist caused greater reduction of beating rate of the SA node and prolongation of AV node conduction time. Thus, parasympathetic regulation of nodal function is critically regulated by modifying the transducer function of G_i.

Higher Centers Also Influence Cardiac Performance

Stimulation of various regions of the brain induces dramatic alterations in cardiac rate, rhythm, and contractility. In the cerebral cortex, the centers that regulate cardiac function are mostly in the anterior half of the brain—principally in the frontal lobe, the orbital cortex, the motor and premotor cortex, the anterior part of the temporal lobe, the insula, and the cingulate gyrus. In the thalamus, tachycardia may be induced by stimulation of the midline, ventral, and medial groups of nuclei. Variations in heart rate also may be evoked by stimulating the posterior and posterolateral regions of the hypothalamus.

Stimuli applied to the H_2 fields of Forel in the diencephalon elicit various cardiovascular responses, including tachycardia; such changes closely resemble those observed during muscular exercise. Undoubtedly the cortical and diencephalic centers are responsible for initiating the cardiac reactions that occur during excitement, anxiety, and other emotional states. Hypothalamic centers are also involved in the cardiac response to alterations in environmental temperature. Localized temperature changes in the preoptic anterior hypothalamus alter heart rate and peripheral resistance.

Stimulation of the parahypoglossal area of the medulla activates cardiac sympathetic and inhibits cardiac parasympathetic pathways. In certain dorsal regions of the medulla, distinct cardiac accelerator and augmentor sites have been detected in animals with transected vagi. Stimulation of accelerator sites raises heart rate, whereas stimulation of augmentor sites increases cardiac contractility. The accelerator regions

were found to be more abundant on the right and the augmentor sites more prevalent on the left. A similar distribution also exists in the hypothalamus. Therefore it appears that for the most part the sympathetic fibers descend the brainstem ipsilaterally.

Heart Rate Can Be Regulated via the Baroreceptor Reflex

Acute changes in arterial blood pressure reflexly elicit inverse changes in heart rate (Figure 5-9) via the baroreceptors located in the aortic arch and carotid sinuses (see also Chapter 9). The inverse relation between heart rate and arterial blood pressure is usually most pronounced over an intermediate range of arterial blood pressures. In the experiment shown in Figure 5-9, this range varied between about 70 and 160 mm Hg. Below the intermediate range of pressures, the heart rate maintains a constant, high value, whereas above this pressure range, it maintains a constant, low value.

The effects of changes in carotid sinus pressure on the activity in the cardiac autonomic nerves of an anesthetized dog are shown in Figure 5-10. Alterations in heart rate are achieved by reciprocal changes in vagal and sympathetic neural activity over an

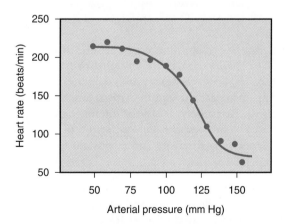

FIGURE 5-9 ▨ Heart rate as a function of mean arterial pressure in a group of five conscious, chronically instrumented monkeys. The mean control arterial pressure was 114 mm Hg. Pressure was increased above the control value by infusion of phenylephrine and was decreased below the control value by infusion of nitroprusside. *(Adapted from Cornish KG, Barazanji MW, Yong T, et al: Volume expansion attenuates baroreflex sensitivity in the conscious nonhuman primate. Am J Physiol 257:r595, 1989.)*

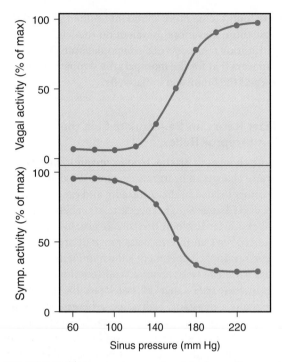

FIGURE 5-10 ▨ Changes in neural activity in cardiac vagal and sympathetic (Symp.) nerve fibers induced by changes in pressure in the isolated carotid sinuses in an anesthetized dog. *(Adapted from Kollai M, Koizumi K: Cardiac vagal and sympathetic nerve responses to baroreceptor stimulation in the dog. Pflugers Arch 413:365, 1989.)*

intermediate range of arterial pressures (from about 100 to 200 mm Hg). Below this range of arterial blood pressures, the high heart rate is achieved by intense sympathetic activity and the virtual absence of vagal activity. Conversely, above the intermediate range of arterial blood pressures, the low heart rate is achieved by intense vagal activity and a constant low level of sympathetic activity.

The Bainbridge Reflex and Atrial Receptors Regulate Heart Rate

In 1915 Bainbridge reported that infusions of blood or saline accelerated the heart rate in dogs. This increase in heart rate occurred whether arterial blood pressure did or did not rise. Tachycardia was observed whenever central venous pressure rose sufficiently to distend the right side of the heart, and the effect was abolished by bilateral transection of the vagi.

The magnitude and direction of the heart rate changes evoked by the Bainbridge reflex depend on the prevailing heart rate. When the heart rate is slow, intravenous infusions usually accelerate the heart. At more rapid heart rates, however, infusions ordinarily slow the heart. Increases in blood volume not only evoke the Bainbridge reflex but also activate other reflexes (notably the baroreceptor reflex) that tend to change the heart rate in the opposite direction. The actual change in heart rate evoked by an alteration of blood volume is, therefore, the result of these antagonistic reflex effects (Figure 5-11).

In unanesthetized dogs, infusions of blood increased heart rate and cardiac output proportionately (Figure 5-12); consequently, stroke volume remained virtually constant. Conversely, reductions in blood volume diminished the cardiac output but increased heart rate. Undoubtedly, the Bainbridge reflex prevailed over the baroreceptor reflex when the blood volume was raised, but the baroreceptor reflex prevailed over the Bainbridge reflex when the blood volume was diminished.

Both atria have receptors that influence heart rate. They are located principally in the venoatrial junctions—in the right atrium at its junctions with the venae cavae and in the left atrium at its junctions with the pulmonary veins. Distention of these atrial receptors sends impulses centrally in the vagi. The efferent impulses are carried by fibers from both autonomic divisions to the SA node. The cardiac response is highly selective. Even when the reflex increase in heart rate is large, changes in ventricular contractility are negligible. Furthermore, the increase in sympathetic activity is restricted to the heart rate; there is no increase of sympathetic activity to the peripheral arterioles.

Stimulation of the atrial receptors also increases the urine volume. Reduced activity in the renal sympathetic nerve fibers might be partially responsible for this diuresis. However, the principal mechanism appears to be a neurally mediated reduction in the secretion of **vasopressin (antidiuretic hormone)** by the posterior pituitary gland.

Atrial natriuretic peptide (ANP) is released from storage granules within atrial myocytes in response to increases in blood volume by virtue of the resulting stretch of the atrial walls. ANP, a

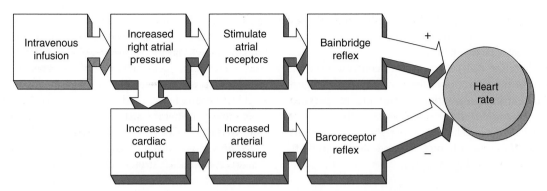

FIGURE 5-11 ▦ Intravenous infusions of blood or electrolyte solutions tend to increase heart rate via the Bainbridge reflex and to decrease heart rate via the baroreceptor reflex. The actual change in heart rate induced by such infusions is the result of these two opposing effects.

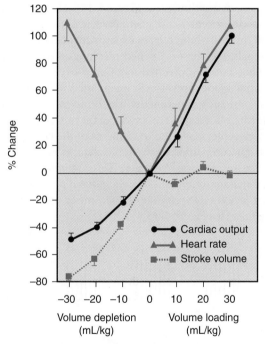

FIGURE 5-12 ▦ Effects of blood transfusion and of bleeding on cardiac output, heart rate, and stroke volume in unanesthetized dogs. *(From Vatner SF, Boettcher DH: Regulation of cardiac output by stroke volume and heart rate in conscious dogs. Circ Res 42:557, 1978.)*

28–amino acid peptide, has potent diuretic and natriuretic effects on the kidneys, and it dilates the resistance and capacitance of blood vessels. Thus, ANP is an important regulator of blood volume and blood pressure.

CLINICAL BOX

In **congestive heart failure,** sodium chloride (NaCl) and water are retained, mainly because of the increased release of aldosterone from the adrenal cortex consequent to stimulation by the renin-angiotensin system. The plasma level of ANP is also increased in congestive heart failure. This peptide acts to enhance the renal excretion of NaCl and water and thereby attenuates the fluid retention and consequent elevations of central venous pressure and cardiac preload.

Respiration Induces a Common Cardiac Dysrhythmia

Rhythmic variations in heart rate, occurring at the frequency of respiration, are detectable in most individuals and tend to be more pronounced in children. Typically, the cardiac rate accelerates during inspiration and decelerates during expiration (see Figure 5-13).

Recordings from cardiac autonomic nerves reveal that activity increases in the sympathetic nerve fibers during inspiration, whereas activity in the vagal nerve fibers increases during expiration (Figure 5-14). Acetylcholine released at the vagal endings is hydrolyzed so rapidly that the rhythmic changes in activity are able to elicit rhythmic variations in heart rate. Conversely, norepinephrine released at the sympathetic endings is removed more slowly, thus damping out the effects of rhythmic variations in norepinephrine release on heart rate. Hence rhythmic changes in heart rate arise almost entirely from oscillations in vagal activity. Respiratory sinus dysrhythmia is exaggerated when vagal tone is enhanced.

Both reflex and central factors contribute to the genesis of the respiratory cardiac dysrhythmia (Figure 5-15). During inspiration, intrathoracic pressure decreases, and therefore venous return to the right side of the heart is accelerated and right atrial pressure increases (see also Chapter 10) and elicits the Bainbridge reflex (see Figure 5-15). After the time delay

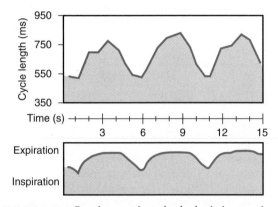

FIGURE 5-13 ▦ Respiratory sinus dysrhythmia in a resting, unanesthetized dog. Note that the cardiac cycle length increases during expiration and decreases during inspiration. *(Modified from Warner MR, de Tarnowsky JM, Whitson CC, et al: Beat-by-beat modulation of AV conduction. II. Autonomic neural mechanisms. Am J Physiol 251:H1134, 1986.)*

required for the increased venous return to reach the left side of the heart, left ventricular output increases and raises arterial blood pressure. This greater pressure, in turn, reduces heart rate reflexly through baroreceptor stimulation (see Figure 5-15).

Fluctuations in sympathetic activity to the arterioles cause peripheral resistance to vary at the respiratory frequency. Consequently, arterial blood pressure fluctuates rhythmically, affecting heart rate via the baroreceptor reflex. Stretch receptors in the lungs may also affect heart rate (see Figure 5-15). Moderate pulmonary inflation may increase heart rate reflexly. The afferent and efferent limbs of this reflex are located in the vagus nerves.

Central factors are also responsible for respiratory cardiac dysrhythmia (see Figure 5-15). The medullary respiratory center influences cardiac autonomic centers. In heart-lung bypass experiments conducted on animals, the chest is opened, the lungs are collapsed, venous return is diverted to a pump-oxygenator, and arterial blood pressure is maintained at a constant level. In such experiments, rhythmic movements of the rib cage attest to the activity of the medullary respiratory centers, and the movements of the rib cage are often accompanied by rhythmic changes in heart rate at the respiratory frequency. *This respiratory cardiac dysrhythmia is almost certainly induced by an interaction between the respiratory and cardiac centers in the medulla* (see Figure 5-15).

FIGURE 5-14 ▦ Respiratory fluctuations in efferent neural activity in the cardiac nerves of an anesthetized dog. Note that the sympathetic nerve activity occurs synchronously with the phrenic nerve discharges (which initiate diaphragmatic contraction), whereas the vagus nerve activity occurs between the phrenic nerve discharges. *(From Kollai M, Koizumi K: Reciprocal and non-reciprocal action of the vagal and sympathetic nerves innervating the heart. J Auton Nerv Syst 1:33, 1979.)*

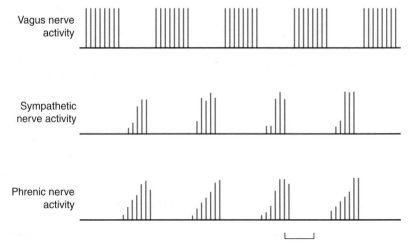

Activation of the Chemoreceptor Reflex Affects Heart Rate

The cardiac response to peripheral (or arterial) chemoreceptor stimulation merits special consideration because it illustrates the complexity that may be introduced when one stimulus excites two organ systems simultaneously. In intact animals, stimulation of the arterial chemoreceptors consistently increases ventilatory rate and depth, but heart rate usually changes only slightly. The directional change in heart rate evoked by the peripheral chemoreceptors is related to the enhancement of pulmonary ventilation (Figure 5-16). When respiratory stimulation is mild, heart rate usually diminishes; when the increase in pulmonary ventilation is more pronounced, heart rate usually accelerates.

The cardiac response to arterial chemoreceptor stimulation is the result of primary and secondary reflex mechanisms (Figure 5-17). The primary reflex effect of arterial chemoreceptor excitation is to stimulate the medullary vagal center and thereby to decrease heart rate. Secondary effects are mediated by the respiratory system. Respiratory stimulation by the arterial chemoreceptors tends to inhibit the medullary vagal center. This inhibitory effect varies with concomitant stimulation of respiration.

An example of the primary inhibitory influence of arterial chemoreceptor stimulation is displayed in Figure 5-18. In this experiment, the lungs were completely collapsed and blood oxygenation was accomplished with an artificial oxygenator. When the carotid chemoreceptors were stimulated, an intense bradycardia and some degree of AV block ensued. These effects are mediated primarily by efferent vagal fibers.

The hyperventilation that is ordinarily evoked by carotid chemoreceptor stimulation influences heart rate secondarily, both by initiating more pronounced pulmonary inflation reflexes and by producing hypocapnia (see Figure 5-17). Each of these influences tends to depress the primary cardiac response to

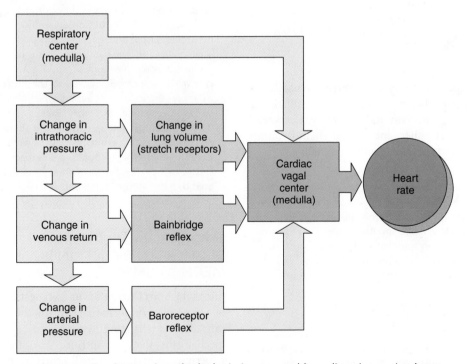

FIGURE 5-15 ■ Respiratory sinus dysrhythmia is generated by a direct interaction between the respiratory and cardiac centers in the medulla as well as by reflexes originating from stretch receptors in the lungs, stretch receptors in the right atrium (Bainbridge reflex), and baroreceptors in the carotid sinuses and aortic arch.

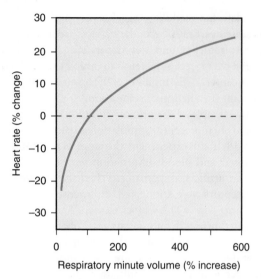

FIGURE 5-16 ■ Relationship between the change in heart rate and the change in respiratory minute volume during carotid chemoreceptor stimulation in spontaneously breathing cats and dogs. When respiratory stimulation was relatively slight, heart rate usually diminished; when respiratory stimulation was more pronounced, heart rate usually increased. *(Modified from Daly MD, Scott MJ: An analysis of the reflex systemic vasodilator response elicited by lung inflation in the dog.* J Physiol 144:148, 958.)

chemoreceptor stimulation and thereby to accelerate the heart. Hence, when pulmonary hyperventilation is not prevented, the primary and secondary effects tend to neutralize each other, and carotid chemoreceptor stimulation affects heart rate only minimally.

The identical primary vagal inhibitory effect also operates in humans. The electrocardiogram shown in Figure 5-19 was recorded from a quadriplegic patient who could not breathe spontaneously but required tracheal intubation and artificial respiration. When the tracheal catheter was briefly disconnected to permit nursing care, profound bradycardia quickly developed. The heart rate was 65 beats/min just before the tracheal catheter was disconnected. In less than 10 s after cessation of artificial respiration, the heart rate fell to about 20 beats/min. This bradycardia could be prevented by blocking of the effects of efferent vagal activity with atropine, and its onset could be delayed considerably by hyperventilation of the patient before disconnection of the tracheal catheter.

Ventricular Receptor Reflexes Play a Minor Role in the Regulation of Heart Rate

Sensory receptors near the endocardial surfaces of the ventricular walls initiate reflexes similar to those elicited by the arterial baroreceptors. Excitation of these endocardial receptors diminishes heart rate and peripheral resistance. Other sensory receptors have been identified in the epicardial regions of the ventricles. Ventricular receptors are excited by a variety of mechanical and chemical stimuli, but their physiological functions are not clear.

Ventricular receptors are suspected of being involved in the initiation of **vasovagal syncope,** which is lightheadedness or brief loss of consciousness that may be triggered by psychological or orthostatic stress. The ventricular receptors are thought to be stimulated by a reduced ventricular filling volume combined with a vigorous ventricular contraction. In a person standing quietly, ventricular filling is diminished because blood tends to pool in the veins in the abdomen and legs, as explained in Chapter 10. Consequently, the reduction in cardiac output and arterial blood pressure leads to a generalized increase in sympathetic neural activity via the baroreceptor reflex (see Figure 5-10). The enhanced sympathetic activity to the heart evokes a vigorous ventricular contraction, which thereby stimulates the ventricular receptors. Excitation of the ventricular receptors appears to initiate the autonomic neural changes that evoke vasovagal syncope, namely, a combination of a profound, vagally mediated bradycardia and a generalized arteriolar vasodilation mediated by a diminution in sympathetic neural activity.

MYOCARDIAL PERFORMANCE IS REGULATED BY INTRINSIC MECHANISMS

Just as the heart can initiate its own beat in the absence of any nervous or hormonal control, the myocardium can adapt to changing hemodynamic conditions by mechanisms that are intrinsic to cardiac muscle. Experiments on denervated hearts reveal that this organ adjusts remarkably well to stress. For example, racing greyhounds with denervated hearts perform almost as well as those with intact innervation. Their

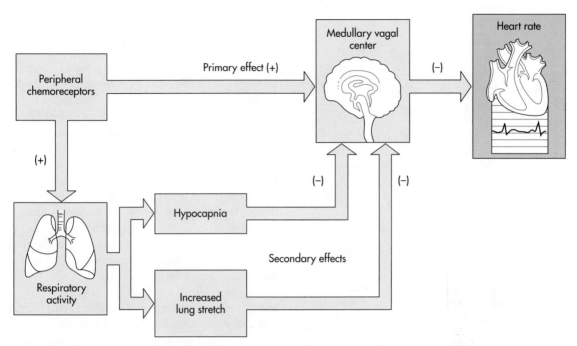

FIGURE 5-17 ■ The primary effect of stimulation of the peripheral chemoreceptors on heart rate is to excite the cardiac vagal center in the medulla and thus to decrease heart rate. Peripheral chemoreceptor stimulation also excites the respiratory center in the medulla. This effect produces hypocapnia and increases lung inflation, both of which secondarily inhibit the medullary vagal center. Thus, these secondary influences attenuate the primary reflex effect of peripheral chemoreceptor stimulation of the heart rate.

maximal running speed was found to be only 5% less after complete cardiac denervation. In these dogs the threefold to fourfold increase in cardiac output during exertion was achieved principally by an increase in stroke volume. In normal dogs the increase of cardiac output with exercise is accompanied by a proportionate increase of heart rate; stroke volume does not change much (see Chapter 13). The cardiac adaptation in the denervated animals is not achieved entirely by intrinsic mechanisms; circulating catecholamines undoubtedly contribute. If the β-adrenergic receptors are blocked in greyhounds with denervated hearts, their racing performance is severely impaired.

The intrinsic cardiac adaptation that has received the greatest attention involves changes in the resting length of the myocardial fibers. This adaptation is designated **Starling's law of the heart** or the **Frank-Starling mechanism.** The mechanical, ultrastructural, and physiological bases for this mechanism are explained in Chapter 4.

The Frank-Starling Mechanism Is an Important Regulator of Myocardial Contraction Force

Isolated Hearts

In 1895, Otto Frank described the response of the isolated heart of the frog to alterations in the load on the myocardial fibers just before ventricular contraction. He noted that as the load was increased, the heart responded with a more forceful contraction.

In 1914, Ernest Starling described the intrinsic response of the heart to changes in right atrial and aortic pressure in the canine isolated heart-lung preparation. In this preparation the right ventricular filling pressure is varied by altering the height of a reservoir connected to the right atrium. The ventricular filling pressure just before ventricular contraction constitutes the **preload** for the myocardial fibers in the ventricular wall (see also Chapter 4). The right ventricle then pumps this blood through the pulmonary vessels to the left atrium. The lungs are artificially ventilated.

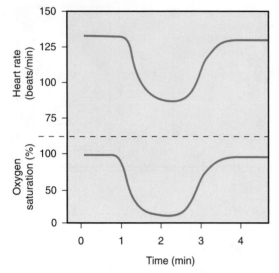

FIGURE 5-18 ■ Changes in heart rate during carotid chemo-receptor stimulation in an anesthetized dog on total heart bypass (*upper tracing*). The lungs remain deflated, and respiratory gas exchange is accomplished by an artificial oxygenator. The *lower tracing* represents the oxygen saturation of the blood perfusing the carotid chemoreceptors. The blood perfusing the remainder of the animal, including the myocardium, was fully saturated with oxygen throughout the experiment. *(Modified from Levy MN, Degeest H, Zieske H: Cardiac response to cephalic ischemia.* Circ Res *18:67, 1966.)*

Blood is pumped by the left ventricle into the aortic arch and then through some external tubing back to the right atrial reservoir. A resistance device in the external tubing allows the investigator to control the aortic pressure; this pressure constitutes the **afterload** for left ventricular ejection (see also Chapter 4).

One of Starling's recordings of the changes in ventricular volume evoked by a sudden increase in right atrial pressure is shown in Figure 5-20. Aortic pressure in this experiment was permitted to increase only slightly when the right atrial pressure (preload) was increased. In the top tracing, the upper border of the tracing represents the systolic ventricular volume, the lower border indicates the diastolic ventricular volume, and the width of the tracing reflects the **stroke volume** (i.e., the volume of blood ejected by a ventricle during each heartbeat).

For several beats after the rise in preload, the ventricular volume progressively increased. This indicates that a disparity must have existed between ventricular inflow during diastole and ventricular outflow during systole. During a given systole, the volume of blood expelled by the ventricles was not as great as the volume that had entered the ventricles during the preceding diastole. This progressive accumulation of blood

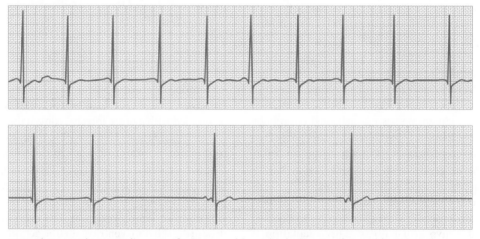

FIGURE 5-19 ■ Electrocardiogram of a 30-year-old quadriplegic man who could not breathe spontaneously and required tracheal intubation and artificial respiration. The two strips are continuous. The tracheal catheter was temporarily disconnected from the respirator at the beginning of the top strip. *(Modified from Berk JL, Levy MN: Profound reflex bradycardia produced by transient hypoxia or hypercapnia in man.* Eur Surg Res *9:75, 1977.)*

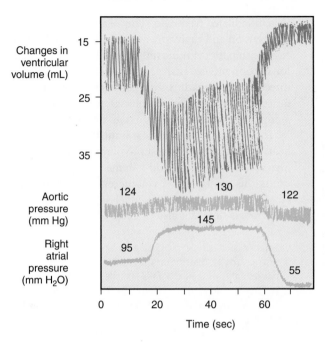

Changes in ventricular volume (mL)

15

25

35

Aortic pressure (mm Hg)

124   130   122

145

Right atrial pressure (mm H₂O)

95

55

0   20   40   60

Time (sec)

FIGURE 5-20 ■ Changes in ventricular volume in a canine heart-lung preparation when the right atrial pressure was suddenly increased from 95 to 145 mm H₂O and subsequently lowered to 55 mm H₂O. Note that an increase in ventricular volume is registered as a downward shift in the volume tracing. *(Redrawn from Patterson SW, Piper H, Starling EH: The regulation of the heart beat.* J Physiol *(Lond) 48:465, 1914.)*

dilated the ventricles and lengthened the individual myocardial fibers in the walls of the ventricles. The increased diastolic fiber length somehow facilitates ventricular contraction and enables the ventricles to pump a greater stroke volume, so that cardiac output exactly matches the augmented venous return at steady state. Increased fiber length alters the structure of cardiac constituents. In particular, the structural protein titin may serve as a mechanotransducer because it forms a scaffold around and binds to actin and myosin. As cardiac muscle is stretched, actin and myosin are brought into closer apposition. Thus, length dependence of cardiac performance is achieved mainly by changing the Ca^{++} sensitivity of the myofilaments and, in part, by changing the number of myofilament crossbridges that can interact (see also Chapter 4). Beyond an optimal fiber length, contraction is actually impaired. Therefore, excessively high filling pressures may depress rather than enhance the pumping capacity of the ventricles by overstretching the myocardial fibers (see Figure 4-4). Such excessive degrees of stretch are rarely encountered under normal conditions.

Changes in diastolic fiber length also permit the isolated heart to compensate for an increase in peripheral resistance. In a Starling preparation, when the arterial resistance is abruptly increased but ventricular filling rate is held constant, the stroke volume diminishes initially in response to the sudden increase in arterial resistance. However, after a brief period, the stroke volume enlarges to equal the constant ventricular filling volume. Concomitantly, the arterial pressure and end-diastolic ventricular volume are greater than the values that prevailed before the experimentally induced increase in afterload. Thus, when the afterload is first increased, the stroke volume ejected by the ventricles during systole is less than the filling volume that enters the ventricles during diastole. The consequent excess of volume in the ventricles stretches the myocardial fibers in the ventricular walls. This increase in myocardial fiber length enables the ventricles to eject a given stroke volume against a greater afterload.

Changes in ventricular volume are also involved in the cardiac adaptation to alterations in heart rate. During bradycardia, for example, the longer duration of diastole permits greater ventricular filling. The consequent augmentation of myocardial fiber length increases stroke volume. Therefore, the reduction in heart rate may be fully compensated by the increase in

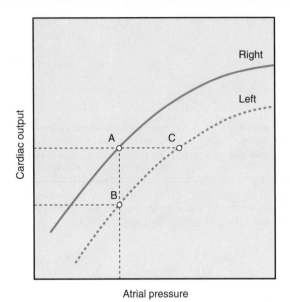

FIGURE 5-21 ■ Outputs of the right and left ventricles as functions of the mean right and left atrial pressure, respectively. At a given level of cardiac output, mean left atrial pressure (e.g., point C) exceeds mean right atrial pressure (point A).

stroke volume, such that cardiac output may remain constant (see Figure 10-22).

The curves that relate cardiac output to mean atrial pressure for the two ventricles are not coincident; the curve for the left ventricle usually lies below that of the right, as shown in Figure 5-21. At equal right and left atrial pressures (points A and B), right ventricular output would exceed left ventricular output. Hence venous return to the left ventricle (a function of right ventricular output) would exceed left ventricular output, and therefore left ventricular diastolic volume and pressure would rise. By the Frank-Starling mechanism, left ventricular output would increase (from point B toward point C). Only when the outputs of both ventricles are identical (points A and C) would the equilibrium be stable. Under such conditions, however, left atrial pressure (point C) would exceed right atrial pressure (point A), and this is precisely the relationship that ordinarily prevails in normal subjects.

When cardiac compensation involves ventricular dilation, the force required by each myocardial fiber to generate a given intraventricular systolic pressure must be appreciably greater than that developed by the fibers in a nondilated ventricle. The relationship between wall tension and cavity pressure resembles the Laplace relationship for cylindric tubes (see Chapter 8), in that, for a constant internal pressure, wall tension varies directly with the radius. As a consequence, the dilated heart requires considerably more O_2 to perform a given amount of external work than does the normal heart.

The relatively rigid pericardium that encloses the heart determines the pressure-volume relationship at high levels of pressure and volume. The pericardium exerts this limitation of volume even under normal conditions—when an individual is at rest and the heart rate is slow (see also Chapter 4).

In the cardiac dilation and hypertrophy that accompanies chronic heart failure, the pericardium is stretched considerably (Figure 5-22). The pericardial limitation of cardiac filling is exerted at pressures and volumes entirely different from those in normal individuals.

Intact Preparations

The major problem in assessing the role of the Frank-Starling mechanism in intact animals and humans is the difficulty of measuring end-diastolic myocardial fiber length. The Frank-Starling mechanism has been represented graphically by plotting an index of ventricular performance along the ordinate and an index of fiber length along the abscissa. The most commonly used indexes of ventricular performance are cardiac output, stroke volume, and stroke work. The indexes of fiber length include ventricular end-diastolic volume, ventricular end-diastolic pressure, ventricular circumference, and mean atrial pressure.

The Frank-Starling mechanism is better represented by a family of so-called ventricular function curves than by a single curve. To construct a control ventricular function curve, one must alter the blood volume of an experimental animal over a range of values, and then measure stroke work and end-diastolic pressure at each step. One then makes similar observations during the desired experimental intervention. For example, the ventricular function curve obtained during a nor-epinephrine infusion lies above and to the left of a control ventricular function curve (Figure 5-23). For a

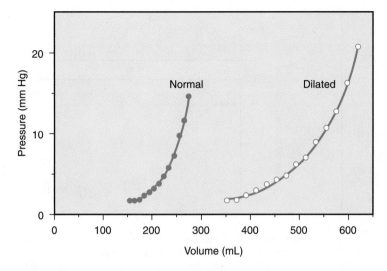

FIGURE 5-22 ▪ Pericardial pressure-volume relations in a normal dog and in a dog with experimentally induced chronic cardiac hypertrophy. *(Modified from Freeman GL, Le Winter MM: Pericardial adaptations during chronic cardiac dilation in dogs. Circ Res 54:294, 1984.)*

given level of left ventricular end-diastolic pressure, the left ventricle performs more work during a norepinephrine infusion than under control conditions. Hence a shift of the ventricular function curve to the left usually signifies an increase of ventricular **contractility** (see Chapter 4); a shift to the right usually indicates a reduction of contractility and a consequent tendency toward **cardiac failure.** Contractility is a measure of cardiac performance at a given level of preload and afterload. The end-diastolic pressure is ordinarily used as an index of preload; the aortic systolic pressure is used as an index of afterload.

The Frank-Starling mechanism is ideally suited for matching cardiac output to venous return. Any sudden, excessive output by one ventricle soon increases the venous return to the other ventricle. The consequent increase in diastolic fiber length in the second ventricle augments the output of that ventricle to correspond with the output of its mate. *Therefore, it is the Frank-Starling mechanism that maintains a precise balance between the outputs of the right and left ventricles.* Because the two ventricles are arranged in series in a closed circuit, even a small, maintained imbalance in the outputs of the two ventricles would be catastrophic.

> This difference in atrial pressures accounts for the observation that in congenital atrial septal defects, in which the two atria communicate, the direction of the shunt flow is usually from left to right.

Changes in Heart Rate Affect Contractile Force

The effects of the frequency of contraction on the force developed in an isometrically contracting cat papillary muscle are shown in Figure 5-24. Initially, the strip of cardiac muscle was stimulated to contract once every 20 s (Figure 5-24A). When the muscle was suddenly made to contract once every 0.63 s, the developed force increased progressively over the next several beats. This progressive increase in developed force induced by a change in contraction frequency is known as the **staircase,** or **Treppe, phenomenon.** At the new steady-state level, the developed force was more than five times as great as it was during stimulation at the longer contraction interval. A return to the longer interval (20 s) had the opposite influence on developed force.

The effect of the interval between contractions on the steady-state level of developed force is shown in Figure 5-24B for a wide range of intervals. As the interval is reduced from 300 s down to about 20 s, developed force changes only slightly. As the interval is reduced further, to a value of about 0.5 s, force increases sharply. Further reduction of the interval to 0.2 s has little additional effect on developed force.

The initial progressive rise in developed force when the interval between beats is suddenly decreased (e.g., from 20 to 0.63 s in Figure 5-24A) is achieved by a gradual increase in intracellular Ca^{++} content. Two mechanisms contribute to the rise in Ca^{++} content: (1)

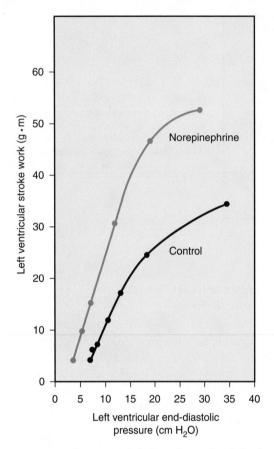

FIGURE 5-23 ■ A constant infusion of norepinephrine in a dog shifts the ventricular function curve to the left. This shift signifies an enhancement of ventricular contractility. *(Redrawn from Sarnoff SJ, Brockman SK, Gilmore JP, et al: Regulation of ventricular contraction: Influence of cardiac sympathetic and vagal nerve stimulation on atrial and ventricular dynamics. Circ Res 8:1108, 1960.)*

an increase in the number of depolarizations per minute and (2) an increase in the inward Ca^{++} current per depolarization.

With respect to the first mechanism, Ca^{++} enters the myocardial cell during each action potential plateau (see Figure 2-20). As the interval between beats is diminished, the number of plateaus per minute increases. Even though the duration of each action potential (and of each plateau) decreases as the interval between beats is reduced (see Figure 2-20), the overriding effect of the higher number of plateaus per minute on the influx of Ca^{++} would increase the intracellular content of Ca^{++}.

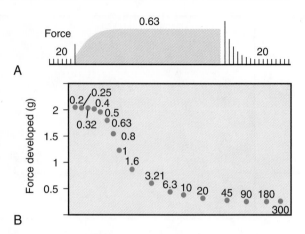

FIGURE 5-24 ■ Changes in force development in an isolated papillary muscle from a cat as the interval between contractions is varied. The numbers in both panels denote the interval (in seconds) between beats. *(Redrawn from Koch-Weser J, Blinks JR: The influence of the interval between beats on myocardial contractility. Pharmacol Rev 15:601, 1963.)*

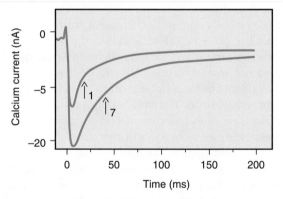

FIGURE 5-25 ■ Calcium currents induced in a guinea pig myocyte during the first and seventh depolarizations in a sequence of depolarizations. *Arrows* indicate the half-times of inactivation. Note that during the seventh depolarization, the maximal inward Ca^{++} current and the half-time of inactivation were greater than the respective values for the first depolarization. *(Modified from Lee KS: Potentiation of the calcium-channel currents of internally perfused mammalian heart cells by repetitive depolarization. Proc Natl Acad Sci U S A 84:3941, 1987.)*

With respect to the second mechanism, as the interval between beats is suddenly diminished, the inward Ca^{++} current (I_{Ca}) progressively increases with each successive beat until a new steady-state level is attained at the new basic cycle length. Figure 5-25 shows that in

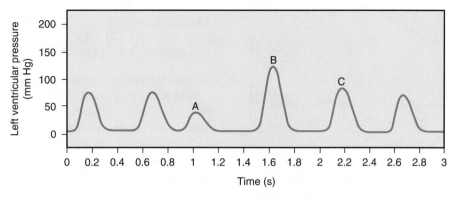

FIGURE 5-26 ■ In an isovolumic canine left ventricle preparation, a premature ventricular systole (beat A) is typically feeble, whereas the postextrasystolic contraction (beat B) is characteristically strong, and the enhanced contractility may persist to a diminishing degree over a few beats (e.g., contraction C). In this preparation the animal is on total heart-lung bypass, and a balloon filled with saline is positioned in the left ventricle. *(From Levy MN: Unpublished tracing.)*

an isolated ventricular myocyte that was subjected to repetitive depolarizations, the Ca^{++} current into the myocyte increased on successive beats. Thus, the maximal I_{Ca} was considerably greater during the seventh depolarization than it was during the first depolarization. Furthermore, the decay of current (i.e., its inactivation) was substantially slower during the seventh depolarization than during the first depolarization. Both of these characteristics of the I_{Ca} would result in a greater Ca^{++} influx of the myocyte during the seventh depolarization than during the first depolarization. The greater influx of Ca^{++} would strengthen the contraction by increasing the Ca^{++} content of the sarcoplasmic reticulum.

Transient changes in the intervals between beats also affect the strength of contraction. When a premature ventricular systole (Figure 5-26, beat A) occurs, the premature contraction (extrasystole) itself is feeble, whereas the beat after the subsequent pause (B) is very strong. In intact animals, this response depends partly on the Frank-Starling mechanism. Inadequate ventricular filling just before the premature beat accounts partly for the weak premature contraction. The exaggerated degree of filling associated with the subsequent pause explains in part the vigorous postextrasystolic contraction.

The Frank-Starling mechanism is not the exclusive mechanism involved in the usual ventricular adaptation

to a premature beat. Directionally similar results are obtained even from isovolumically contracting ventricles. In the experiment shown in Figure 5-26 the coronary circulation was perfused with oxygenated blood; then a balloon was inserted into the left ventricle and filled with enough saline to fill the entire ventricle. Thus, the left ventricle contracts against an incompressible fluid; that is, the ventricle contracts isovolumically. Figure 5-26 shows the changes in pressure that were recorded from this balloon during a series of contractions. Note that the premature beat (A) was much weaker than the preceding beat, and that the postextrasystolic beat (B) that immediately followed the premature beat was very strong. Such enhanced contractility in contraction B is an example of **postextrasystolic potentiation,** and it may persist for one or more additional beats (e.g., contraction C).

The weakness of the premature beat is directly related to the degree of prematurity. Conversely, as the time (**coupling interval**) between the premature beat and the preceding beat is increased, the strength of the premature beat is more nearly normal. The curve that relates the strength of contraction of a premature beat to the coupling interval is called a **mechanical restitution curve.** Figure 5-27 shows the restitution curve obtained by varying the coupling intervals of test beats in an isolated ventricular muscle preparation from a guinea pig.

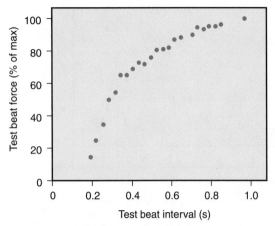

FIGURE 5-27 ▥ Force generated during premature contractions in a guinea pig isolated ventricular muscle preparation. The muscle was driven to contract once per second. Periodically, the muscle was stimulated to contract prematurely. The scale along the abscissa denotes the time between the driven and premature beat. The ordinate denotes the ratio of the contractile force of the premature beat to that of the driven beat. *(Modified from Seed WA, Walker JM: Review: Relation between beat interval and force of the heartbeat and its clinical implications.* Cardiovasc Res 22:303, 1988.)

The restitution of contractile strength depends on the time course of intracellular Ca^{++} circulation during the contraction and relaxation process (see Figure 4-8). During relaxation, the Ca^{++} that dissociates from the contractile proteins is rapidly taken up by the sarcoplasmic reticulum for subsequent release. However, the ryanodine receptor recovers slowly from adaptation or inactivation such that about 500 to 800 ms are required before the Ca^{++} that had been taken up becomes available for release in response to the next depolarization.

The premature beat itself (Figure 5-26, beat A) is weak because not enough time has elapsed to allow much of the Ca^{++} taken up by the sarcoplasmic reticulum during the preceding relaxation to become available for release in response to the premature depolarization. Conversely, the postextrasystolic beat (Figure 5-26, beat B) is considerably stronger than normal. The reason is that after the pause between beats A and B, the sarcoplasmic reticulum had available for release the Ca^{++} that had been taken up during two heartbeats: the extrasystole (beat A) and the preceding normal beat.

MYOCARDIAL PERFORMANCE IS REGULATED BY NERVOUS AND HUMORAL FACTORS

Although the completely isolated heart can adapt well to changes in preload and afterload, various extrinsic factors also influence the heart in the intact animal. Under many normal conditions, these extrinsic regulatory mechanisms may overwhelm the intrinsic mechanisms. These extrinsic regulatory factors may be subdivided into nervous and chemical components.

Nervous Control

Sympathetic Influences

Sympathetic nervous activity enhances atrial and ventricular contractility. The effects of increased cardiac sympathetic activity on the ventricular myocardium are asymmetrical. The cardiac sympathetic nerves on the left side of the body usually have a much greater effect on left ventricular contraction than do those on the right side (see Figure 5-6).

Electrical stimulation of the left stellate ganglion markedly raised both the peak pressure and the maximal rate of pressure rise (dP/dt) during systole in an isovolumic left ventricle preparation (Figure 5-28). Also, the duration of systole is reduced and the rate of ventricular relaxation is increased during the early phases of diastole. The shortening of systole and more rapid ventricular relaxation can enhance ventricular filling in the intact circulatory system. For a given cardiac cycle length, the briefer systole allows more time for diastole and hence for ventricular filling. In the experiment shown in Figure 5-29, for example, the animal's heart was paced at a constant rapid rate. Sympathetic stimulation (*right panel*) shortened systole, allowing substantially more time for ventricular filling.

Sympathetic nervous activity enhances myocardial performance. Neurally released norepinephrine or circulating catecholamines interact with β-adrenergic receptors on the cardiac cell membranes (see Figure 5-5). This reaction activates adenylyl cyclase, which raises the intracellular cAMP levels. Consequently, protein kinases are activated that promote the phosphorylation of various proteins within the myocyte. Phosphorylation of specific sarcolemmal proteins activates the calcium channels in the myocardial cell

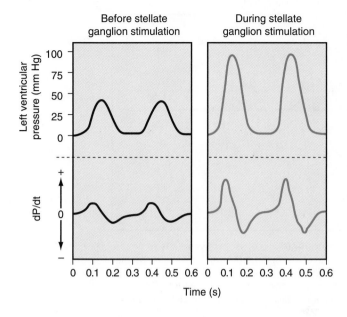

FIGURE 5-28 ■ In a canine isovolumic left ventricle preparation, stimulation of cardiac sympathetic nerves evokes a substantial rise in peak left ventricular pressure and in the maximal rates of intraventricular pressure rise and fall (dP/dt). *(From Levy MN: Unpublished tracing.)*

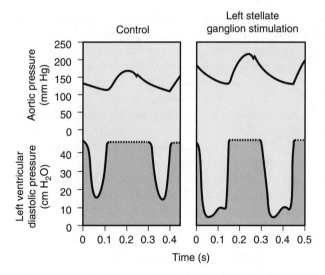

FIGURE 5-29 ■ Stimulation of the left stellate ganglion of a dog increases arterial pressure, stroke volume, and stroke work despite a concomitant reduction in ventricular end-diastolic pressure. Systole is also abbreviated, thereby allowing more time for ventricular filling; the heart was paced at a constant rate. In the ventricular pressure tracings, the pen excursion is limited at 45 mm Hg; actual ventricular pressures during systole can be estimated from the aortic pressure tracings. *(Redrawn from Mitchell JH, Linden RJ, Sarnoff SJ: Influence of cardiac sympathetic and vagal nerve stimulation on the relation between left ventricular diastolic pressure and myocardial segment length. Circ Res 8:1100, 1960.)*

membranes. Phosphorylation of **phospholamban** facilitates the reuptake of systolic Ca^{++} by the sarcoplasmic reticulum, and phosphorylation of troponin I reduces Ca^{++} sensitivity. These effects accelerate the relaxation of myocardial cells (see also Chapter 4).

Activation of Ca^{++} channels increases Ca^{++} influx during the action potential plateau, and more Ca^{++} is released from the sarcoplasmic reticulum in response to each cardiac excitation. The contractile strength of the heart is thereby increased. Figure 5-30 shows the correlation between the contractile force developed by a thin strip of ventricular muscle and the Ca^{++} concentration (as reflected by the aequorin light signal) in the myocytes as the concentration of isoproterenol (a β-adrenergic agonist) was increased in the tissue bath.

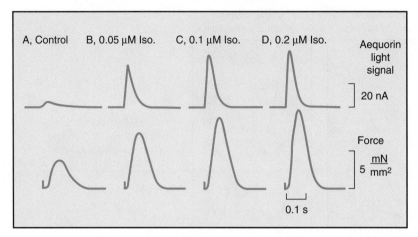

FIGURE 5-30 ▪ Effects of various concentrations of isoproterenol (Iso) on the aequorin light signal (in nA) and contractile force (in mN/mm²) in a rat ventricular muscle injected with aequorin. The aequorin light signal reflects the instantaneous changes in intracellular Ca^{++} concentration. *(Modified from Kurihara S, Konishi M: Effects of beta-adrenoceptor stimulation on intracellular Ca transients and tension in rat ventricular muscle. Pflugers Arch 409:427, 1987.)*

The overall effect of increased cardiac sympathetic activity in intact animals can best be appreciated in terms of families of ventricular function curves. When stepwise increases in the frequency of electrical stimulation are applied to the left stellate ganglion, the ventricular function curves shift progressively to the left. The changes parallel those produced by catecholamine infusions (see Figure 5-23). Hence for any given left ventricular end-diastolic pressure, the ventricle is capable of performing more work as the level of sympathetic nervous activity is raised.

During cardiac sympathetic stimulation, the enhanced cardiac response is usually accompanied by a reduction in left ventricular end-diastolic pressure (see Figure 5-29). This reduction in end-diastolic pressure represents a decrease in the preload. The reason for the reduction in ventricular preload is explained in Chapter 10.

Parasympathetic Influences
The vagus nerves inhibit the cardiac pacemaker, atrial myocardium, and AV conduction tissue. The vagus nerves also depress the ventricular myocardium, albeit less markedly. In the isovolumic left ventricle preparation, vagal stimulation decreases the peak left ventricular pressure, maximal rate of pressure development

(dP/dt), and maximal rate of pressure decline during diastole (Figure 5-31). In pumping heart preparations, vagal stimulation affects the relation between ventricular performance and preload such that the ventricular function curve shifts to the right.

The vagal effects on the ventricular myocardium are achieved by at least two mechanisms, as shown in Figure 5-5. The acetylcholine (ACh) released from the vagal endings can interact with muscarinic (M) receptors in the cardiac cell membrane to inhibit adenylyl cyclase and the cAMP/protein kinase A (PKA) cascade. This inhibition diminishes the Ca^{++} conductance of the cardiac cell membrane, reduces phosphorylation of the Ca^{++} channel, and hence decreases myocardial contractility. The ACh released from vagal endings can also inhibit norepinephrine release from neighboring sympathetic nerve endings (see Figures 5-5 and 5-7).

Baroreceptor Reflex
Stimulation of the carotid sinus and aortic arch baroreceptors changes the heart rate (see Figure 5-9) and also alters myocardial performance. Evidence of reflex alterations of ventricular contractility is presented in Figure 5-32. Ventricular function curves were obtained at four levels of carotid sinus pressure. With each

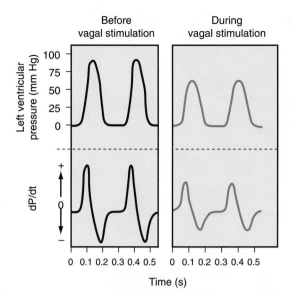

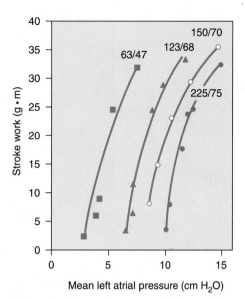

FIGURE 5-31 ■ In an isovolumic left ventricle preparation, when the ventricle is paced at a constant frequency, vagal stimulation decreases the peak left ventricular pressure and diminishes the maximal rates of pressure rise and fall (dP/dt). *(From Levy MN: Unpublished Tracing.)*

FIGURE 5-32 ■ As the pressure in the isolated carotid sinus is progressively raised, the ventricular function curves shift to the right. The *numbers* at the tops of each curve represent the systolic/diastolic perfusion pressures (in millimeters of mercury) in the carotid sinus regions of the dog. *(Redrawn from Sarnoff SJ, Gilmore JP, Brockman SK, et al: Regulation of ventricular contraction by the carotid sinus: its effect on atrial and ventricular dynamics.* Circ Res 8:1123, 1960.*)*

successive rise in pressure, the ventricular function curves were displaced farther and farther to the right, denoting a progressively greater reflex depression of ventricular performance.

Cardiac Performance Is Also Regulated by Hormonal Substances

Hormones

Adrenomedullary Hormones The adrenal medulla is essentially a component of the autonomic nervous system. Epinephrine is the principal hormone secreted by the adrenal medulla, although it also releases some norepinephrine. The rate of secretion of catecholamines by the adrenal medulla is largely regulated by the same mechanisms that control sympathetic nervous activity. The catecholamine concentrations in the blood rise under the same conditions that activate the sympathoadrenal system. However, the cardiovascular effects of circulating catecholamines are probably minimal under normal resting conditions.

The changes in myocardial contractility induced by norepinephrine infusions have been tested in resting,

unanesthetized dogs. The maximal rate of rise of left ventricular pressure (dP/dt), an index of myocardial contractility, was proportional to the norepinephrine concentration in the blood (Figure 5-33). In these same animals, moderate exercise increased the maximal dP/dt by almost 100%, but it raised the circulating catecholamines by only 500 pg/mL. Such a rise in blood norepinephrine concentration, by itself, would have had only a negligible effect on left ventricular dP/dt (see Figure 5-33). Hence the pronounced change in dP/dt observed during exercise must have been achieved mainly by the norepinephrine released from cardiac sympathetic nerve fibers rather than by catecholamines released from the adrenal medulla.

Adrenocortical Hormones The influence of adrenocortical steroids on cardiac function is not well understood. Cardiac muscle removed from adrenalectomized animals and placed in a tissue bath is more likely to fatigue than that obtained from normal animals. In some species the adrenocortical hormones enhance contractility. Furthermore, hydrocortisone

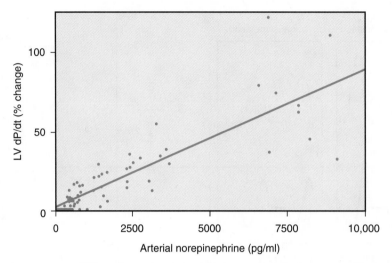

FIGURE 5-33 ▪ Effect of norepinephrine infusions on ventricular contractility in a group of resting, unanesthetized dogs. The plasma concentrations of norepinephrine (pg/mL) plotted along the abscissa are the increments above the control values. The maximal rate of rise of left ventricular pressure (Lv dP/dt) is plotted along the ordinate as percentage change from the control value; it is an index of contractility. *(Redrawn from Young MA, Hintze TH, Vatner SF: Correlation between cardiac performance and plasma catecholamine levels in conscious dogs. Am J Physiol 248:H82, 1985.)*

potentiates the cardiotonic effects of the catecholamines. This potentiation may be mediated in part by an inhibition of the extraneuronal uptake mechanisms for the catecholamines by the adrenocortical steroids. The adrenocortical hormone aldosterone is synthesized locally in the heart. Aldosterone promotes cardiac hypertrophy in heart failure and, when applied over the long term in large doses, also augments the L-type Ca^{++} current. How it functions under physiological conditions is not clear.

CLINICAL BOX

Cardiovascular problems are common in adrenocortical insufficiency **(Addison' disease).** The blood volume tends to fall, possibly leading to severe hypotension and cardiovascular collapse, the so-called **addisonian crisis.**

Thyroid Hormones Thyroid hormones (levothyroxine, T_4; triiodothyronine, T_3) enhance heart rate and myocardial contractility in humans. Triiodothyronine is

the principal agent responsible for cardiac effects. Some of the effects of thyroid hormone arise from changes in gene expression via activation of transcription factors. Increased activity of sarcoplasmic reticulum Ca^{++}-ATPase and of Na^+,K^+-ATPase are among these genomic effects. The rates of Ca^{++} uptake and of adenosine triphosphate (ATP) hydrolysis by the sarcoplasmic reticulum are increased in response to thyroid hormones (hyperthyroidism). Expressions of α-myosin heavy chain with high ATPase activity and of β-adrenergic receptor are also greater and contribute to the higher rate and greater contractility of the heartbeat. Systemically, these effects contribute to increased cardiac output. When in excess, thyroid hormone also reduces systemic vascular resistance and changes preload. Nongenomic effects on ion channels in vascular smooth muscle and heart contribute to this action. Opposite effects occur when thyroid hormones are present at inadequate levels (hypothyroidism). For example, preferential synthesis of β-myosin heavy chains and of phospholamban occurs in thyroid hormone deficiency. *Thus, a balanced or euthyroid state is very important in the regulation of cardiovascular function.*

The cardiovascular changes in thyroid dysfunction also depend on indirect mechanisms. Thyroid hyperactivity increases the body's metabolic rate, and this in turn results in arteriolar vasodilation. The consequent reduction in total peripheral resistance increases cardiac output (see Chapter 10). Substantial evidence indicates that hyperthyroidism increases the density of β-adrenergic receptors in cardiac tissue and that it increases the responsiveness of the heart to sympathetic neural activity. Cardiac activity is sluggish in patients with inadequate thyroid function (**hypothyroidism**); that is, the heart rate is slow and cardiac output is diminished. The converse is true in patients with overactive thyroid glands (**hyperthyroidism**). Characteristically, hyperthyroid patients exhibit tachycardia, high cardiac output, palpitations, and dysrhythmias (such as atrial fibrillation).

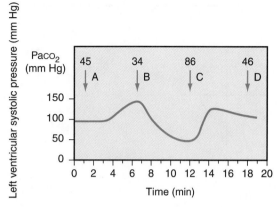

FIGURE 5-34 ■ Decrease in Pa_{CO_2} increases left ventricular systolic pressure (*arrow B*) in an isovolumic left ventricle preparation; a rise in Pa_{CO_2} (*arrow C*) has the reverse effect. when Pa_{CO_2} is returned to the control level (*arrow D*), left ventricular systolic pressure returns to its original value (*arrow A*). (*From Levy MN: Unpublished tracing.*)

Insulin Insulin has a prominent, direct, positive inotropic effect on the human heart. This acute, nongenomic action of insulin appears, in part, to be due to increased Ca^{++} entry secondary to stimulation of Na^+-Ca^{++} exchange. In addition to increased intracellular Ca^{++} transients, myofilament sensitivity to Ca^{++} increases when glucose is present. The effect of insulin is evident even when hypoglycemia is prevented by glucose infusions.

Glucagon Glucagon has potent positive inotropic and chronotropic effects on the heart. This endogenous hormone probably plays no significant role in the normal regulation of the cardiovascular system, but it has been used to treat various cardiac conditions. The effects of glucagon on the heart closely resemble those of the catecholamines, and certain of their metabolic effects are similar. Both glucagon and catecholamines activate adenylyl cyclase to raise the myocardial tissue levels of cAMP. The catecholamines activate adenylyl cyclase by interacting with β-adrenergic receptors, but glucagon activates this enzyme through a different mechanism.

Blood Gases Oxygen Changes in O_2 tension (Pa_{O_2}) of the blood perfusing the brain and the peripheral chemoreceptors affect the heart through nervous mechanisms, as described earlier in this chapter. These indirect cardiac effects of hypoxia are usually greater than those caused by the direct effect of hypoxia. Moderate degrees of systemic hypoxia characteristically increase heart rate, cardiac output, and myocardial contractility. These changes are largely mediated by the sympathetic nervous system, and they are effectively abolished by β-adrenergic receptor blockade.

The Pa_{O_2} of the blood perfusing the myocardium also influences myocardial performance directly. Moderate to severe degrees of hypoxia depress myocardial contractility. One mechanism for the diminished contractility is reduced sensitivity of the contractile proteins to Ca^{++}. The impaired contractility has also been attributed to higher intracellular concentrations of inorganic phosphate and of H^+. Indeed, it is difficult to separate the effect of reduced Pa_{O_2} from the acidosis caused by hypoxia.

CARBON DIOXIDE AND ACIDOSIS Changes in Pa_{CO_2} may also affect the myocardium directly and indirectly. The indirect, neurally mediated effects produced by increased Pa_{CO_2} are similar to those evoked by a decrease in Pa_{O_2}.

With respect to the direct effects on the heart, alterations in myocardial performance elicited by changes of Pa_{CO_2} in the coronary arterial blood are illustrated in Figure 5-34. In intact animals, systemic hypercapnia activates the sympathoadrenal system, which tends to compensate for the direct depressant effect of the greater Pa_{CO_2} on the heart.

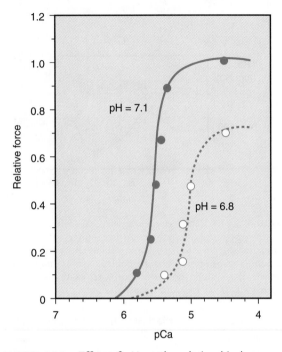

FIGURE 5-35 ■ Effect of pH on the relationship between relative force and pCa (the negative logarithm of the intracellular Ca^{++} concentration) in a "skinned" ventricular fiber from a rat. Relative force is the force developed by the preparation under the various experimental conditions, expressed as a percentage of the maximal force developed by the preparation when intracellular pH was normal (i.e., 7.1) and pCa was less than 4.6. The "skinned" fiber was prepared by treating the preparation with a detergent to solubilize the cell membranes, thus exposing the contractile proteins in the fiber to the concentrations of H^+ and Ca^{++} that prevailed in the bathing solution. *(Modified from Mayoux E, Coutry N, Lechêne P, et al: Effects of acidosis and alkalosis on mechanical properties of hypertrophied rat heart fiber bundles. Am J Physiol 266:H2051, 1994.)*

Neither the Pa_{CO_2} nor the blood pH is a primary determinant of myocardial function. The associated change in intracellular pH is the critical factor. The reduced intracellular pH diminishes the the L-type Ca^{++} current and the amount of Ca^{++} released from the sarcoplasmic reticulum in response to excitation. The diminished pH also decreases myofilament sensitivity to Ca^{++} by reducing TnC affinity for Ca^{++}. This effect of acidosis on sensitivity to Ca^{++} is reflected by a shift in the relationship between developed force and pCa (the negative logarithm of the intracellular Ca^{++} concentration). Figure 5-35 illustrates such a shift in an experiment on isolated ventricular fibers immersed in a tissue bath. When the pH of the bath was changed from 7.1 to 6.8, the curve of contractile force as a function of pCa was shifted substantially to the right (normal intracellular pH is about 7.1). Furthermore, in this same preparation, at high intracellular Ca^{++} concentrations (i.e., at values of pCa below about 4.6), a reduction in pH diminishes the maximal developed force. This reduction in maximal force suggests that the low pH depresses the actomyosin interactions by reducing crossbridge efficiency.

SUMMARY

- Cardiac function is regulated by intrinsic and extrinsic mechanisms.
- Sympathetic nervous activity increases heart rate, whereas parasympathetic (vagal) activity decreases heart rate. When both systems are active, the vagal effects usually dominate.
- The baroreceptor, chemoreceptor, pulmonary inflation, atrial receptor (Bainbridge), and ventricular receptor reflexes regulate heart rate. The efferent

path for the reflexes is the autonomic nervous system.
- A change in the resting length of the muscle alters the distance between actin and myosin and thereby influences the subsequent contraction in part by altering the affinity of the myofilaments for Ca^{++}; this is called the Frank-Starling mechanism.
- A sustained change in contraction frequency affects the strength of contraction by altering the influx of

Ca^{++} into the cell per minute. A transient change in contraction frequency alters contractile strength because an appreciable delay exists between the time that Ca^{++} is taken up by the sarcoplasmic reticulum and the time that it becomes available again for release.

■ The autonomic nervous system regulates myocardial performance mainly by varying the phosphorylation state of proteins (L-type Ca^{++} channel, phospholamban, troponin I) that regulate the entry and intracellular disposition of Ca^{++}.

■ Various hormones, including epinephrine, adrenocortical steroids, thyroid hormones, insulin, glucagon, and anterior pituitary hormones, regulate myocardial performance.

■ Changes in the blood concentrations of O_2, CO_2, and H^+ alter cardiac function directly (by interacting with ion channels and proteins associated with contraction/relaxation) and reflexly (via the central and peripheral chemoreceptors).

ADDITIONAL READING

Bernardi L, Porta C, Gabutti A, Spicuzza L, Sleight P: Modulatory effects of respiration, *Auton Neurosci* 90:47, 2001.

Bers DM: *Excitation-Contraction Coupling and Cardiac Contractile Force*, ed 2, Boston, 2001, Kluwer Academic Publishers.

Chapleau MW, Li Z, Meyrelles SS, Ma X, Abboud FM: Mechanisms determining sensitivity of baroreceptor afferents in health and disease, *Ann N Y Acad Sci* 940:1, 2001.

Cini G, Carpi A, Mechanick J, et al: Thyroid hormones and the cardiovascular system: Pathophysiology and interventions, *Biomed Pharmacother* 63:742, 2009.

Dillmann WH: Cellular action of thyroid hormone on the heart, *Thyroid* 12:447, 2002.

Fu Y, Huang X, Piao L, et al: Endogenous RGS proteins modulate SA and AV nodal functions in isolated heart: implications for sick sinus syndrome and AV block, *Am J Physiol* 292:H2532, 2007.

Iancu RV, Jones SW, Harvey RD: Compartmentation of cAMP signaling in cardiac myocytes, *Biophys J* 92:3317, 2007.

Jiang C, Rojas A, Wang R, Wang X: CO_2 central chemosensitivity: Why are there so many sensing molecules? *Respir Physiol Neurobiol* 145:115, 2005.

Klein I, Danzi S: Thyroid disease and the heart, *Circ* 116:1725, 2007.

Lewinski D, Rainer PP, Gasser R, et al: Glucose-transporter-mediated positive inotropic effects in human myocardium of diabetic and nondiabetic patients, *Metabolism* 59:1020, 2010.

Posokova E, Wydeven N, Allen KL: RGS6/Gβ5 complex accelerates I_{KACh} gating kinetics in atrial myocytes and modulates parasympathetic regulation of heart rate, *Circ Res* 107:1350, 2010.

Potts JT: Neural circuits controlling cardiorespiratory responses: Baroreceptor and somatic afferents in the nucleus tractus solitarius, *Clin Exp Pharmacol Physiol* 29:103, 2002.

Scott JD, Santana LF: A-kinase anchoring proteins, *Circ* 121:1264, 2011.

Shepherd JT, Vatner SF, editors: *Nervous Control of the Heart*, Amsterdam, 1996, Harwood Academic Press.

Shimizu J, Todaka K, Burkhoff D: Load dependence of ventricular performance explained by model of calcium-myofilament interactions, *Am J Physiol Heart Circ Physiol* 282:H1081, 2002.

Stangherlin A, Gesellchen F, Zoccarato A, et al: cGMP signals modulate cAMP levels in a compartment-specific manner to regulate catecholamine-dependent signaling in cardiac myocytes, *Circ Res* 108:929, 2011.

Taggart P, Critchley H, Lambiase PD: Heart-brain interactions in cardiac arrhythmia, *Br Med J* 97:698, 2011.

Yang J, Huang J, Mait B, et al: GRS6, a modulator of parasympathetic activation in heart, *Circ Res* 107:1345, 2010.

Zhang P, Mende U: Regulators of G-protein signaling in the heart and their potential as therapeutic targets, *Circ Res* 109:320, 2011.

CASE 5-1

HISTORY

A 48-year-old woman was susceptible to occasional, usually brief, episodes of light-headedness. She noticed that her heart rate was very rapid during these episodes and that the light-headedness disappeared when the heart rate returned to normal. Her doctor noted no significant abnormalities on physical examination. Review of a 24-hour recording of the patient's electrocardiogram revealed a 7-minute period during which the patient's heart rate increased abruptly from a resting value of about 75 beats/min to a steady level of about 145 beats/min. At the end of the 7-minute period of tachycardia, the heart rate decreased within 1 minute to the resting value of about 75 beats/min. The patient's problem was diagnosed as paroxysmal supraventricular tachycardia, which is a sudden, pronounced increase in heart rate. This problem is mediated usually by a reentry circuit in the atrioventricular junction.

During a subsequent visit to her doctor, the patient's paroxysmal tachycardia appeared spontaneously. The doctor was able to terminate the tachycardia promptly with carotid sinus massage (i.e., massaging the patient's neck just below the angles of the jaw, in the region of the bifurcations of the common carotid arteries). The physician noted that the patient's arterial blood pressure during tachycardia was 95 mm Hg systolic/75 mm Hg diastolic and that it returned to a value of 130/85 mm Hg (the patient's usual resting blood pressure) soon after the termination of the tachycardia.

QUESTIONS

1. A reduction in the patient's mean arterial pressure during the paroxysmal tachycardia would cause a reflex:
   a. decrease in myocardial contractility.
   b. increase in cardiac cycle duration.
   c. decrease in AV conduction velocity.
   d. increase in norepinephrine release from the cardiac sympathetic nerves.
   e. decrease in Ca^{++} conductance of myocytes during the action potential plateau.

2. A sudden, substantial increase in efferent vagal activity (induced by carotid sinus massage, for example) would:
   a. strengthen the contraction of atrial myocytes.
   b. strengthen the stimulatory action of any concurrent sympathetic activity.
   c. increase the speed of impulse conduction in the ventricular Purkinje fibers.
   d. decrease the heart rate within one or two cardiac cycles.
   e. shorten the AV conduction time.

3. When the subject was in a normal sinus rhythm, administration of a drug that antagonizes the muscarinic cholinergic receptors would:
   a. dampen any changes in heart rate that occur at the subject's respiratory frequency.
   b. weaken the contractions of the atrial myocytes.
   c. delay AV conduction.

   d. decrease the action potential duration in atrial myocytes.
   e. hyperpolarize the atrial myocytes during the resting phase (phase 4) of the action potential.

4. If the patient had a prominent respiratory sinus dysrhythmia when she was not experiencing paroxysmal tachycardia, the following functional change would take place:
   a. Efferent vagal activity would decrease during inspiration.
   b. Efferent cardiac sympathetic activity would decrease during inspiration.
   c. The slope of the slow diastolic depolarization of the sinoatrial cells would decrease during inspiration.
   d. The respiratory sinus dysrhythmia would become more pronounced in response to hemorrhage.
   e. Propranolol would abolish the respiratory sinus dysrhythmia.

5. When neural activity in the vagus nerves suddenly ceases, the heart rate response to that vagal activity disappears rapidly because:
   a. the cardiac cells gradually become more responsive to acetylcholine.
   b. the vagus nerve endings rapidly take up the released acetylcholine.
   c. the cardiac myocytes rapidly take up the released acetylcholine.
   d. the acetylcholine in the nerve endings is rapidly depleted.
   e. the abundant acetylcholinesterase rapidly degrades the released acetylcholine.

6

HEMODYNAMICS

OBJECTIVES

1. Define the relation between the velocity of blood flow and vascular cross-sectional area.

2. Describe the factors that govern the relationship between blood flow and pressure gradient.

3. Distinguish between resistances in series and resistances in parallel.

4. Distinguish between laminar flow and turbulent flow.

5. Describe the influence of the particulates in blood on blood flow.

The precise mathematical expression of the pulsatile flow of blood through the cardiovascular system remains to be solved. The heart is a complicated pump, and its behavior is affected by a variety of physical and chemical factors. The blood vessels are multibranched, elastic conduits of continuously varying dimensions. The blood itself is not a simple, homogeneous solution but is instead a complex suspension of red and white corpuscles, platelets, and lipid globules dispersed in a colloidal solution of proteins.

Despite these complex factors, considerable insight may be gained from an understanding of the elementary principles of fluid mechanics as they pertain to simple physical systems. Such principles are elaborated in this chapter to explain the interrelationships among the blood flow, the blood pressure, and the dimensions of the various components of the systemic circulation.

VELOCITY OF THE BLOODSTREAM DEPENDS ON BLOOD FLOW AND VASCULAR AREA

In describing the variations in blood flow in different vessels, the terms **velocity** and **flow** must first be distinguished. The former term, sometimes designated as **linear velocity,** means the rate of displacement with respect to time and it has the dimensions of distance per unit time, for example, cm/s. The flow, often designated as **volume flow,** has the dimensions of volume per unit time, for example, cm^3/s. In a conduit of varying cross-sectional dimensions, velocity, v, flow, Q, and cross-sectional area, A, are related by the following equation:

$$v = Q/A \qquad (1)$$

The interrelationships among velocity, flow, and area are portrayed in Figure 6-1. The flow of an incompressible fluid past successive cross-sections of a rigid tube must be constant. For a given constant flow, the velocity varies inversely as the cross-sectional area (see Figure 1-3). Thus for the same volume of fluid per second passing from section a into section b, where the cross-sectional area is five times greater, the velocity diminishes to one fifth of its previous value. Conversely, when the fluid proceeds from section b to section c, where the cross-sectional area is one tenth as great, the velocity of each particle of fluid must increase tenfold.

The velocity at any point in the system depends not only on the cross-sectional area but also on the flow, Q. This in turn depends on the pressure gradient, properties of the fluid, and dimensions of the entire hydraulic system, as discussed in the next section. For any given flow, however, the ratio of the velocity past one cross-section relative to that past a second cross-section depends only on the inverse ratio of the respective areas; that is,

$$v_1 / v_2 = A_2 / A_1 \qquad (2)$$

This rule pertains regardless of whether a given cross-sectional area applies to a system that consists of a single large tube or to a system made up of several smaller tubes in parallel.

As shown in Figure 1-3, velocity decreases progressively as the blood traverses the aorta, its larger primary branches, the smaller secondary branches, and the arterioles. Finally, a minimal value is reached in the capillaries. As the blood then passes through the venules and continues centrally toward the venae cavae, the velocity progressively increases again. The relative velocities in the various components of the circulatory system are related only to the respective cross-sectional areas. Thus each point on the cross-sectional

area curve is inversely proportional to the corresponding point on the velocity curve (see Figure 1-3).

BLOOD FLOW DEPENDS ON THE PRESSURE GRADIENT

In that portion of a hydraulic system in which the total energy remains virtually constant, changes in velocity may be accompanied by appreciable alterations in the measured pressure. Consider three sections (A, B, and C) of the hydraulic system depicted in Figure 6-2. Six pressure probes, or **Pitot tubes,** have been inserted. The openings of three of these (2, 4, and 6) are tangential to the direction of flow and hence measure the **lateral,** or **static,** pressure within the tube. The openings of the remaining three Pitot tubes (1, 3, and 5) face upstream. Therefore they detect the **total pressure,** which is the lateral pressure plus a dynamic pressure component that reflects the kinetic energy of the flowing fluid. This dynamic component, P_{dyn}, of the total pressure may be calculated from the following equation:

$$P_{dyn} = \rho v^2 / 2 \qquad (3)$$

where ρ is the density of the fluid and v is the velocity. If the midpoints of segments A, B, and C are at the

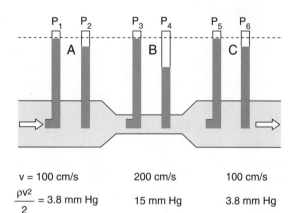

v = 100 cm/s	200 cm/s	100 cm/s
$\dfrac{\rho v^2}{2}$ = 3.8 mm Hg	15 mm Hg	3.8 mm Hg

FIGURE 6-2 ■ In a narrow section, B, of a tube, the linear velocity, v, and hence the dynamic component of pressure, $\rho v^2/2$, are greater than in the wide sections, A and C, of the same tube. If the total energy is virtually constant throughout the tube (i.e., if the energy loss due to viscosity is negligible), the total pressures (P_1, P_3, and P_5) are not detectably different, but the lateral pressure, P_4, in the narrow section is less than the lateral pressures (P_2 and P_6) in the wide sections of the tube.

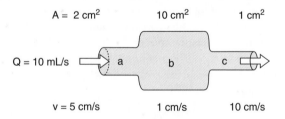

FIGURE 6-1 ■ As fluid flows through a tube of variable cross-sectional area, A, the linear velocity, v, varies inversely with the cross-sectional area.

same hydrostatic level, the corresponding total pressures, P_1, P_3, and P_5, will be equal, provided that the energy loss from viscosity in these segments is negligible. However, because of the changes in cross-sectional area, the concomitant velocity changes alter the dynamic component.

In sections A and C, let $\rho = 1$ g/cm^3 and $v = 100$ cm/s. From equation 3:

$$P_{dyn} = 5000 \text{ dynes} / \text{cm}^2$$
$$= 3.8 \text{ mm Hg}$$

because 1330 dynes/cm^2 = 1 mm Hg. In the narrow section, B, let the velocity be twice as great as in sections A and C. Therefore:

$$P_{dyn} = 20,000 \text{ dynes} / \text{cm}^2$$
$$= 15 \text{ mm Hg}$$

Hence in the wide sections of the conduit, the lateral pressures (P_2 and P_6) will be only 3.8 mm Hg less than the respective total pressures (P_1 and P_5), whereas in the narrow section, the lateral pressure (P_4) is 15 mm Hg less than the total pressure (P_3).

The peak velocity of flow in the ascending aorta of normal dogs is about 150 cm/second (s). Therefore the measured pressure at this site may vary significantly, depending on the orientation of the pressure probe. In the descending thoracic aorta the peak velocity is substantially less than that in the ascending aorta (Figure 6-3), and lesser velocities have been recorded in still more distal arterial sites. In most arterial locations the dynamic component is a negligible fraction of the total pressure, and the orientation of the pressure probe

does not materially influence the pressure recorded. At the site of a constriction, however, the dynamic pressure component may attain substantial values. In **aortic stenosis,** for example, the entire output of the left ventricle is ejected through a narrow aortic valve orifice. The high flow velocity is associated with a large kinetic energy, and therefore the lateral pressure is correspondingly reduced.

CLINICAL BOX

The pressure tracings shown in Figure 6-4 were obtained from two pressure transducers inserted into the left ventricle of a patient with aortic stenosis. The transducers were located on the same catheter and were 5 cm apart. When both transducers were well within the left ventricular cavity (Figure 6-4A), they both recorded the same pressures. However, when the proximal transducer was positioned in the aortic valve orifice (Figure 6-4B), the lateral pressure recorded during ejection was much less than that recorded by the transducer in the ventricular cavity. This pressure difference was associated almost entirely with the much greater velocity of flow in the narrowed valve orifice than in the ventricular cavity. The pressure difference reflects mainly the conversion of some potential energy to kinetic energy. When the catheter was withdrawn still farther, so that the proximal transducer was in the aorta (Figure 6-4C), the pressure difference was even more pronounced, because substantial energy was lost through friction (viscosity) as blood flowed rapidly through the narrow aortic valve.

The reduction of lateral pressure in the region of the stenotic valve orifice influences coronary blood flow in patients with aortic stenosis. The orifices of the right and left coronary arteries are located in the sinuses of Valsalva, just behind the valve leaflets. The initial segments of these vessels are oriented at right angles to the direction of blood flow through the aortic valves. Therefore the lateral pressure is that component of total pressure that propels the blood through the two major coronary arteries. During the ejection phase of the cardiac cycle, the lateral pressure is diminished by the conversion of potential energy to kinetic energy. This process is greatly exaggerated in aortic stenosis because of the high flow velocities.

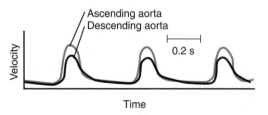

FIGURE 6-3 ■ Velocity of the blood in the ascending and descending aorta of a dog. *(Redrawn from Falsetti HL, Kiser KM, Francis GP, et al: Sequential velocity development in the ascending and descending aorta of the dog. Circ Res 31:328, 1972.)*

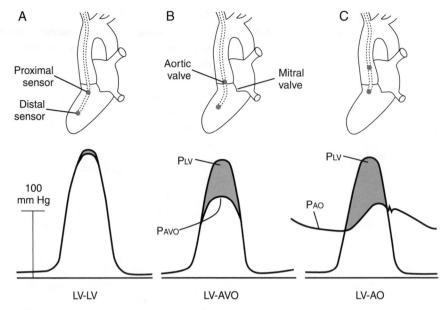

FIGURE 6-4 ■ Pressures (P) recorded by two transducers in a patient with aortic stenosis. **A,** Both transducers were in the left ventricle (LV-LV). **B,** One transducer was in the left ventricle and the other was in the aortic valve orifice (LV-AVO). **C,** One transducer was in the left ventricle and the other was in the ascending aorta (LV-AO). P_{AO}, pressure in ascending aorta; P_{AVO}, aortic valve orifice; P_{LV}, pressure in left ventricle. *(Redrawn from Pasipoularides A, Murgo JP, Bird JJ, et al: Fluid dynamics of aortic stenosis: mechanisms for the presence of subvalvular pressure gradients.* Am J Physiol *246:H542, 1984.)*

RELATIONSHIP BETWEEN PRESSURE AND FLOW DEPENDS ON THE CHARACTERISTICS OF THE CONDUITS

The most fundamental law that governs the flow of fluids through cylindrical tubes was derived empirically by the French physiologist Jean Poiseuille. He was primarily interested in the physical determinants of blood flow, but he replaced blood with simpler liquids for his measurements of flow through glass capillary tubes. His work was so precise and important that his observations have been designated **Poiseuille's law.** Subsequently, this same law has been derived theoretically.

Poiseuille's law is applicable to the flow of fluids through cylindrical tubes only under special conditions, namely, in the case of steady, laminar flow of newtonian fluids. The term **steady flow** signifies the absence of variations of flow in time, that is, a nonpulsatile flow. **Laminar flow** is the type of motion in

which the fluid moves as a series of individual layers, with each stratum moving at a different velocity from its neighboring layers (Figure 6-5). In the case of flow through a tube, the fluid consists of a series of infinitesimally thin concentric tubes sliding past one another. Laminar flow is described in greater detail later, where it is distinguished from turbulent flow. Also, a **newtonian fluid** is defined more precisely. For the present discussion, it may be considered to be a homogeneous fluid, such as water, in contradistinction to a suspension, such as blood.

Pressure is one of the principal determinants of the rate of flow. The pressure, P, in dynes/cm^2, at a distance h, in centimeters, below the surface of a liquid is:

$$P = h\rho g \qquad (4)$$

where ρ is the density of the liquid in g/cm^3 and g is the acceleration of gravity in cm/s^2. For convenience, however, pressure is frequently expressed simply in

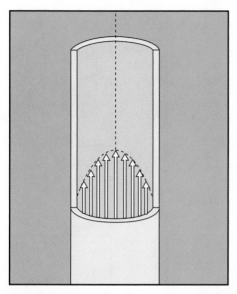

FIGURE 6-5 ■ In laminar flow, all elements of the fluid move in streamlines that are parallel to the axis of the tube; movement does not occur in a radial or circumferential direction. The layer of fluid in contact with the wall is motionless; the fluid that moves along the axis of the tube has the maximal velocity.

terms of the height of the column of liquid above some arbitrary reference point.

Consider the tube connecting reservoirs R_1 and R_2 in Figure 6-6A. Let reservoir R_1 be filled with liquid to height h_1, and let reservoir R_2 be empty, as in Figure 6-6A. The outflow pressure, P_o, is therefore equal to the atmospheric pressure, which shall be designated as the zero, or reference, level. The inflow pressure, P_i, is then equal to the same reference level plus the height, h_1, of the column of liquid in reservoir R_1. Under these conditions, let the flow, Q, through the tube be 5 mL/s.

If reservoir R_1 is filled to height h_2, which is twice h_1, and reservoir R_2 is again empty (as in panel B), the flow is twice as great, that is, 10 mL/s. Thus with reservoir R_2 empty, the flow is directly proportional to the inflow pressure, P_i.

If reservoir R_2 is now allowed to fill to height h_1, and the fluid level in R_1 is maintained at h_2 (as in panel C), the flow again becomes 5 mL/s. Thus, flow is directly proportional to the difference between inflow and outflow pressures:

$$Q \propto P_i - P_o \qquad (5)$$

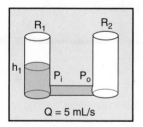

A When R_2 is empty, fluid flows from R_1 to R_2 at a rate proportional to the pressure in R_1.

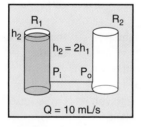

B When the fluid level in R_1 is increased twofold, the flow increases proportionately.

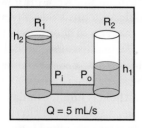

C Flow from R_1 to R_2 is proportional to the difference between the pressures in R_1 and R_2.

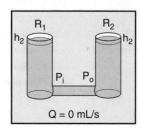

D When pressure in R_2 rises to equal the pressure in R_1, flow ceases in the connecting tube.

FIGURE 6-6 ■ A to D, The flow, Q, of fluid through a tube connecting two reservoirs, R_1 and R_2, is proportional to the difference between the pressure at the inflow end (P_i) and the pressure at the outflow end (P_o) of the tube. h_1 and h_2, heights of liquid in the reservoir.

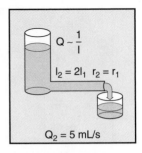

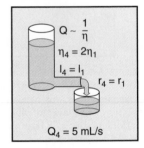

A Reference condition: for a given pressure, length, radius, and viscosity, let the flow (V_1) equal 10 ml/s.

B If tube length doubles, flow decreases by 50%.

FIGURE 6-7 ■ **A** to **D,** The flow, Q, of fluid through a tube is inversely proportional to the length, l, and the viscosity, η, and is directly proportional to the fourth power of the radius, r. h_1 and h_2, heights of liquid in the reservoir.

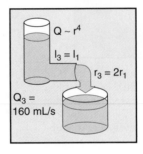

C If tube radius doubles, flow increases 16-fold.

D If viscosity doubles, flow decreases by 50%.

If the fluid level in R_2 attains the same height as in R_1, flow ceases (panel D).

For any given pressure difference between the two ends of a tube, the flow depends on the dimensions of the tube. Consider the tube connected to the reservoir in Figure 6-7A. With length l_1 and radius r_1, the flow Q_1 is observed to be 10 mL/s.

The tube connected to the reservoir in panel B has the same radius but is twice as long. Under those conditions the flow Q_2 is found to be 5 mL/s, or only half as great as Q_1. Conversely, for a tube half as long as l_1, the flow would be twice as great as Q_1. In other words, flow is inversely proportional to the length of the tube:

$$Q \propto 1/l \qquad (6)$$

The tube connected to the reservoir in Figure 6-7C is the same length as l_1, but the radius is twice as great. Under these conditions, the flow Q_3 is found to increase to a value of 160 mL/s, which is 16 times greater than Q_1. The precise measurements of Poiseuille revealed

that flow varies directly as the fourth power of the radius:

$$Q \propto r^4 \qquad (7)$$

Because $r_3 = 2r_1$ in the example above (Figure 6-7C), Q_3 will be proportional to $(2r_1)^4$, or $16r_1^4$; therefore Q_3 will equal $16Q_1$.

Finally, for a given pressure difference and for a cylindrical tube of given dimensions, the flow varies as a function of the nature of the fluid itself. This flow-determining property of fluids is termed **viscosity,** η, which Newton defined as the ratio of **shear stress** to the **shear rate** of the fluid. Those fluids for which the shear rate is proportional to the shear stress are known as **newtonian fluids.** If the shear rate is not proportional to the shear stress, the fluid is **nonnewtonian.**

These terms may be comprehended more clearly if one considers the flow of a homogeneous fluid between parallel plates. In Figure 6-8, let the bottom plate (the bottom of a large basin) be stationary, and let the upper plate move at a constant velocity along the upper surface

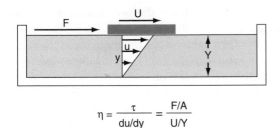

$$\eta = \frac{\tau}{du/dy} = \frac{F/A}{U/Y}$$

FIGURE 6-8 ■ For a newtonian fluid, the viscosity, η, is defined as the ratio of shear stress, τ, to shear rate, du/dy. For a plate of contact area, A, moving across the surface of a liquid, τ equals the ratio of the force, F, applied in the direction of motion to the contact area, and du/dy equals the ratio of the velocity of the plate, U, to the depth of the liquid, Y.

of the fluid. The **shear stress**, η, is defined as the ratio of F:A, where *F* is the force applied to the upper plate in the direction of its motion along the upper surface of the fluid, and *A* is the area of the upper plate in contact with the fluid. The **shear rate** is du/dy, where *u* is the velocity of a minute element of the fluid in the direction parallel to the motion of the upper plate, and *y* is the distance of that fluid element above the bottom, stationary plate.

For a movable plate traveling at constant velocity across the surface of a homogeneous fluid, the velocity profile of the fluid will be linear. The fluid layer in contact with the upper plate will adhere to it and therefore will move at the same velocity, *U*, as the plate. Each minute element of fluid between the plates will move at a velocity, *u*, proportional to its distance, *y*, from the lower plate. Therefore the shear rate will be U/Y, where *Y* is the total distance between the two plates. Because viscosity, η, is defined as the ratio of shear stress, τ, to the shear rate, du/dy, in the example illustrated in Figure 6-8:

$$\eta = (F/A)/(U/Y) \qquad (8)$$

Thus the dimensions of viscosity are $dynes/cm^2$ divided by $(cm/s)/cm$, or $dynes \cdot s/cm^2$. In honor of Poiseuille, 1 $dyne \cdot s/cm^2$ has been termed a **poise**. The viscosity of water at 20° C is approximately 0.01 poise, or 1 centipoise.

With regard to the flow of newtonian fluids through cylindrical tubes, the flow varies inversely as the viscosity. Thus in the example of flow from the reservoir in Figure 6-7D, if the viscosity of the fluid in the reser-

voir were doubled, the flow would be halved (5 mL/s instead of 10 mL/s).

In summary, for the steady, laminar flow of a newtonian fluid through a cylindrical tube, the flow, Q, varies directly as the pressure difference, $P_i - P_o$, and the fourth power of the radius, r, of the tube, and it varies inversely as the length, l, of the tube and the viscosity, η, of the fluid. The full statement of Poiseuille's law is

$$Q = \pi (P_i - P_o)r^4 / 8 \eta l \qquad (9)$$

where $\pi/8$ is the constant of proportionality.

RESISTANCE TO FLOW

In electrical theory the resistance, R, is defined as the ratio of voltage drop, E, to current flow, I. Similarly, in fluid mechanics the hydraulic resistance, R, may be defined as the ratio of pressure drop, $P_i - P_o$, to flow, Q; P_i and P_o are the pressures at the inflow and outflow ends, respectively, of the hydraulic system. For the steady, laminar flow of a newtonian fluid through a cylindrical tube, the physical components of hydraulic resistance may be appreciated by rearranging Poiseuille's law to give the **hydraulic resistance equation:**

$$R = P_i - P_o / Q = 8\eta l / \pi r^4 \qquad (10)$$

Thus when Poiseuille's law applies, the resistance to flow depends only on the dimensions of the tube and on the characteristics of the fluid.

The principal determinant of the resistance to blood flow through any vessel within the circulatory system is its caliber because resistance varies with the fourth power of the tube radius. The resistance to flow through small blood vessels in cat mesentery has been measured, and the resistance per unit length of vessel (R/l) is plotted against the vessel diameter in Figure 6-9. The resistance is highest in the capillaries (diameter 7 µm), and it diminishes as the vessels increase in diameter on the arterial and venous sides of the capillaries. The values of R/l were found to be virtually proportional to the fourth power of the diameter (or radius) for the larger vessels on both sides of the capillaries.

Figure 1-3 shows that the greatest upstream to downstream drop in internal pressure occurs in the arterioles and small arteries. It follows that the greatest

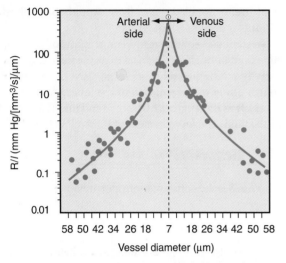

resistance to flow resides in the arterioles because the
total flow is the same through the various series components of the circulatory system. For example, if R_a
represents the resistance of the arterioles, and R_x represents the resistance of any other component of the
vascular system in series with the arterioles, then by
the definition of hydraulic resistance (equation 10),

$$R_a = (P_i - P_o)_a / Q_a \qquad (11)$$

for the arterioles, and

$$R_x = (P_i - P_o)_x / Q_x \qquad (12)$$

for the other vascular component.

However, the two components are in series, $Q_a = Q_x$ as stated previously. Therefore:

$$R_a / R_x = (P_i - P_o)_a / (P_i - P_o)_x \qquad (13)$$

That is, the ratio of the pressure drop across the
length of the arterioles to the pressure drop across the
length of any other series component of the vascular
system is equal to the ratio of the hydraulic resistances
of these two vascular components.

The reason that the highest resistance does not
reside in the capillaries (as might otherwise be suspected from Figure 6-9) is related to the relative numbers of parallel capillaries and parallel arterioles, as
explained later (see Figure 6-11). The arterioles are
vested with a thick coat of circularly arranged smooth
muscle fibers, by means of which the lumen radius
may be varied. From the hydraulic resistance equation,
wherein R varies inversely with r^4, it is clear that small
changes in radius will alter resistance greatly.

Resistances in Series and in Parallel

In the cardiovascular system, the various types of vessels listed along the horizontal axis in Figure 1-3 lie in
series with one another. For two vessels arranged in
series, a red blood cell that flows through the upstream
vessel will also flow through the downstream
vessel. Furthermore, the individual members of a given cate-
gory of vessels are ordinarily arranged in parallel with
one another (see Figure 1-1). For two vessels arranged
in parallel, a red blood cell will pass through one of
these vessels but not through the other during one circuit around the body. For example, the capillaries
throughout the body are in most instances parallel elements. However, notable exceptions are the renal vasculature (wherein the peritubular capillaries are in
series with the glomerular capillaries) and the splanchnic vasculature (wherein the intestinal and hepatic
capillaries are aligned in series). Formulas for the total
hydraulic resistance of tubes arranged in series and in
parallel have been derived in the same manner as those
for similar combinations of electrical resistances.

Three hydraulic resistances, R_1, R_2, and R_3, are
arranged in series in the schema depicted in Figure
6-10. The pressure drop across the entire system—that
is, the difference between inflow pressure, P_i, and outflow pressure, P_o—consists of the sum of the pressure
drops across each of the individual resistances (equation a in Figure 6-10). Under steady-state conditions,
the flow, Q, through any given cross-section must
equal the flow through any other cross-section. When

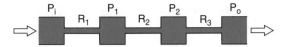

(a) $P_i - P_o = (P_i - P_1) + (P_1 - P_2) + (P_2 - P_o)$

(b) $\dfrac{P_i - P_o}{Q} = \dfrac{(P_i - P_1)}{Q} + \dfrac{(P_1 - P_2)}{Q} + \dfrac{(P_2 - P_o)}{Q}$

(c) $R_t = R_1 + R_2 + R_3$

FIGURE 6-10 ■ For resistances (R_1, R_2, and R_3) arranged in series, the total resistance, R_t, equals the sum of the individual resistances.

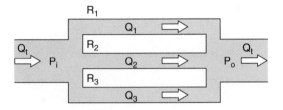

A $Q_t = Q_1 + Q_2 + Q_3$

B $\dfrac{Q_t}{P_i - P_o} = \dfrac{Q_1}{(P_i - P_o)} + \dfrac{Q_2}{(P_i - P_o)} + \dfrac{Q_3}{(P_i - P_o)}$

C $\dfrac{1}{R_t} = \dfrac{1}{R_1} + \dfrac{1}{R_2} + \dfrac{1}{R_3}$

FIGURE 6-11 ■ For resistances (R_1, R_2, and R_3) arranged in parallel, the reciprocal of the total resistance, R_t, equals the sum of the reciprocals of the individual resistances.

each component in equation a is divided by Q (equation b), it becomes evident from the definition of resistance (equation c) that *the total resistance, R_t, of the entire system of tubes in series equals the sum of the individual resistances*: that is,

$$R_t = R_1 + R_2 + R_3 \tag{14}$$

For resistances in parallel, as illustrated in Figure 6-11, the inflow and outflow pressures are the same for all tubes. Under steady-state conditions, the total flow, Q_t, through the system equals the sum of the flows through the individual parallel elements (equation a in Figure 6-10). Because the pressure gradient ($P_i - P_o$) is identical for all parallel elements, each term in equation a may be divided by that pressure gradient to yield equation b. From the definition of resistance, equation c may

be derived. This equation states that *the reciprocal of the total resistance, R_t, of tubes in parallel equals the sum of the reciprocals of the individual resistances*; that is,

$$1/R_t = 1/R_1 + 1/R_2 + 1/R_3 \tag{15}$$

Stated in another way, if we define hydraulic **conductance** as the reciprocal of resistance, it becomes evident that, *for tubes in parallel, the total conductance is the sum of the individual conductances.*

Considering a few simple illustrations helps some of the fundamental properties of parallel hydraulic systems become apparent. For example, if the resistance of the three parallel elements in Figure 6-11 were all equal, then

$$R_1 = R_2 = R_3 \tag{16}$$

Therefore

$$1/R_t = 3/R_1 \tag{17}$$

and

$$R_t = R_1/3 \tag{18}$$

Thus the total resistance is less than any of the individual resistances. Furthermore, it becomes evident that for any parallel arrangement, the total resistance must be less than that of any individual component. For example, consider a system in which a very high-resistance tube is added in parallel to a low-resistance tube. The total resistance must be less than that of the low-resistance component by itself, because the high-resistance component affords an additional pathway, or conductance, for fluid flow.

FLOW MAY BE LAMINAR OR TURBULENT

Under certain conditions, the flow of a fluid in a cylindrical tube is **laminar** (sometimes called **streamlined**), as illustrated in Figure 6-5. The thin layer of fluid in contact with the wall of the tube adheres to the wall and thus is motionless. The layer of fluid just central to this external lamina must shear against this motionless layer and therefore moves slowly, but with a finite velocity. Similarly, the adjacent, more central layer travels still more rapidly. The longitudinal velocity profile is that of a paraboloid (see Figure 6-5). The velocity of the fluid adjacent to the wall is zero, whereas

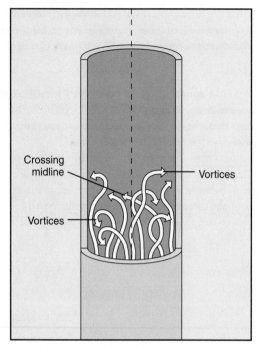

FIGURE 6-12 ■ In turbulent flow the elements of the fluid move irregularly in axial, radial, and circumferential directions. Vortices frequently develop.

the velocity at the center of the stream is maximum and equal to twice the mean velocity of flow across the entire cross-section of the tube. In laminar flow, fluid elements remain in one lamina, or streamline, as the fluid progresses longitudinally along the tube.

Irregular motions of the fluid elements may develop in the flow of fluid through a tube; this flow is called **turbulent.** Under such conditions, fluid elements do not remain confined to definite laminae, but rapid, radial mixing occurs (Figure 6-12). A much greater pressure is required to force a given flow of fluid through the same tube when the flow is turbulent than when it is laminar. In turbulent flow the pressure drop is approximately proportional to the square of the flow rate, whereas in laminar flow the pressure drop is proportional to the first power of the flow rate. Hence to produce a given flow, a pump such as the heart must do considerably more work to generate a given flow if turbulence develops.

Whether turbulent or laminar flow will exist in a tube under given conditions may be predicted on the basis of a dimensionless number called the **Reynold number,** N_R. This number represents the ratio of inertial to viscous forces. For a fluid flowing through a cylindric tube,

$$N_R = \rho D \bar{v} / \eta \qquad (19)$$

where D is the tube diameter, $\bar{v}$ is the mean velocity, ρ is the density, and η is the viscosity. For $N_R = 2000$, the flow is usually laminar; for $N_R > 3000$, the flow is turbulent. Various possible conditions may develop in the transition range of N_R between 2000 and 3000. The definition of N_R indicates that large diameters, high velocities, and low viscosities predispose to turbulence because flow tends to be laminar at low N_R and turbulent at high N_R.

Turbulence is usually accompanied by audible vibrations. When turbulent flow exists within the cardiovascular system, it is usually detected as a **murmur.** The factors listed previously that predispose to turbulence may account for murmurs heard clinically. In severe anemia, **functional cardiac murmurs** (murmurs not caused by structural abnormalities) are frequently detectable. The physical basis for such murmurs resides in (1) the reduced viscosity of blood in anemia and (2) the high flow velocities associated with the high cardiac output that usually prevails in anemic patients. Turbulence also occurs when the cross-sectional area of the bloodstream suddenly changes, as when the blood passes through a narrowed (stenotic) cardiac valve or when it passes through an abnormal widening (aneurysm) of a large artery. Such abrupt changes in dimensions of the bloodstream cause audible murmurs.

Blood clots, or **thrombi,** are much more likely to develop in turbulent than in laminar flow. One of the problems with the use of artificial valves in the surgical treatment of valvular heart disease is that thrombi may occur in association with the prosthetic valve. The thrombi may be dislodged and occlude a crucial artery. It is thus important to design such valves to avert turbulence.

SHEAR STRESS ON THE VESSEL WALL

In Figure 6-8, an external force is applied to a plate floating on the surface of a liquid in a large basin. This force, exerted parallel to the surface, causes a shearing stress on the liquid below and thereby produces a differential motion of each layer of liquid relative to the adjacent layers. At the bottom of the basin, the flowing liquid exerts a shearing stress on the surface of the basin in contact with the liquid. If the equation for viscosity stated in Figure 6-8 is rearranged, it is apparent that the shear stress, τ, equals η (du/dy); that is, the shear stress equals the product of the viscosity and the shear rate. Hence *the greater the rate of flow, the greater the shear stress that the liquid exerts on the walls of the container in which it flows.*

For precisely the same reasons, the rapidly flowing blood in a large artery tends to pull the endothelial lining of the artery along with it. This force (**viscous drag**) is proportional to the shear rate (*du/dy*) of the layers of blood very close to the wall. For a flow regimen that obeys Poiseuille's law,

$$\tau = 4\eta Q/\pi r^3 \qquad (20)$$

The greater the rate of blood flow (Q) in the artery, the greater will be du/dy near the arterial wall, and the greater will be the viscous drag (τ). Under physiological conditions, shear stress is 1 to 6 dynes/cm^2 in veins and 10 to 70 dynes/cm^2 in arteries. Also, shear stress is linked to biochemical changes in blood vessel function. Thus, laminar flow with high shear can protect against atherosclerosis by reducing the synthesis of atherogenic genes and increasing the production of atheroprotective genes. Turbulent flow patterns, seen at vessel bifurcations and curvatures, are likely to increase synthesis of genes that promote inflammation, the cause of atherosclerotic plaque formation. For example, angiotensin II, an endogenous substance, is implicated in inflammation that underlies atherosclerosis. Physiological shear stress may be atherprotective by causing a reduction (downregulation) of angiotensin type 1 receptors (AT_1Rs) on the surface of endothelial cells.

CLINICAL BOX

In certain types of arterial disease, particularly in patients with hypertension, the subendothelial layers tend to degenerate locally, and small regions of the endothelium may lose their normal support. The viscous drag on the arterial wall may cause a tear between a normally supported region and an unsupported region of the endothelial lining. Blood may then flow from the vessel lumen through the rift in the lining and dissect between the various layers of the artery. Such a lesion is called a **dissecting aneurysm.** It occurs most commonly in the proximal portions of the aorta and is extremely serious. One reason for its predilection for this site is the high velocity of blood flow, with the associated large values of du/dy at the endothelial wall. The shear stress at the vessel wall also influences many other vascular functions, such as the permeability of the vascular walls to large molecules, the biosynthetic activity of the endothelial cells, the integrity of the formed elements in the blood, and the coagulation of the blood.

RHEOLOGIC PROPERTIES OF BLOOD

The viscosity of a newtonian fluid, such as water, may be determined by measuring the rate of flow of the fluid at a given pressure gradient through a cylindrical tube of known length and radius. As long as the fluid flow is laminar, the viscosity may be computed by substituting these values into Poiseuille's equation. The viscosity of a given newtonian fluid at a specified temperature will be constant over a wide range of tube dimensions and flows. However, for a nonnewtonian fluid, the viscosity calculated by substituting into Poiseuille's equation may vary considerably as a function of tube dimensions and flows. Therefore, the term **viscosity** does not have a unique meaning in considering the rheologic properties of a suspension such as blood. The terms **anomalous viscosity** and **apparent viscosity** are frequently applied to the value of viscosity obtained for blood under the particular conditions of measurement.

Rheologically, blood is a suspension of formed elements, principally erythrocytes, in a relatively homogeneous liquid, the blood plasma. For this reason, the apparent viscosity of blood varies as a function of the **hematocrit ratio** (ratio of volume of red blood cells to volume of whole blood). In Figure 6-13 the upper curve represents the ratio of the apparent viscosity of whole blood to that of plasma over a range of hematocrit ratios from 0% to 80%, measured in a tube 1 mm in diameter. The viscosity of plasma is 1.2 to 1.3 times that of water. Figure 6-13 (*upper curve*) shows that blood, with a normal

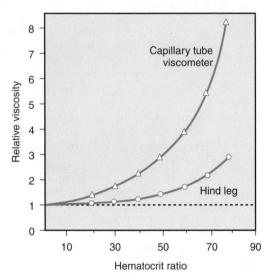

FIGURE 6-13 ■ The viscosity of whole blood, relative to that of plasma, increases at a progressively greater rate as the hematocrit ratio increases. For any given hematocrit ratio, the apparent viscosity of blood is less when measured in a biological viscometer (such as the hind leg of a dog) than in a conventional capillary tube viscometer. *(Redrawn from Levy MN, Share L: The influence of erythrocyte concentration upon the pressure-flow relationships in the dog's hind limb.* Circ Res *1:247, 1953.)*

hematocrit ratio of 45%, has an apparent viscosity 2.4 times that of plasma.

For any given hematocrit ratio, the apparent viscosity of blood depends on the dimensions of the tube employed in estimating the viscosity. Figure 6-14 demonstrates that the apparent viscosity of blood diminishes progressively as tube diameter decreases below a value of about 0.3 mm. The diameters of the highest-resistance blood vessels, the arterioles, are considerably less than this critical value. This phenomenon therefore reduces the resistance to flow in the blood vessels that possess the greatest resistance.

CLINICAL BOX

In severe anemia, blood viscosity is low. With greater hematocrit ratios, the relative viscosity increases (see Figure 6-13). This effect is especially profound at the upper range of erythrocyte concentrations. A rise in hematocrit ratio from 45% to 70%, which occurs in

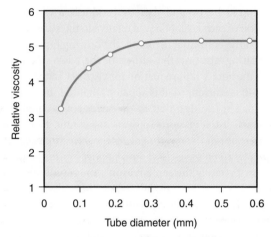

FIGURE 6-14 ■ The viscosity of blood, relative to that of water, increases as a function of tube diameter up to a diameter of about 0.3 mm. *(Redrawn from Fåhraeus R, Lindqvist T: The viscosity of the blood in narrow capillary tubes.* Am J Physiol *96:562, 1931.)*

polycythemia, increases the relative viscosity more than twofold, with a proportionate effect on the resistance to blood flow. The effect of such a change in hematocrit ratio on peripheral resistance may be appreciated when it is recognized that even in the most severe cases of **essential hypertension,** total peripheral resistance rarely increases by more than a factor of two. In essential hypertension, the increase in peripheral resistance is achieved by arteriolar vasoconstriction.

The apparent viscosity of blood, when measured in living tissues, is considerably less than when it is measured in a conventional capillary tube viscometer with a diameter greater than 0.3 mm. In the lower curve of Figure 6-13, the apparent viscosity of blood was assessed by using the hind leg of an anesthetized dog as a biological viscometer. Over the entire range of hematocrit ratios, the apparent viscosity was less when measured in the living tissue than in the capillary tube viscometer (*upper curve*), and the disparity was greater the higher the hematocrit ratio.

The influence of tube diameter on apparent viscosity depends in part on the change in actual composition of the blood as it flows through small tubes. The composition changes because the red blood cells tend

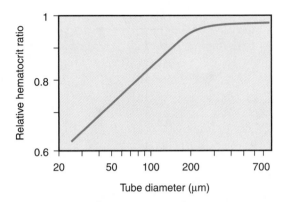

FIGURE 6-15 ■ The relative hematocrit ratio of blood flowing from a feed reservoir through capillary tubes of various calibers, as a function of the tube diameter. The relative hematocrit is the ratio of the hematocrit of the blood in the tubes to that of the blood in the feed reservoir. *(Redrawn from Barbee JH, Cokelet GR: The Fahraeus effect.* Microvasc Res *3:6, 1971.)*

to accumulate in the faster axial stream in the blood vessels, whereas the blood component that flows in the slower marginal layers is mainly plasma.

To illustrate this phenomenon, a reservoir such as R_1 in Figure 6-6C has been filled with blood possessing a given hematocrit ratio. The blood in R_1 was constantly agitated to prevent settling and was permitted to flow through a narrow capillary tube into reservoir R_2. As long as the tube diameter was substantially greater than the diameter of the red blood cells, the hematocrit ratio of the blood in R_2 was not detectably different from that in R_1. Surprisingly, however, the hematocrit ratio of the blood contained *within* the tube was found to be considerably lower than the hematocrit ratio of the blood in either reservoir.

In Figure 6-15, the relative hematocrit is the ratio of the hematocrit in the tube to that in the reservoir at either end of the tube. For tubes of 300 μm diameter or greater, the relative hematocrit ratio was close to 1. However, as the tube diameter was reduced below 300 μm, the relative hematocrit ratio progressively diminished; for a tube diameter of 30 μm, the relative hematocrit ratio was only 0.65.

This effect, called the Fahraeus-Lindqvist phenomenon, results from a disparity in the relative velocities of the red blood cells and plasma. The red blood cells tend to traverse the tube in less time than the plasma because the axial portions of the bloodstream contain a greater proportion of red blood cells and move with a greater velocity. Measurement of transit times through various organs has shown that red blood cells do travel faster than the plasma. Furthermore, the hematocrit ratios of the blood contained in the smallest vessels in various tissues are lower than those in blood samples withdrawn from large arteries or veins in the same animal (Figure 6-16).

The physical forces causing the drift of the erythrocytes toward the axial stream and away from the vessel walls are not fully understood. One factor is the great flexibility of the red blood cells. At low flow (or shear) rates, comparable with those in the microcirculation, flexible particles migrate toward the axis of a tube, whereas rigid particles do not. The concentration of flexible particles near the tube axis is enhanced by an increase in the shear rate.

The apparent viscosity of blood diminishes as the shear rate is increased (Figure 6-17), a phenomenon called **shear thinning.** The greater tendency of the erythrocytes to accumulate in the axial laminae at higher flow rates is partly responsible for this nonnewtonian behavior. However, a more important factor is that at very slow rates of shear, the suspended cells tend to form aggregates, which would increase viscosity. As the flow is increased, this aggregation would decrease and so would the apparent viscosity (see Figure 6-17).

The tendency for the erythrocytes to aggregate at low flows depends on the concentration in the plasma of the larger protein molecules, especially fibrinogen. For this reason, the changes in blood viscosity with shear rate are much more pronounced when the concentration of fibrinogen is high. Also, at low flow rates, leukocytes tend to adhere to the endothelial cells of the microvessels and thereby increase the apparent viscosity.

The deformability of erythrocytes is also a factor in shear thinning, especially at high hematocrit ratios. The mean diameter of human red blood cells is about 8 μm, yet they are able to pass through openings with a diameter of only 3 μm. As blood that is densely packed with erythrocytes is made to flow at progressively greater rates, the erythrocytes become more and more deformed, diminishing the apparent viscosity of the blood. The flexibility of human erythrocytes is enhanced as the concentration of fibrinogen in the plasma increase (Figure 6-18).

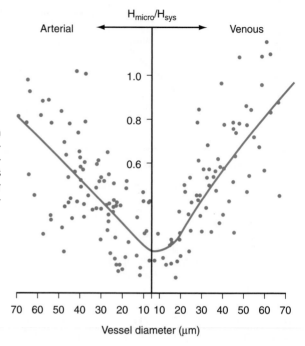

FIGURE 6-16 ■ The hematocrit ratio (H_{micro}) of the blood in various-sized arterial and venous microvessels in the cat mesentery, relative to the hematocrit ratio (H_{sys}) in the large systemic vessels. The hematocrit ratio is least in the capillaries and tiny venules. *(Modified from Lipowsky HH, Usami S, Chien S: In vivo measurements of "apparent viscosity" and microvessel hematocrit in the mesentery of the cat.* Microvasc Res *19:297, 1980.)*

CLINICAL BOX

If the red blood cells become hardened, as they are in certain **spherocytic anemias,** shear thinning may become much less prominent. When erythrocytes are extremely deformed, especially in **sickle cell anemia,** they tend to aggregate and completely block flow in small vessels; the tissues supplied by those vessels frequently become infarcted.

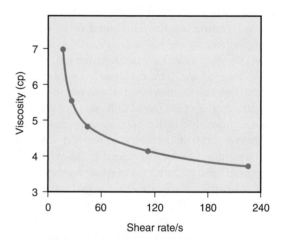

FIGURE 6-17 ■ Decrease in the viscosity of blood (in centipoise) at increasing rates of shear. The shear rate refers to the velocity of one layer of fluid relative to that of the adjacent layers and is directionally related to the rate of flow. *(Redrawn from Amin TM, Sirs JA: The blood rheology of man and various animal species.* Q J Exp Physiol *70:37, 1985.)*

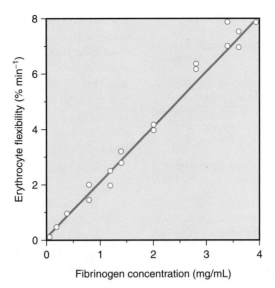

FIGURE 6-18 ■ The effect of the plasma fibrinogen concentration on the flexibility of human erythrocytes. *(Redrawn from Amin TM, Sirs JA: The blood rheology of man and various animal species.* Q J Exp Physiol *70:37, 1985.)*

S U M M A R Y

- The vascular system is composed of two major subdivisions in series with each other—the systemic circulation and the pulmonary circulation.
- Each subdivision consists of several types of vessels (e.g., arteries, arterioles, capillaries) aligned in series with one another. In general, the vessels of a given type are arranged in parallel with each other.
- The mean velocity ($\bar{v}$) of blood flow in a given type of vessel is directly proportional to the total blood flow (Q_t) being pumped by the heart, and it is inversely proportional to the cross-sectional area (A) of all the parallel vessels of that type; i.e., $\bar{v} = Q_t / A$.
- The laterally directed pressure in the bloodstream decreases as the flow velocity increases; the decrement in lateral pressure is proportional to the square of the velocity.
- When blood flow is steady and laminar in vessels larger than arterioles, the flow (Q) is proportional to the pressure drop down the vessel ($P_i - P_o$) and to the fourth power of the radius (r), and it is inversely proportional to the length (l) of the vessel and to the viscosity (η) of the fluid; i.e., $Q = \pi(P_i - P_o)r^4/8\eta l$ (Poiseuille's law).

- For resistances aligned in series, the total resistance equals the sum of the individual resistances.
- For resistances aligned in parallel, the reciprocal of the total resistance equals the sum of the reciprocals of the individual resistances.
- Flow tends to become turbulent when flow velocity is high, when fluid viscosity is low, when tube diameter is large, or when the wall of the vessel is very irregular.
- Blood flow is nonnewtonian in very small vessels; i.e., Poiseuille's law is not applicable. The apparent viscosity of blood diminishes as shear rate (flow) increases and as the tube dimensions decrease.

ADDITIONAL READING

Baskurt OK, Meiselman HJ: Blood rheology and hemodynamics, *Semin Thromb Hemost* 29:435, 2003.

Cecchi E, Gigioli C, Valente S, et al: Role of hemodynamic shear stress in cardiovascular disease, *Atheroclerosis* 214:249, 2011.

Chiu J-J, Chien S: Effects of disturbed flow on vascular endothelium: pathophysiological basis and clinical perspectives, *Physiol Rev* 91:327, 2011.

Helmke BP: Molecular control of cytoskeletal mechanics by hemo-dynamic forces, *Physiology* 20:43, 2005.

Hoeks APG, Samijo SK, Brands PJ, et al: Noninvasive determination of shear-rate distribution across the arterial wall, *Hypertension* 26:26, 1995.

Kwaan HC, Wang J: Hyperviscosity in polycythemia vera and other red cell abnormalities, *Semin Thromb Hemost* 29:451, 2003.

Long DS, Smith ML, Pries A, et al: Microviscometry reveals reduced blood viscosity and altered shear rate and shear stress profiles in microvessels after hemodilution, *Proc Natl Acad Sci U S A* 101:10060, 2004.

McCue S, Noria S, Langille BL: Shear-induced reorganization of endothelial cell cytoskeleton and adhesion complexes, *Trends Cardiovasc Med* 14:143, 2004.

Pries AR, Secomb TW: Microvascular blood viscosity in vivo and the endothelial surface layer, *Am J Physiol* 289:H2657, 2005.

Pries AR, Secomb TW, Gaetgens P: Design principles of vascular beds, *Circ Res* 77:1017, 1995.

Resnick N, Yahav H, Shay-Salit A, et al: Fluid shear stress and the vascular endothelium: for better and for worse, *Prog Biophys Mol Biol* 81:177, 2003.

Tyml K, Anderson D, Lidington D, Ladak HM: A new method for assessing arteriolar diameter and hemodynamic resistance using image analysis of vessel lumen, *Am J Physiol* 284:H1721, 2003.

CASE 6-6

HISTORY

A 70-year-old man complained of severe pain in his right leg whenever he walked briskly; the pain disappeared soon after he stopped walking. His doctor referred him to a vascular surgeon, who carried out several hemodynamic tests. Angiography showed partial obstruction by large arteriosclerotic plaques about 3 cm distal to the origin of the right femoral artery. The left femoral artery appeared to be normal. The mean arterial pressure in the left femoral artery with the patient at rest was 100 mm Hg, and the blood flow in this artery was 500 mL/min. The mean arterial pressure in the right femoral artery proximal to the obstruction was 100 mm Hg, and just distal to the obstruction, it was 80 mm Hg. The blood flow in this artery was 300 mL/min. The mean venous pressure was 10 mm Hg in the left and right femoral veins.

QUESTIONS

1. The resistance to blood flow in the vascular bed perfused by the right femoral artery was:
   a. 0.03 mm Hg/mL/min.
   b. 0.30 mm Hg/mL/min.
   c. 3.00 mm Hg/mL/min.
   d. 3.33 mm Hg/mL/min.
   e. 33.3 mm Hg/mL/min.

2. The resistance to blood flow (R_t) in the combined vascular beds perfused by both femoral arteries was:
   a. 0.48 mm Hg/mL/min.
   b. 0.84 mm Hg/mL/min.
   c. 1.10 mm Hg/mL/min.
   d. 0.11 mm Hg/mL/min.
   e. 11.1 mm Hg/mL/min.

3. The resistance to flow imposed by the arteriosclerotic obstruction in the right femoral artery amounted to:
   a. 0.066 mm Hg/mL/min.
   b. 0.660 mm Hg/mL/min.
   c. 0.15 mm Hg/mL/min.
   d. 1.50 mm Hg/mL/min.
   e. 15.0 mm Hg/mL/min.

7

THE ARTERIAL SYSTEM

OBJECTIVES

1. Explain how the pulsatile blood flow in the large arteries is converted into a steady flow in the capillaries.

2. Discuss arterial compliance and its relation to stroke volume and pulse pressure.

3. Explain the factors that determine the mean, systolic, and diastolic arterial pressures and the arterial pulse pressure.

4. Describe the common procedure for measuring the arterial blood pressure in humans.

THE HYDRAULIC FILTER CONVERTS PULSATILE FLOW TO STEADY FLOW

The principal functions of the systemic and pulmonary arterial systems are to distribute blood to the capillary beds throughout the body. The arterioles, which are the terminal components of the arterial system, regulate the distribution of flow to the various capillary beds. In the region between the heart and the arterioles, the aorta and pulmonary artery, and their major branches constitute a system of conduits of considerable volume and distensibility. This system of elastic conduits and high-resistance terminals constitutes a **hydraulic filter** that is analogous to the resistance-capacitance filters of electrical circuits.

Hydraulic filtering converts the intermittent output of the heart to a steady flow through the capillaries. This important function of the large elastic arteries has been likened to the **Windkessels** of antique fire engines. The Windkessel in such a fire engine contains

a large volume of trapped air. The compressibility of the air trapped in the Windkessel converts the intermittent inflow of water to a steady outflow of water at the nozzle of the fire hose.

The analogous function of the large elastic arteries is illustrated in Figure 7-1. The heart is an intermittent pump. The cardiac stroke volume is discharged into the arterial system during systole. The duration of the discharge usually occupies about one third of the cardiac cycle. In fact, as shown in Figure 4-13, most of the stroke volume is pumped during the rapid ejection phase. This phase constitutes about half of systole. Part of the energy of cardiac contraction is dissipated as forward capillary flow during systole. The remaining energy in the distensible arteries is stored as potential energy (Figure 7-1A and B). During diastole, the elastic recoil of the arterial walls converts this potential energy into capillary blood flow. If the arterial walls had been rigid, capillary flow would have ceased during diastole.

Compliant arteries

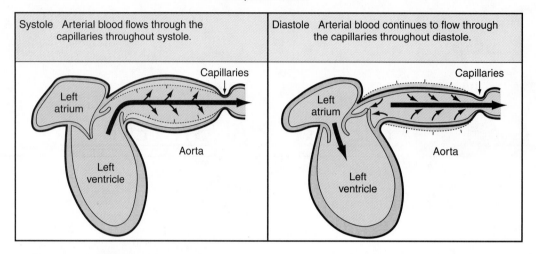

A When the arteries are normally compliant, a substantial fraction of the stroke volume is stored in the arteries during ventricular systole. The arterial walls are stretched.

B During ventricular diastole the previously stretched arteries recoil. The volume of blood that is displaced by the recoil furnishes continuous capillary flow diastole.

Rigid arteries

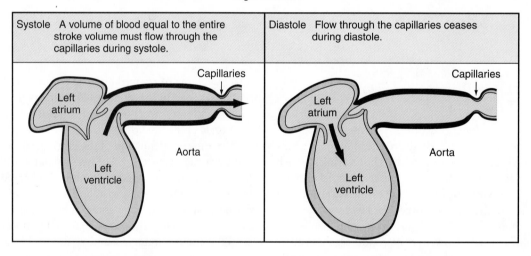

C When the arteries are rigid, virtually none of the stroke volume can be stored in the arteries.

D Rigid arteries cannot recoil appreciably during diastole.

FIGURE 7-1 ■ A to D, When the arteries are normally compliant, blood flows through the capillaries throughout the cardiac cycle. When the arteries are rigid, blood flows through the capillaries during systole, but flow ceases during diastole.

Hydraulic filtering minimizes the cardiac workload. More work is required to pump a given flow intermittently than steadily; the steadier the flow, the less is the excess work. A simple example illustrates this point.

Consider first that a fluid flows at the steady rate of 100 mL per second (s) through a hydraulic system that has a resistance of 1 mm Hg/mL/s. This combination of flow and resistance would result in a constant pressure of 100 mm Hg, as shown in Figure 7-2A. Neglecting any inertial effect, hydraulic work, W, may be defined as:

$$W = \int_{t_2}^{t_1} P dV \qquad (1)$$

that is, each small increment of volume, dV, pumped is multiplied by the pressure, P, that exists at that time. The products are integrated over the time interval, $t_2 - t_1$, to yield the total work. When flow is steady,

$$W = PV \qquad (2)$$

In the example in Figure 7-2A, the work done in pumping the fluid for 1 s would be 10,000 mm Hg mL (or 1.33×10^7 dyne-cm). Next, consider an intermittent pump that generates a constant flow of fluid for 0.5 s, and then pumps nothing during the next 0.5 s. Hence, flow is generated at the rate of 200 mL/s for 0.5 s, as shown in Figure 7-2B and C. In panel B, the conduit is rigid, and the fluid is incompressible. However, the system has the same resistance to flow as in panel A. During the pumping phase of the cycle (systole), the flow of 200 mL/s through a resistance of 1 mm Hg/mL/s would produce a pressure of 200 mm Hg. During the filling phase (diastole) of the pump, the pressure in this rigid system would be 0 mm Hg. The work done during systole would be 20,000 mm Hg mL. This value is twice that required in the example shown in Figure 7-2A.

If the system were very distensible, hydraulic filtering would be very effective and the pressure would remain virtually constant throughout the entire cycle (Figure 7-2C). Of the 100 mL of fluid pumped during the 0.5 s of systole, only 50 mL would be emitted through the high-resistance outflow end of the system during systole. The remaining 50 mL would be stored by the distensible conduit during systole, and it would flow out during diastole. Hence the pressure would be

virtually constant at 100 mm Hg throughout the cycle. The fluid pumped during systole would be ejected at only half the pressure that prevailed in Figure 7-2B. Therefore, the work would be only half as great. If filtering were nearly perfect, as in Figure 7-2C, the work would be identical to that for steady flow (Figure 7-2A).

Naturally, the filtering accomplished by the systemic and pulmonic arterial systems is intermediate between the examples in Figures 7-2B and C. The additional work imposed by the intermittent pumping, in excess of that for steady flow, is about 35% for the right ventricle and about 10% for the left ventricle. These fractions change, however, with variations in heart rate, peripheral resistance, and arterial distensibility.

The greater cardiac energy requirement imposed by a rigid arterial system is illustrated in Figure 7-3. In a group of anesthetized dogs, the cardiac output pumped by the left ventricle was allowed to flow either through the natural route (the aorta) or through a stiff plastic tube to the peripheral arteries. The total peripheral resistance (TPR) values were virtually identical, regardless of which pathway was selected. The data (see Figure 7-3) from a representative animal show that, for any given stroke volume, the myocardial oxygen consumption ($M\dot{V}_{O_2}$) was substantially greater when the blood was diverted through the plastic tubing than when it flowed through the aorta. This increase in $M\dot{V}_{O_2}$ indicates that the left ventricle had to expend more energy to pump blood through a less compliant conduit than through a more compliant conduit.

ARTERIAL ELASTICITY COMPENSATES FOR THE INTERMITTENT FLOW DELIVERED BY THE HEART

The elastic properties of the arterial wall are determined by the composition and mechanical properties of the vessel. Two important constituents of the arterial wall are elastic fibers, composed of elastin and microfibrils, and collagen. Elastin is elaborated by endothelial cells and is found in the tunica intima, whereas collagen is derived from myofibroblasts and located in the tunica adventitia.

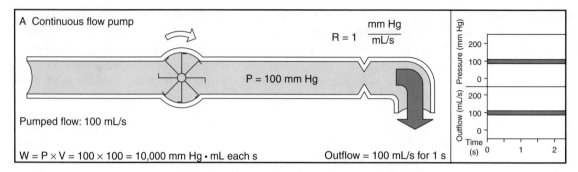

A, The pump flow is steady, and pressure will remain constant regardless of the distensibility of the conduit.

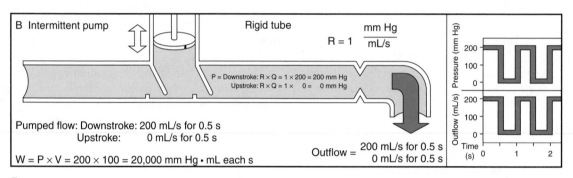

B, The flow *(Q)* produced by the pump is intermittent; it is steady for half the cycle and ceases for the remainder of the cycle. The conduit is rigid and therefore, the flow produced by the pump during its downstroke must exit through the resistance during the same 0.5 s that elapses during the downstroke. The pump must do twice as much work as the pump in **A.**

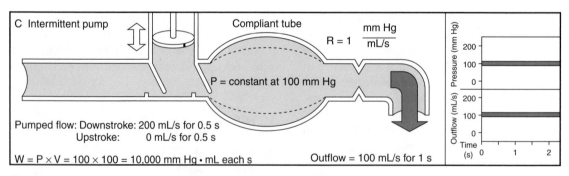

C, The pump operates as in B, but the conduit is infinitely distensible. This results in perfect filtering of the pressure; that is, the pressure is steady, and the outflow through the resistance is also steady. The work equals that in A.

FIGURE 7-2 ■ **A** to **C,** The relationships between pressure and flow for three hydraulic systems. In each the overall flow is 100 mL/s and the resistance is 1 mm Hg/mL/s.

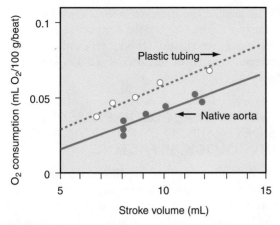

FIGURE 7-3 ■ The relationship between myocardial oxygen consumption (mL/100 g/beat) and stroke volume (mL) in an anesthetized dog whose cardiac output could be pumped by the left ventricle either through the aorta or through a stiff plastic tube to the peripheral arteries. *(Modified from Kelly RP, Tunin R, Kass DA: Effect of reduced aortic compliance on cardiac efficiency and contractile function of in situ canine left ventricle.* Circ Res *71:490, 1992.)*

The elastic properties of the arterial wall may be appreciated by considering first the **static pressure-volume relationship** for the aorta. To derive the curves shown in Figure 7-4, aortas were obtained at autopsy from individuals in different age groups. All branches of each aorta were ligated and successive volumes of liquid were injected into this closed elastic system. After each increment of volume, the internal pressure was measured. In Figure 7-4, the curve that relates pressure to volume in the youngest age group (curve a) is sigmoidal. Although the curve is nearly linear, the slope decreases at the upper and lower ends. At any point on the curve, the slope (dV/dP) represents the **aortic compliance.** Thus, in young individuals the aortic compliance is least at very high at low pressures and greatest at intermediate pressures. This sequence of compliance changes resembles the familiar compliance changes encountered in inflating a balloon. The greatest difficulty in introducing air into the balloon is experienced at the beginning of inflation and again at near-maximal volume, just before the balloon ruptures. At intermediate volumes, the balloon is relatively easy to inflate; that is, it is more compliant.

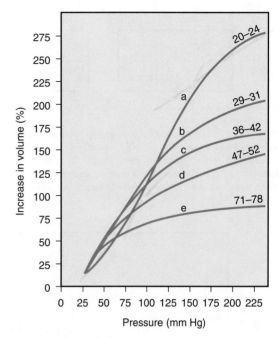

FIGURE 7-4 ■ Pressure-volume relationships for aortas obtained at autopsy from humans in different age groups (ages in years denoted by the numbers at the right end of each of the curves). *(Redrawn from Hallock P, Benson IC: Studies on the elastic properties of human isolated aorta.* J Clin Invest *16:595, 1937.)*

Figure 7-4 reveals that the pressure-volume curves derived from subjects in different age groups are displaced downwards, and the slopes diminish as a function of advancing age. Thus, for any pressure above about 80 mm Hg, the aortic compliance decreases with age. This manifestation of greater rigidity (arteriosclerosis) is caused by progressive changes in the collagen and elastin contents of the arterial walls.

The previously described effects of the subject's age on the elastic characteristics of the arterial system were derived from aortas removed at autopsy (see Figure 7-4). Such age-related changes have been confirmed in living subjects by ultrasound imaging techniques. These studies disclosed that the increase in the diameter of the aorta produced by each cardiac contraction is much less in elderly persons than in young persons (Figure 7-5). The effects of aging on the elastic modulus of the aorta in healthy subjects are

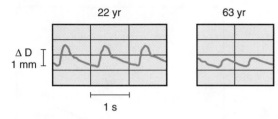

FIGURE 7-5 ■ The pulsatile changes in diameter (ΔD), measured ultrasonically, in a 22-year-old man and a 63-year-old man. *(Modified from Imura T, Yamamoto K, Kanamori K, et al: Non-invasive ultrasonic measurement of the elastic properties of the human abdominal aorta. Cardiovasc Res 20:208, 1986.)*

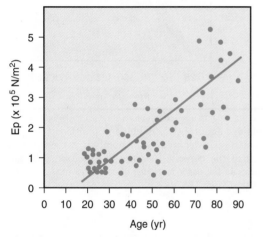

FIGURE 7-6 ■ The effects of age on the elastic modulus (Ep) of the abdominal aorta in a group of 61 human subjects. *(Modified from Imura T, Yamamoto K, Kanamori K, et al: Non-invasive ultrasonic measurement of the elastic properties of the human abdominal aorta. Cardiovasc Res 20:208, 1986.)*

shown in Figure 7-6. The elastic modulus, E_p, is defined as:

$$E_p = \Delta P / (\Delta D / D) \qquad (3)$$

where ΔP is the aortic pulse pressure, (Figure 7-7), D is the mean aortic diameter during the cardiac cycle, and ΔD is the maximal change in aortic diameter during the cardiac cycle.

The fractional change in diameter (ΔD/D) of the aorta during the cardiac cycle reflects its change in volume (ΔV) as the left ventricle ejects its stroke volume into the aorta each systole. Thus E_p is **inversely** related to compliance, which is the ratio of ΔV to ΔP.

Consequently, the **increase** in elastic modulus with aging (see Figure 7-6) and the **decrease** in compliance with aging (see Figure 7-4) both reflect the stiffening (**arteriosclerosis**) of the arterial walls as individuals age.

THE ARTERIAL BLOOD PRESSURE IS DETERMINED BY PHYSICAL AND PHYSIOLOGICAL FACTORS

The determinants of the pressure within the arterial system of intact subjects cannot be evaluated precisely. Nevertheless, arterial blood pressure is routinely measured in patients, and it provides a useful clue to cardiovascular status. We therefore take a simplified approach to explain the principal determinants of arterial blood pressure. To accomplish this, the determinants of the **mean arterial pressure,** defined in the next section, are analyzed first. **Systolic** and **diastolic arterial pressures** are then considered as the upper and lower limits of the periodic oscillations about this mean pressure.

The determinants of the arterial blood pressure may be subdivided arbitrarily into "physical" and "physiological" factors (Figure 7-8). The arterial system is assumed to be a static, elastic system. The only two "physical" factors are considered to be the **blood volume** within the arterial system and the **elastic characteristics (compliance)** of the system. The following "physiological" factors will be considered: namely, (1) the cardiac output, which equals **heart rate × stroke volume,** and (2) the **peripheral resistance.** *Such physiological factors operate through one or both of the physical factors.*

Mean Arterial Pressure

The mean arterial pressure is the pressure in the large arteries, averaged over time. The mean pressure may be obtained from an arterial pressure tracing, by measuring the area under the pressure curve. This area is divided by the time interval involved, as shown in Figure 7-7. The mean arterial pressure, $\overline{P}_a$, can usually be determined satisfactorily from the measured values of the systolic (P_s) and diastolic (P_d) pressures, by means of the following empirical formula:

$$\overline{P}_a \cong P_d + \frac{1}{3}(P_s - P_d) \qquad (4)$$

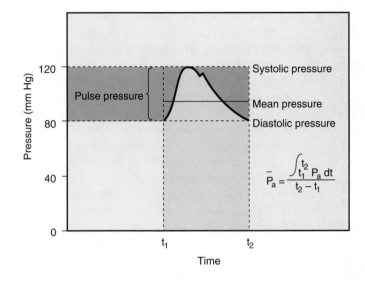

$$\overline{P}_a = \frac{\int_{t_1}^{t_2} P_a\, dt}{t_2 - t_1}$$

FIGURE 7-7 ■ Arterial systolic, diastolic, pulse, and mean pressures. The mean arterial pressure ($\overline{P}_a$) represents the area under the arterial pressure curve (*colored area*) divided by the cardiac cycle duration ($t_2 - t_1$).

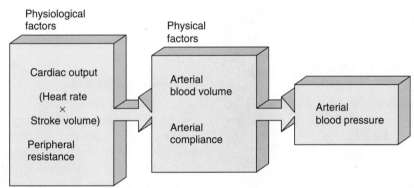

FIGURE 7-8 ■ Arterial blood pressure is determined directly by two major physical factors, the arterial blood volume and the arterial compliance. These physical factors are affected in turn by certain physiological factors, primarily the heart rate, stroke volume, cardiac output (heart rate × stroke volume), and peripheral resistance.

The mean arterial pressure depends mainly on the mean blood volume in the arterial system and on the arterial compliance (see Figure 7-8). The arterial volume, V_a, in turn depends (1) on the rate of inflow, Q_h, from the heart into the arteries (**cardiac output**), and (2) on the rate of outflow, Q_r, from the arteries through the resistance vessels. This constitutes the **peripheral runoff.** Expressed mathematically,

$$dV_a / dt = Q_h - Q_r \qquad (5)$$

This equation is an expression of the law of **conservation of mass.** The equation states that the change in arterial blood volume per unit time (dV_a/dt) represents the difference between the rate (Q_h) at which blood is pumped into the arterial system by the heart, and the rate (Q_r) at which the blood leaves the arterial system through the resistance vessels.

If the arterial inflow exceeds the outflow, the arterial volume increases, the arterial walls are stretched, and the arterial pressure rises. The converse happens when the arterial outflow exceeds the inflow. When the inflow equals the outflow, the arterial pressure remains constant.

Cardiac Output

The change in pressure in response to an alteration of cardiac output can be appreciated better by considering some simple examples. Under control conditions, let cardiac output be 5 L/min and let mean arterial pressure ($\bar{P}_a$) be 100 mm Hg (Figure 7-9A). From the definition of total peripheral resistance,

$$R = (\bar{P}_a - P_{ra}) / Q_r \qquad (6)$$

where P_{ra} is right atrial pressure. If $\bar{P}_{ra}$ (mean right atrial pressure) is negligible compared with $\bar{P}_a$,

$$R \cong \bar{P}_a / Q_r \qquad (7)$$

Therefore in the example, R is 100/5, or 20 mm Hg/L/min.

Now let cardiac output, Q_h, suddenly increase to 10 L/min (Figure 7-9B). $\bar{P}_a$ will remain unchanged. Because the outflow, Q_r, from the arteries depends on $\bar{P}_a$ and R, Q_r will also remain unchanged. Therefore Q_h, now 10 L/min, will exceed Q_r, still only 5 L/min. This will increase the mean arterial blood volume ($\bar{V}_a$). From equation 5, when $Q_h > Q_r$, $d\bar{V}_a / dt > 0$; that is, volume is increasing.

Because $\bar{P}_a$ depends on the mean arterial blood volume, $\bar{V}_a$ and on the arterial compliance, C_a, an increase in $\bar{V}_a$ will raise the $\bar{P}_a$. By definition,

$$C_a = d\bar{V}_a / d\bar{P}_a \qquad (8)$$

Therefore,

$$d\bar{V}_a = C_a d\bar{P}_a \qquad (9)$$

and

$$d\bar{V}_a / dt = C_a d\bar{P}_a / dt \qquad (10)$$

From equation 5,

$$d\bar{P}_a / dt = (Q_h - Q_r) / C_a \qquad (11)$$

Hence $\bar{P}_a$ will rise when $Q_h > Q_r$, it will fall when $Q_h < Q_r$, and it will remain constant when $Q_h = Q_r$.

In this example, Q_h suddenly increased to 10 L/min, and $\bar{P}_a$ continued to rise as long as Q_h exceeded Q_r. Equation 7 shows that Q_r will not attain a value of 10 L/min until $\bar{P}_a$ reaches a level of 200 mm Hg. Thereafter, R will remain constant at 20 mm Hg/L/min. Hence, as $\bar{P}_a$ approaches 200, Q_r will approach the value of Q_h, and $\bar{P}_a$ will rise very slowly. When Q_h begins to rise, however, Q_h exceeds Q_r, and therefore $\bar{P}_a$ will rise sharply. The pressure-time tracing in Figure 7-10 indicates that, regardless of the value of C_a, the slope gradually diminishes as pressure rises, and thus the final value is approached asymptomatically.

Furthermore, the **height** to which $\bar{P}_a$ will rise does not depend on the elastic characteristics of the arterial walls. $\bar{P}_a$ must rise to a level such that the peripheral runoff will equal the cardiac output; that is, $Q_r = Q_h$. Equation 6 shows that Q_r depends only on the pressure gradient and the resistance to flow. Hence C_a determines only the rate at which the new equilibrium value of P_a will be approached, as illustrated in Figure 7-10. When C_a is small (as in rigid vessels), a relatively slight increment in V_a would increase $\bar{P}_a$ greatly. This increment in $\bar{P}_a$ is caused by a transient excess of Q_h over Q_r. Hence $\bar{P}_a$ attains its new equilibrium level quickly. Conversely, when C_a is large, considerable volumes can be accommodated with relatively small pressure changes. Therefore the new equilibrium value of $\bar{P}_a$ is reached at a slower rate.

Peripheral Resistance

Similar reasoning may now be applied to explain the changes in $\bar{P}_a$ that accompany alterations in peripheral resistance. Let the control conditions be identical to those of the preceding example, that is, $Q_h = 5$, $P_a = 100$, and $R = 20$ (see Figure 7-9A). Then, let R suddenly be increased to 40 (see Figure 7-9D). $\bar{P}_a$ would not change appreciably. When $\bar{P}_a = 100$ and $R = 40$, Q_r would equal $\bar{P}_a / R$, which would then equal 2.5 L/min. Thus, the peripheral runoff would be only 2.5 L/min, even though cardiac output equals 5 L/min. If Q_h remains constant at 5 L/min, Q_h would exceed Q_r and $\bar{V}_a$ would increase; and therefore $\bar{P}_a$ would rise. $\bar{P}_a$ will continue to rise until it reaches 200 mm Hg (see Figure 7-9, E). At this pressure level, $Q_r = 200/40 = 5$ L/min, which equals Q_h. $\bar{P}_a$ will remain at this new, elevated level, as long as Q_h and R do not change.

It is evident, therefore, that the level of the mean arterial pressure depends on cardiac output and peripheral resistance. This dependency applies regardless of whether the change in cardiac output is accomplished by an alteration of heart rate or of stroke volume. Any change in heart rate that is balanced by a concomitant, oppositely directed change in stroke volume, will not alter Q_h. Hence $\bar{P}_a$ will not be affected.

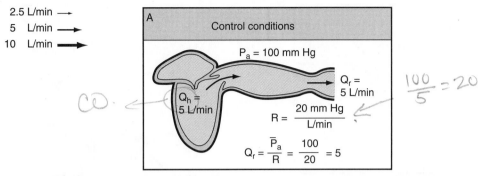

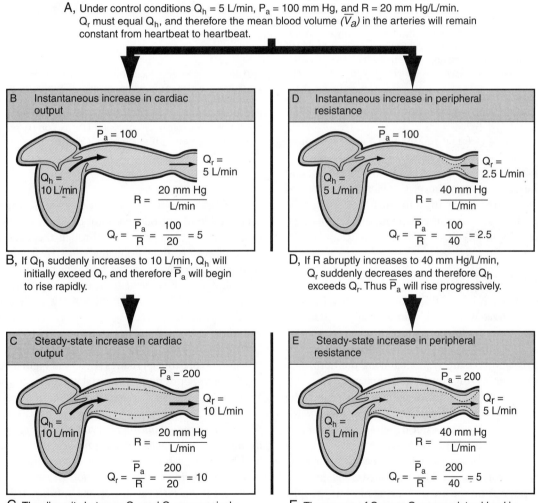

2.5 L/min ⟶
5 L/min ⟶
10 L/min ➤

A Control conditions

$\bar{P}_a$ = 100 mm Hg

CO. ⟵

Q_h = 5 L/min

Q_r = 5 L/min

$\dfrac{100}{5} = 20$

$R = \dfrac{20 \text{ mm Hg}}{\text{L/min}}$

$Q_r = \dfrac{\bar{P}_a}{R} = \dfrac{100}{20} = 5$

A, Under control conditions Q_h = 5 L/min, $\bar{P}_a$ = 100 mm Hg, and R = 20 mm Hg/L/min. Q_r must equal Q_h, and therefore the mean blood volume $(\overline{V_a})$ in the arteries will remain constant from heartbeat to heartbeat.

B Instantaneous increase in cardiac output

$\bar{P}_a$ = 100

Q_h = 10 L/min

Q_r = 5 L/min

$R = \dfrac{20 \text{ mm Hg}}{\text{L/min}}$

$Q_r = \dfrac{\bar{P}_a}{R} = \dfrac{100}{20} = 5$

B, If Q_h suddenly increases to 10 L/min, Q_h will initially exceed Q_r, and therefore $\bar{P}_a$ will begin to rise rapidly.

D Instantaneous increase in peripheral resistance

$\bar{P}_a$ = 100

Q_h = 5 L/min

Q_r = 2.5 L/min

$R = \dfrac{40 \text{ mm Hg}}{\text{L/min}}$

$Q_r = \dfrac{\bar{P}_a}{R} = \dfrac{100}{40} = 2.5$

D, If R abruptly increases to 40 mm Hg/L/min, Q_r suddenly decreases and therefore Q_h exceeds Q_r. Thus $\bar{P}_a$ will rise progressively.

C Steady-state increase in cardiac output

$\bar{P}_a$ = 200

Q_h = 10 L/min

Q_r = 10 L/min

$R = \dfrac{20 \text{ mm Hg}}{\text{L/min}}$

$Q_r = \dfrac{\bar{P}_a}{R} = \dfrac{200}{20} = 10$

C, The disparity between Q_h and Q_r progressively increases arterial blood volume. The volume continues to increase until $\bar{P}_a$ reaches a level of 200 mm Hg.

E Steady-state increase in peripheral resistance

$\bar{P}_a$ = 200

Q_h = 5 L/min

Q_r = 5 L/min

$R = \dfrac{40 \text{ mm Hg}}{\text{L/min}}$

$Q_r = \dfrac{\bar{P}_a}{R} = \dfrac{200}{40} = 5$

E, The excess of Q_h over Q_r accumulates blood in the arteries. Blood continues to accumulate until $\bar{P}_a$ rises to a level of 200 mm Hg.

FIGURE 7-9 ▮ The relationship of mean arterial blood pressure ($\bar{P}_a$) to cardiac output (Q_h), peripheral runoff (Q_r), and peripheral resistance (R) under control conditions (**A**), in response to an increase in cardiac output (**B** and **C**), and in response to an increase in peripheral resistance (**D** and **E**).

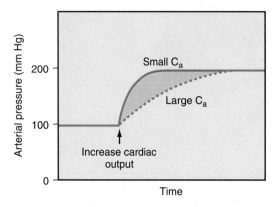

FIGURE 7-10 ■ When cardiac output is suddenly increased, the arterial compliance (C_a) determines the rate at which the mean arterial pressure will attain its new, elevated value but will not determine the magnitude of the new pressure.

Pulse Pressure

Let us assume (see Figure 7-8) that the arterial pressure, P_a, at any moment depends on the two physical factors, namely (1) the arterial blood volume, V_a, and (2) the arterial compliance, C_a. Hence, the arterial **pulse pressure** (that is, the difference between systolic and diastolic pressures) is principally a function of the **stroke volume** and the **arterial compliance.**

Stroke Volume

The effect of a change in stroke volume on pulse pressure may be analyzed when C_a remains virtually constant. C_a is constant over any linear region of the pressure-volume curve (see Figure 7-11). Volume is plotted along the vertical axis, and pressure is plotted along the horizontal axis; the slope, dV/dP, equals the compliance, C_a.

In an individual with such a linear $P_a:V_a$ curve, the arterial pressure would oscillate about a mean value ($\overline{P}_a$ in Figure 7-11). This value depends entirely on cardiac output and peripheral resistance, as explained above. The mean pressure reflects a specific mean arterial blood volume, $\overline{V}_a$. The coordinates, $\overline{P}_a$ and $\overline{V}_a$, define point A on the graph. During diastole, peripheral runoff from the arterial system occurs in the absence of the ventricular ejection of blood. Furthermore, P_a and V_a diminish to the minimal values, P_1 and V_1, just before the next ventricular ejection. P_1 defines the diastolic pressure.

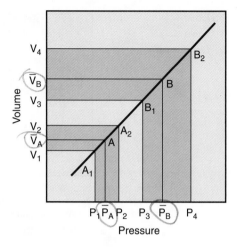

FIGURE 7-11 ■ Effect of a change in stroke volume on pulse pressure in a system in which arterial compliance is constant over the range of pressures and volumes involved. A larger volume increment ($V_4 - V_3$ as compared with $V_2 - V_1$) results in a greater mean pressure ($\overline{P}_B$ as compared with ($\overline{P}_A$) and a greater pulse pressure ($P_4 - P_3$ as compared with $P_2 - P_1$).

During the rapid ejection phase of systole, the volume of blood introduced into the arterial system exceeds the volume that exits through the arterioles. Arterial pressure and volume therefore rise from point A_1 toward point A_2 in Figure 7-11. The maximal arterial volume, V_2, is reached at the end of the rapid ejection phase (see Figure 4-13); this volume corresponds to the peak pressure, P_2, which is the **systolic pressure.**

The pulse pressure is the difference between the systolic and diastolic pressures ($P_2 - P_1$ in Figure 7-11), and it corresponds to some arterial volume increment, $V_2 - V_1$. *This increment equals the volume of blood discharged by the left ventricle during the rapid ejection phase, minus the volume that has run off to the periphery during this same phase of the cardiac cycle.* When a healthy heart beats at a normal frequency, the volume increment during the rapid ejection phase is a large fraction (about 80%) of the stroke volume. It is this increment that raises the arterial volume rapidly from V_1 to V_2. Consequently, the arterial pressure will rise from the diastolic to the systolic level (P_1 to P_2 in Figure 7-11). During the remainder of the cardiac cycle, peripheral runoff will exceed cardiac ejection. During diastole, the heart ejects no blood. Consequently, the arterial blood volume decrement will cause volumes and pressures to fall from point A_2 back to point A_1 in Figure 7-11.

If stroke volume is suddenly doubled while heart rate and peripheral resistance remain constant, the mean arterial pressure will be doubled, to point B, in Figure 7-11. Thus the arterial pressure will now oscillate with each heartbeat about this new value of the mean arterial pressure. A normal, vigorous heart will eject this greater stroke volume during a fraction of the cardiac cycle. This fraction approximately equals the fraction that prevailed at the lower stroke volume. Therefore the arterial volume increment, $V_4 - V_3$, will be a large fraction of the new stroke volume. Hence, the increment will be about *twice as great* as the previous volume increment $(V_2 - V_1)$. If the P_a:V_a curve were linear, the greater volume increment would be reflected by a pulse pressure $(P_4 - P_3)$ that was approximately twice as great as the original pulse pressure $(P_2 - P_1)$. Inspection of Figure 7-11 reveals that when both mean and pulse pressures rise, the increment in systolic pressure (from P_2 to P_4) exceeds the rise in diastolic pressure (from P_1 to P_3). Thus an increase in stroke volume raises systolic pressure more than it raises diastolic pressure.

CLINICAL BOX

The arterial pulse pressure affords valuable clues about a person's stroke volume, provided that the arterial compliance is essentially normal. Patients who have severe **congestive heart failure**, or who have had a **severe hemorrhage**, are likely to have very small arterial pulse pressures, because their stroke volumes are abnormally small. Conversely, individuals with large stroke volumes, as in **aortic regurgitation**, are likely to have increased arterial pulse pressures. For example, **well-trained athletes** at rest tend to have low heart rates. The prolonged ventricular filling times in these subjects induce the ventricles to pump a large quantity of blood per heartbeat, and thus their pulse pressures are large.

Arterial Compliance

To assess how arterial compliance affects pulse pressure, the relative effects of a given volume increment

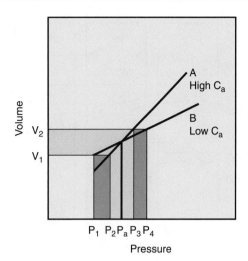

FIGURE 7-12 ■ For a given volume increment ($V_2 - V_1$), a reduced arterial compliance (curve B as compared with curve A) results in an increased pulse pressure ($P_4 - P_1$ as compared with $P_3 - P_2$).

($V_2 - V_1$ in Figure 7-12) in a young person (curve A) and in an elderly person (curve B) are compared. Let cardiac output and TPR be the same in both people; therefore $\overline{P}_a$ will be the same in both subjects. Figure 7-12 shows that the same volume increment ($V_2 - V_1$) will cause a greater pulse pressure ($P_4 - P_1$) in the less distensible arteries of the elderly individual than in the more compliant arteries of the young person ($P_3 - P_2$). Hence, the workload on the left ventricle of the elderly person would exceed that on the workload of the young person, even if the stroke volumes, TPR values, and mean arterial pressures were equivalent.

Figure 7-13 displays the effects of changes in arterial compliance and in peripheral resistance, R_p, on the arterial pressure in an isolated cat heart preparation. As the compliance was reduced from 43 to 14 to 3.6 units, the pulse pressure increased significantly. Changes of pulse pressure are greater when compliance changes at constant R_p than when R_p changes at constant compliance. In this preparation, the stroke volume decreased as the arterial compliance was diminished. This relationship accounts for the failure of the mean arterial pressure to remain constant at the different levels of arterial compliance. The effects of changes in peripheral resistance

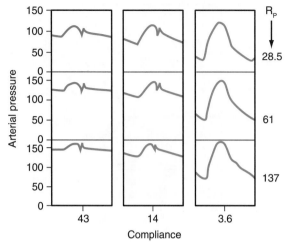

FIGURE 7-13 ▦ The changes in aortic pressure induced by changes in arterial compliance and peripheral resistance (R_p) in an isolated cat heart preparation. Note that at a constant R_p of 28.5 units, reducing compliance from 43 to 3.6 units increases systolic and decreases diastolic pressures, resulting in a widened pulse pressure. When compliance is kept constant at 14 units, increasing R_p from 28.5 to 137 units increases systolic and diastolic pressures. *(Modified from Elzinga G, Westerhof N: Pressure and flow generated by the left ventricle against different impedances.* Circ Res *32:178, 1973.)*

in this same preparation are described in the next section.

Total Peripheral Resistance and Arterial Diastolic Pressure

It is often claimed that an increase in TPR affects the diastolic arterial pressure more than it does the systolic arterial pressure. The validity of such an assertion deserves close scrutiny. First, let TPR be increased in an individual with a linear P_a:V_a curve, as depicted in Figure 7-14A. If the subject's heart rate and stroke volume remain constant, an increase in TPR will increase the $\overline{P}_a$ proportionately (from P_2 to P_5). If the volume increments ($V_2 - V_1$ and $V_4 - V_3$) are equal at both levels of TPR, the pulse pressures ($P_3 - P_1$ and $P_6 - P_4$) will also be equal. Hence systolic (P_6) and diastolic (P_4) pressures will have been elevated by exactly the same amounts from their respective control levels (P_3 and P_1).

The combination of an increased resistance and diminished arterial compliance on arterial blood pressure are represented in Figure 7-13 by a shift in direction from the top leftmost panel to the bottom rightmost panel. Both the mean pressure and the pulse pressure would be increased significantly. These results also coincide with the changes predicted by $\overline{P}_a$.

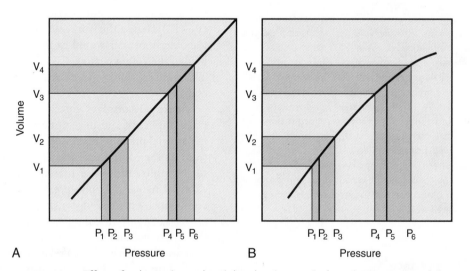

FIGURE 7-14 ▦ Effect of a change in total peripheral resistance (volume increment remaining constant) on pulse pressure when the pressure-volume curve for the arterial system is rectilinear (**A**) or curvilinear (**B**).

CLINICAL BOX

Chronic **hypertension** is characterized by a persistent elevation of TPR. It occurs more commonly in older than in younger persons. The $P_a:V_a$ curve for a hypertensive patient would therefore resemble that shown in Figure 7-14B. In this figure, the slope of the $P_a:V_a$ curve diminishes as pressure and volume are increased. Hence, C_a is less at higher than at lower pressures. If cardiac output remains constant, an increase in TPR would increase P_a proportionally (from P_2 to P_5). For equivalent increases in TPR, the pressure elevation from P_2 to P_5 would be the same in panel A as in panel B (see Figure 7-10). If the volume increment ($V_4 - V_3$ in Figure 7-14B) at elevated TPR were equal to the control increment ($V_2 - V_1$), the pulse pressure ($P_6 - P_4$) in the hypertension range would greatly exceed that ($P_3 - P_1$) at normal pressure levels. In other words, a given volume increment produces a greater pressure increment (i.e., pulse pressure) when the arteries are more rigid than when they are more compliant. Hence the rise in systolic pressure ($P_6 - P_3$) will exceed the increase in diastolic pressure ($P_4 - P_1$). These hypothetical changes in arterial pressure closely resemble those actually observed in **hypertensive** patients. Diastolic pressure is indeed elevated in such persons, but usually not more than 10 to 40 mm Hg above the average normal level (about 80 mm Hg). Conversely, systolic pressures are often found to be elevated by 50 to 150 mm Hg above the average normal level (about 120 mm Hg). *Thus, an increase in peripheral resistance will usually raise systolic pressure more than it will raise the diastolic pressure.*

THE PRESSURE CURVES CHANGE IN ARTERIES AT DIFFERENT DISTANCES FROM THE HEART

The radial stretch of the ascending aorta brought about by left ventricular ejection initiates a pressure wave that is propagated down the aorta and its branches. *The pressure wave travels much faster (~4-12 m/s) than does the blood itself.* It is this pressure wave that one perceives by palpating a peripheral artery (for example, in the wrist).

The velocity of the pressure wave varies inversely with the vascular compliance. Accurate measurement of the transmission velocity has provided valuable information about the elastic characteristics of the arterial

tree. In general, transmission velocity increases with age. This finding confirms the observation that the arteries become less compliant with advancing age (see Figures 7-4 and 7-6). Furthermore, the pulse wave velocity increases progressively as the pulse wave travels from the ascending aorta toward the periphery. This indicates that vascular compliance is less in the more distal than in the more proximal portions of the arterial system. In addition, there is greater overlap between the forward and reflected pulse waves because of the increasing resistance of the vessels as their diameter decreases.

The arterial pressure contour becomes distorted as the wave is transmitted down the arterial system. The changes in configuration of the pulse with distance are shown in Figure 7-15. Aside from the lengthening delay in the onset of the initial pressure rise, three major changes occur in the arterial pulse contour as the pressure wave travels distally. First, the high-frequency components of the pulse, such as the **incisura** (the notch that appears at the end of ventricular ejection), are damped out and soon disappear. Second, the systolic portions of the pressure wave become narrow and elevated. In Figure 7-15, the systolic pressure at the level of the knee was 39 mm Hg greater than that recorded in the aortic arch. Third, a hump may appear on the diastolic portion of the pressure wave. These changes in contour are pronounced in young individuals, but they diminish with age. In elderly patients, the pulse wave may be transmitted virtually unchanged from the ascending aorta to the periphery.

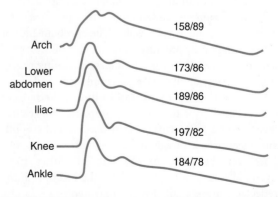

FIGURE 7-15 ▦ Arterial pressure (mm Hg) curves recorded from various sites in an anesthetized dog. *(From Remington JW, O'Brien LJ: Construction of aortic flow pulse from pressure pulse. Am J Physiol 218:437, 1970.)*

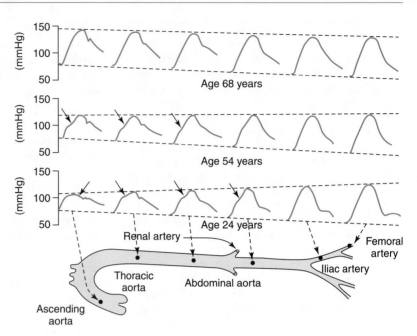

FIGURE 7-16 ■ Pulse pressures recorded from different sites in the arterial trees of humans at different ages. *(Reproduced by permission of Hodder Education from Nichols WW, O'Rourke M, editors: McDonald's blood flow in arteries: theoretical, experimental and clinical principles, ed 5, London, 2005, Arnold.)*

An illustration of all these features as recorded in the human arterial tree is shown in Figure 7-16. In the 24-year-old subject, the arterial pulse propagates slowly and displays changes in the pulse pressure amplitude and contour, as seen in the canine model in Figure 7-15. By contrast, the pulse pressure wave in the 68-year-old subject travels more rapidly than in the younger subject. Also, the pulse pressure wave is relatively unchanged as the pulse travels because there is less wave reflection.

The damping of the high-frequency components of the arterial pulse is caused largely by the viscoelastic properties of the arterial walls. The mechanisms for the peaking of the pressure wave are complex. Several factors contribute to these changes, including reflection, tapering of the arteries, resonance, and pulse wave velocity. The **augmentation index**, the ratio of the reflected wave to the pulse pressure, is a relative measure of arterial stiffness. Thus, as arterial compliance decreases with age, the reflected wave superimposes on the pulse pressure at an earlier time. Eventually, as seen in Figure 7-16, the location of the reflected wave is evident as an increased central pulse pressure in the 68 year-old subject rather than as an inflection detected at various times during the pulse pressure recording in the 24 year- old subject.

BLOOD PRESSURE IS MEASURED BY A SPHYGMOMANOMETER IN HUMAN PATIENTS

In hospital intensive care units, arterial blood pressure can be measured **directly** by introducing a needle or catheter into a peripheral artery. Ordinarily, however, the blood pressure is estimated **indirectly,** by means of a **sphygmomanometer.** This instrument consists of an inextensible cuff that contains an inflatable bag. The

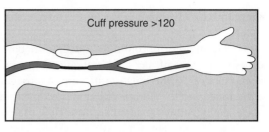

B, When the cuff pressure exceeds the systolic arterial pressure (120 mm Hg), no blood progresses through the arterial segment under the cuff, and no sounds can be detected by a stethoscope bell placed on the arm distal to the cuff.

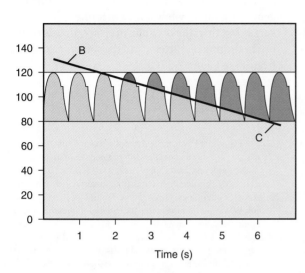

A, Consider that the arterial blood pressure is being measured in a patient whose blood pressure is 120/80 mm Hg. The pressure (represented by the *oblique line*) in a cuff around the patient's arm is allowed to fall from greater than 120 mm Hg (point *B*) to below 80 mm Hg (point *C*) in about 6 seconds.

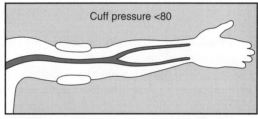

C, When the cuff pressure falls below the diastolic arterial pressure, arterial flow past the region of the cuff is continuous, and no sounds are audible. When the cuff pressure is between 120 and 80 mm Hg, spurts of blood traverse the artery segment under the cuff with each heartbeat, and the Korotkoff sounds are heard through the stethoscope.

FIGURE 7-17 ■ **A** to **C**, Measurement of arterial blood pressure with a sphygmomanometer.

cuff is wrapped around an extremity, usually the arm, so that the inflatable bag lies between the cuff and the skin, directly over the artery to be compressed. The artery is occluded by inflating the bag, by means of a rubber squeeze bulb, to a pressure in excess of the arterial systolic pressure. The pressure in the bag is measured by means of a mercury, or an aneroid, manometer. Pressure is released from the bag, at a rate of 2 or 3 mm Hg per heartbeat, by means of a needle valve in the inflating bulb (see Figure 7-17).

When blood pressure is determined from an arm, the systolic pressure may be estimated by palpating the radial artery at the wrist (**palpatory method**). When pressure in the bag exceeds the systolic level, no pulse is perceived. As the pressure falls just below the systolic level (see Figure 7-17A), a spurt of blood passes through the brachial artery under the cuff during the peak of systole, and a slight pulse is felt at the wrist.

The **auscultatory method** is a more sensitive, and therefore a more precise, method for measuring **systolic pressure**; it also permits estimation of the **diastolic pressure**. The practitioner listens with a stethoscope applied to the skin of the antecubital space, over the **brachial artery**. While the pressure in the bag exceeds the systolic pressure, the brachial artery is occluded, and no sounds are heard (see Figure 7-17B). When the inflation pressure falls just below the systolic level (120 mm Hg in Figure 7-17A), small spurts of blood escape through the cuff and slight tapping sounds (called **Korotkoff sounds**) are heard with each heartbeat. The pressure at which the first sound is detected represents the **systolic pressure.** It usually corresponds closely with the directly measured systolic pressure.

As inflation pressure continues to fall, more blood escapes under the cuff per heartbeat, and the sounds become louder. As the inflation pressure approaches the diastolic level, the Korotkoff sounds become muffled. As the inflation pressure falls just below the diastolic level (80 mm Hg in Figure 7-17A), the sounds disappear; this point identifies the **diastolic pressure.** The origin of the Korotkoff sounds is related to the spurts of blood that pass under the cuff and that meet a static column of blood; the impact and turbulence generate audible vibrations. Once the inflation pressure is less than the diastolic pressure, flow is continuous in the brachial artery, and the sounds are no longer heard (see Figure 7-17C).

SUMMARY

- The arteries not only serve to conduct blood from the heart to the capillaries but also store some of the ejected blood during each cardiac systole. Therefore blood can continue to flow through the capillaries during cardiac diastole.
- The compliance of the arteries diminishes with age.
- The less compliant the arteries, the more work the heart must do to pump a given cardiac output.
- The mean arterial pressure varies directly with the cardiac output and total peripheral resistance.
- The arterial pulse pressure varies directly with the stroke volume, but inversely with the arterial compliance.
- The contour of the systemic arterial pressure wave is distorted as it travels from the ascending aorta to the periphery. The high-frequency components of the wave are damped, the systolic components are narrowed and elevated, and a hump may appear in the diastolic component of the wave.
- When blood pressure is measured by a sphygmomanometer in humans, systolic pressure is manifested by the occurrence of a tapping sound that originates in the artery distal to the cuff as the cuff pressure falls below peak arterial pressure. The diminished cuff pressure permits spurts of blood to pass through the compressed artery. Diastolic pressure is manifested by the disappearance of the sound as the cuff pressure falls below the minimal arterial pressure, permitting flow through the artery to become continuous.

ADDITIONAL READING

Espinola-Klein, Rupprecht Hans J, Bickel C, et al: Different calculations of ankle-brachial index and their impact on cardiovascular risk prediction, *Circ* 118:961, 2008.

Folkow B, Svanborg A: Physiology of cardiovascular aging, *Physiol Rev* 73:725, 1993.

Lakatta EG, Wang J, Najjar SS: Arterial aging and subclinical arterial disease are fundamentally intertwined at macroscopic and molecular levels, *Med Clin N Amer* 93:583, 2009.

London GM, Pannier B: Arterial functions: how to interpret the complex physiology, *Nephrol Dial Transplant* 25:3815, 2010.

Nichols WW: Clinical measurement of arterial stiffness obtained from noninvasive pressure waveforms, *Am J Hypertens* 18:3S, 2005.

Nichols WW, Edwards DG: Arterial elastance and wave reflection augmentation of systolic blood pressure: deleterious effects and implications for therapy, *J Cardiovasc Pharmacol Ther* 6:5, 2001.

O'Rourke M: Mechanical principles in arterial disease, *Hypertension* 26:2, 1995.

Perloff D, Grim C, Flack J, et al: Human blood pressure determination by sphygmomanometry, *Circ* 88:2460, 1993.

Stergiopulos N, Meister JJ, Westerhof N: Evaluation of methods for estimation of total arterial compliance, *Am J Physiol* 268:H1540, 1995.

Wagenseil JE, Mecham RP: Vascular extracellular matrix and arterial mechanics, *Physiol Rev* 89:957, 2009.

CASE 7-1

HISTORY

A 33-year-old man complained about chest pain on exertion. He was referred to a cardiologist, who carried out a number of studies, including right- and left-sided cardiac catheterization (for hemodynamic information) and coronary angiography (to image the status of the coronary arteries). Among the data that were obtained during these studies were the findings that the patient's pulmonary artery and aortic pressures, in mm Hg, were as follows:

Pressures	Pulmonary Artery	Aorta
Systolic	30	120
Diastolic	15	80
Pulse	15	40
Mean	20	93

The hemodynamic and angiographic studies disclosed no serious abnormalities. The patient's physicians recommended certain changes in lifestyle and diet, and the patient continued to do well for about 20 years. At this time, the physician found that the patient's systemic arterial blood pressure was 190 mm Hg systolic/100 mm Hg diastolic, and the mean arterial pressure was estimated to be 130 mm Hg. These and other findings led his physicians to the diagnosis of essential hypertension.

QUESTIONS

1. At the time of the initial examination, the patient's mean aortic pressure (93 mm Hg) was so much higher than the mean pulmonary arterial pressure (20 mm Hg) because:

   a. the systemic vascular resistance was much greater than the pulmonary vascular resistance.

   b. the aortic compliance was much greater than the pulmonary arterial compliance.

   c. the left ventricular stroke volume was much greater than the right ventricular stroke volume.

   d. the total cross-sectional area of the pulmonary capillary bed was much greater than the total cross-sectional area of the systemic capillary bed.

   e. the duration of the rapid ejection phase of the left ventricle exceeded the duration of the rapid ejection phase of the right ventricle.

2. When the patient became hypertensive, his arterial pulse pressure (90 mm Hg) became much greater than his pre-hypertension pulse pressure (40 mm Hg) because:

   a. the systemic vascular resistance is much less than it was before he became hypertensive.

   b. the duration of the reduced ejection phase of the left ventricle decreases as the arterial blood pressure rises.

   c. the arterial compliance was diminished in part by virtue of the hypertension per se, and in part because of the effects of aging.

   d. the total cross-sectional area of the systemic capillary bed increases substantially in hypertensive subjects.

   e. the aortic compliance becomes greater than the pulmonary arterial compliance.

8

THE MICROCIRCULATION AND LYMPHATICS

OBJECTIVES

1. Describe the regulation of regional blood flow by the arterioles.

2. Enumerate the physical and chemical factors that affect the microvessels.

3. Explain the roles of diffusion, filtration, and pinocytosis in transcapillary exchange.

4. Describe the balance between hydrostatic and osmotic forces under normal and abnormal conditions.

5. Describe the lymphatic circulation.

The entire circulatory system is geared to supply the body tissues with blood in amounts that are commensurate with their requirements for O_2 and nutrients. The system also operates to remove CO_2 and other waste products for excretion by the lungs and kidneys. The exchange of gases, water, and solutes between the vascular and interstitial fluid (ISF) compartments occurs mainly across the capillaries. These vessels consist of a single layer of endothelial cells. The arterioles, capillaries, and venules constitute the microcirculation, and blood flow through the microcirculation is regulated by the arterioles, which are also known as the **resistance vessels** (see Chapter 9). The large arteries serve solely as blood conduits, whereas the veins serve as storage or **capacitance vessels** as well as blood conduits.

FUNCTIONAL ANATOMY

Arterioles are the Stopcocks of the Circulation

The arterioles, which range in diameter from about 5 to 100 µm, have a thick smooth muscle layer, a thin adventitial layer, and an endothelial lining (see Figure 1-2). The arterioles give rise directly to the capillaries (5 to 10 µm in diameter) or in some tissues to metarterioles (10 to 20 µm in diameter), which then give rise to capillaries (Figure 8-1). The **metarterioles** can serve either as thoroughfare channels to the venules, which bypass the capillary bed, or as conduits to supply the capillary bed. There are often cross-connections between the arterioles and venules as well as in the capillary network. Arterioles that give rise directly to capillaries regulate flow through their cognate

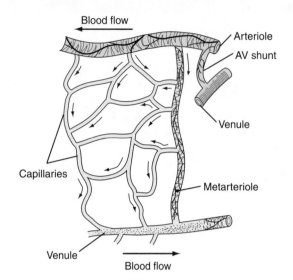

FIGURE 8-1 ■ Composite schematic drawing of the microcirculation. The *circular structures* on the arteriole and venule represent smooth muscle fibers, and the *branching solid lines* represent sympathetic nerve fibers. The *arrows* indicate the direction of blood flow.

capillaries by constriction or dilation. The capillaries form an interconnecting network of tubes of different lengths, with an average length of 0.5 to 1 mm.

Capillaries Permit the Exchange of Water, Solutes, and Gases

Capillary distribution varies from tissue to tissue. In metabolically active tissues, such as cardiac and skeletal muscle and glandular structures, capillaries are numerous. In less active tissues, such as subcutaneous tissue or cartilage, **capillary density** is low. Also, all capillaries do not have the same diameter. It is necessary for the cells to become temporarily deformed in their passage through these capillaries, because some capillaries have diameters less than those of the erythrocytes. Fortunately, normal red blood cells are quite flexible, and they readily change their shape to conform to that of the small capillaries.

Blood flow in the capillaries is not uniform; it depends chiefly on the contractile state of the arterioles. The average velocity of blood flow in the capillaries is approximately 1 mm per second; however, it can vary from zero to several millimeters per second in the same vessel within a brief period. Such changes in capillary

blood flow may be random or they may show rhythmical oscillatory behavior of different frequencies. This behavior is caused by contraction and relaxation (**vasomotion**) of the precapillary vessels. The vasomotion is partially an intrinsic contractile behavior of the vascular smooth muscle, and it is independent of external input. Furthermore, changes in **transmural pressure** (**intravascular minus extravascular pressure**) influence the contractile state of the precapillary vessels. An increase in transmural pressure, whether produced by an increase in venous pressure or by dilation of arterioles, results in contraction of the terminal arterioles at the points of origin of the capillaries. Conversely, a decrease in transmural pressure elicits precapillary vessel relaxation (see **myogenic response,** Chapter 9).

Reduction of transmural pressure relaxes the terminal arterioles. However, **blood flow** through the capillaries cannot increase if the reduction in intravascular pressure is caused by severe constriction of the parent vasculature. Large arterioles and metarterioles also exhibit vasomotion. However, in the contraction phase, they usually do not completely occlude the lumen of the vessel and arrest blood flow as may occur when the terminal arterioles contract (Figure 8-2). *Thus, flow rate may be altered by contraction and relaxation of small arteries, arterioles, and metarterioles.*

Because blood flow through the capillaries provides for exchange of gases and solutes between the blood and tissues, the flow has been termed **nutritional flow.** Conversely, blood flow that bypasses the capillaries in traveling from the arterial to the venous side of the circulation has been termed nonnutritional, or shunt, flow (see Figure 8-1). In some areas of the body (e.g., fingertips and ears), true arteriovenous shunts exist (see Figure 12-1). However, in many tissues, such as muscle, evidence of anatomic shunts is lacking. Nevertheless, nonnutritional flow can occur, and the behavior has been termed **physiological shunting of blood flow.** This shunting is the result of a greater flow of blood through previously open capillaries, along with either no change or an increase in the number of closed capillaries. In tissues that have metarterioles, shunt flow may be continuous from the arterioles to the venules during low metabolic activity, at which time many precapillary vessels are closed. When metabolic activity rises in such tissues and more precapillary vessels open, blood

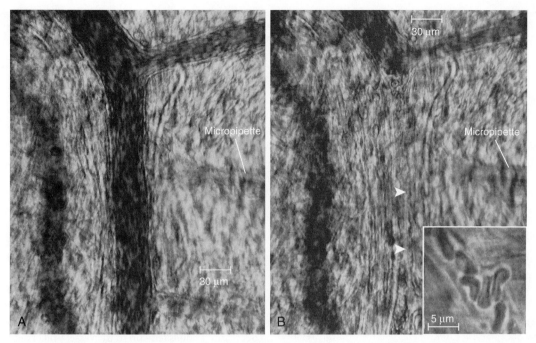

FIGURE 8-2 ■ Arterioles of a hamster cheek pouch before (**A**) and after (**B**) injection of norepinephrine. Note the complete closure of the arteriole between the *arrowheads* and the narrowing of a branch arteriole at the *upper right*. *Inset,* Capillary with red blood cells during a period of complete closure of the feeding arteriole. Scale in **A** and **B,** 30 μm; in *inset,* 5 μm. *(Courtesy David N. Damon.)*

passing through the metarterioles is readily available for capillary perfusion.

The true capillaries are devoid of smooth muscle and are therefore incapable of active constriction. Nevertheless, the endothelial cells that form the capillary wall contain actin and myosin, and they can alter shape in response to certain chemical stimuli. There is no evidence, however, that changes in endothelial cell shape regulate blood flow through the capillaries. *Hence, changes in capillary diameter are passive and are caused by alterations in precapillary and postcapillary resistance.*

The Law of Laplace Explains How Capillaries Can Withstand High Intravascular Pressures

The law of Laplace is illustrated in the following comparison of wall tension in a capillary with that in the aorta (Table 8-1). The Laplace equation is:

$$T = \Delta Pr \tag{1}$$

where T is tension in the vessel wall, ΔP is transmural pressure difference (internal minus external), and r is radius of the vessel.

Wall tension is the force per unit length tangential to the vessel wall. This tension opposes the distending force (ΔPr) that tends to pull apart a theoretical longitudinal slit in the vessel (Figure 8-3). Transmural pressure is essentially equal to intraluminal pressure, because extravascular pressure is usually negligible. The Laplace equation applies to very thin-walled vessels, such as capillaries. Wall thickness must be taken into consideration when the equation is applied to thick-walled vessels such as the aorta. This is done by dividing ΔPr (pressure × radius) by wall thickness (w). The equation now becomes:

$$\sigma \text{ (wall stress)} = \Delta Pr / w \tag{2}$$

Pressure in mm Hg (height of an Hg column) is converted to dynes per square centimeter, according to the following equation:

$$P = h\rho g \tag{3}$$

	TABLE 8-1	
	Vessel Wall Tension in the Aorta and a Capillary	
	AORTA	*CAPILLARY*
r (radius)	1.5 cm	5×10^{-4} cm
h (height of Hg column)	10 cm Hg	2.5 cm Hg
ρ (density of Hg)	13.6 g/cm³	13.6 g/cm³
g (gravitational acceleration)	980 cm/s²	980 cm/s²
P (pressure)	$10 \times 13.6 \times 980 = 1.33 \times 10^5$ dyne/cm²	$2.5 \times 13.6 \times 980 = 3.33 \times 10^4$ dyne/cm²
w (wall thickness)	0.2 cm	1×10^{-4} cm
T = Pr	$(1.33 \times 10^5)\,(1.5) = 2 \times 10^5$ dyne/cm	$(3.33 \times 10^4)\,(5 \times 10^{-4}) = 16.7$ dyne/cm
σ (wall stress) = Pr/w	$2 \times 10^5/0.2 = 1 \times 10^6$ dyne/cm²	$16.7/1 \times 10^{-4} = 1.67 \times 10^5$ dyne/cm²

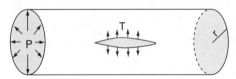

FIGURE 8-3 ■ Diagram of a small blood vessel to illustrate the law of Laplace. T = ΔPr, where ΔP is transmural pressure difference, r is radius of the vessel, and T is wall tension as the force per unit length tangential to the vessel wall, tending to pull apart a theoretical longitudinal slit in the vessel.

where *h* is the height of an Hg column in centimeters, ρ is the density of Hg in g/cm³, *g* is gravitational acceleration in cm/s²; and (σ)wall stress is force per unit area.

Thus, at normal aortic and capillary pressures, the wall tension of the aorta is about 12,000 times greater than that of the capillary (see Table 8-1). In a person who is standing quietly, capillary pressure in the feet may reach 100 mm Hg. Under such conditions, capillary wall tension increases to 66.5 dynes/cm, a value that is still only one three-thousandths that of the wall tension in the aorta at the same internal pressure. However, σ (wall stress), which takes wall thickness into consideration, is only about tenfold greater in the aorta than in the capillary.

In addition to explaining the ability of capillaries to withstand large internal pressures, the preceding calculations also show that in dilated vessels, wall stress increases even when internal pressure remains constant.

The diameter of the resistance vessels is determined by the balance between the contractile force of the vascular smooth muscle and the distending force produced by the intraluminal pressure. The greater the contractile activity of the vascular smooth muscle of an arteriole, the smaller is its diameter, until the small arterioles are completely occluded. This occlusion is caused by infolding of the endothelium and the consequent trapping of the cells in the vessel. With progressive reduction in the intravascular pressure, vessel diameter decreases, as does tension in the vessel wall. This constitutes the **law of Laplace**.

THE ENDOTHELIUM PLAYS AN ACTIVE ROLE IN REGULATING THE MICROCIRCULATION

For many years, the endothelium was considered to be an inert, single layer of cells that served solely as a passive filter that (1) permitted water and small molecules to pass across the blood vessel wall and (2) retained blood cells and large molecules (proteins) within the vascular compartment. However, the endothelium is now recognized as a source of substances that elicit contraction and relaxation of the vascular smooth muscle (see Figures 8-4 and 9-4).

As shown in Figure 8-4, prostacyclin (prostaglandin I₂, PGI₂) can relax vascular smooth muscle via an increase in the cyclic adenosine monophosphate (cAMP) concentration. Prostacyclin is formed in the endothelium from arachidonic acid, and it may be released by the shear stress caused by the pulsatile blood flow. Prostacyclin formation is catalyzed by the enzyme prostacyclin synthase. The primary function of PGI₂ is to inhibit platelet adherence to the endothelium and platelet aggregation, thus preventing intravascular clot formation.

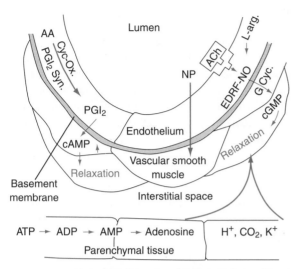

FIGURE 8-4 ■ Endothelially and nonendothelially mediated vasodilation. Prostacyclin (PGI$_2$) is formed from arachidonic acid (AA) by the action of cyclooxygenase (Cyc-Ox.) and prostacyclin synthase (PGI$_2$ Syn.) in the endothelium and elicits relaxation of the adjacent vascular smooth muscle via increases in cyclic adenosine monophosphate (cAMP). Stimulation of the endothelial cells with acetylcholine (ACh) or other agents (see text) results in the formation and release of an endothelium-derived relaxing factor (EDRF) identified as nitric oxide (NO). The NO stimulates guanylyl cyclase (G Cyc.) to increase cyclic guanosine monophosphate (cGMP) in the vascular smooth muscle to cause relaxation. The vasodilator agent nitroprusside (NP) acts directly on the vascular smooth muscle. Substances such as adenosine, hydrogen ions (H$^+$), CO$_2$, and potassium ions (K$^+$) can arise in the parenchymal tissue and elicit vasodilation by direct action on the vascular smooth muscle (see p. 182). ADP, adenosine diphosphate; L-arg., L-arginine.

Of far greater importance in endothelially mediated vascular dilation is the formation and release of the **endothelium-derived relaxing factor** (**EDRF**) (see Figure 8-4), which has been identified as **nitric oxide** (**NO**). Stimulation of the endothelial cells in vivo, in isolated arteries, or in culture by acetylcholine or several other agents (such as adenosine triphosphate [ATP], adenosine diphosphate [ADP], bradykinin, serotonin, substance P, and histamine) produce and release NO. In blood vessels whose endothelium has been removed, these agents do not elicit vasodilation; some, including acetylcholine and ATP, can cause constriction. The NO (synthesized from L-arginine) activates guanylyl cyclase in the vascular smooth muscle. This process raises the cyclic guanosine monophosphate (cGMP) concentration and increases the activity of cGMP-dependent protein kinase (PKG), which in turn activates myosin light-chain phosphatase (MLCP). Myosin light-chain phosphatase induces relaxation by reducing the concentration of phosphorylated myosin regulatory light-chain subunits (MLC$_{20}$) in vascular smooth muscle (see Figure 9-2). NO release can be stimulated by the shear stress of blood flow on the endothelium, but the physiological role of NO in the local regulation of blood flow remains to be elucidated. The drug nitroprusside also increases cGMP, causing vasodilation. Nitroprusside acts directly on the vascular smooth muscle; its action is not endothelially mediated (see Figure 8-4). Vasodilator agents, such as adenosine, H$^+$, CO$_2$, and K$^+$, may be released from parenchymal tissue and act locally on the resistance vessels (see Figure 8-4).

The endothelium can also synthesize **endothelin,** a very potent vasoconstrictor peptide (see Figure 9-4A). Endothelin can affect vascular tone and blood pressure in humans, and it may be involved in such pathological states as atherosclerosis, pulmonary hypertension, congestive heart failure, and renal failure.

THE ENDOTHELIUM IS AT THE CENTER OF FLOW-INITIATED MECHANOTRANSDUCTION

Blood vessels are continuously subjected to cyclic changes of blood pressure and flow. Endothelial cells that form the inner lining of blood vessels are linked with the glycocalyx on their luminal surfaces (see Figure 8-7) and with the basement membrane on their abluminal surfaces (Figure 8-5). These interfaces are important signaling sites for transduction of the mechanical force (shear stress) imparted by the blood, into a signal for the regulation of endothelial cell function. The glycocalyx (composed of proteoglycans and glycoproteins) can extend up to 0.5 μm from the surfaces of endothelial cells. The fibrous network of the glycocalyx serves as a filter at the vessel wall in addition to that of endothelial cells. Also, the glycocalyx serves as a mechanotransducer of shear stress signals to the plasma membrane and cortical cytoskeletons of endothelial cells. For example, shear stress causes flow-mediated release of vasodilators including NO and PGI_2 (see Figure 8-4 and Chapter 9). On the one hand, the ability of endothelial cells to release vasodilators is impeded when glycosaminoglycans in the glycocalyx are degraded enzymatically. On the other hand, when flow is laminar, the synthesis of glycocalyx components is increased, becoming a counterforce that sustains the ability of endothelial cells to sense and react to flow patterns.

The basement membrane also functions in mechanotransduction. Normally, the basement membrane underlying endothelial cells is rich in collagen and laminin. Integrins, a family of cell adhesion receptors, are found in the endothelial cell, where they anchor to the cytoskeleton and intracellular signaling molecules. In addition, integrins bind to collagen (α2β1, α1β1) and laminin (α6β1, α6β4) found in the extracellular

matrix of the basement membrane. The result of this binding is an endothelial cell phenotype that is slow to proliferate. Injury, such as that produced by turbulent flow, promotes the deposition of fibronectin and fibrinogen in the extracellular matrix, where they bind integrins (α5β1, αvβ3). Thus, by having fibronectin and fibrinogen present to bind other integrins, the endothelial cell expresses a phenotype that proliferates and migrates. The change of matrix structure and composition can trigger a reaction cascade that changes endothelial cell function to initiate inflammation and, eventually, atherosclerosis. Thus, the balance between atheroprotective and atherogenic forces on the endothelial cell can be changed by a transition from laminar to turbulent flow.

THE ENDOTHELIUM PLAYS A PASSIVE ROLE IN TRANSCAPILLARY EXCHANGE

Solvent and solute move across the capillary endothelial wall by three processes: diffusion, filtration, and **pinocytosis.** The permeability of the capillary endothelial membrane is not the same in all body tissues. For example, liver capillaries are quite permeable, and albumin escapes from them at a rate several times greater than that from the less permeable muscle capillaries. Also, permeability is not uniform along the whole capillary; the venous ends are more permeable

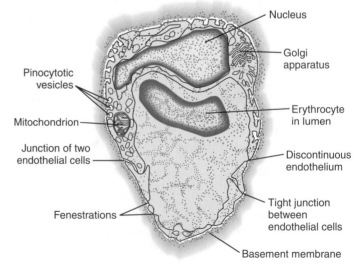

FIGURE 8-5 ■ Diagrammatic sketch of an electron micrograph of a composite capillary in cross-section.

Nucleus

Golgi apparatus

Pinocytotic vesicles

Erythrocyte in lumen

Mitochondrion

Junction of two endothelial cells

Discontinuous endothelium

Fenestrations

Tight junction between endothelial cells

Basement membrane

than the arterial ends, and permeability is greatest in the venules. The greater permeability at the venous ends of the capillaries and in the venules is attributed to the greater number of pores in these regions of the microvessels.

The sites at which filtration occurs have been a controversial subject for many years. Water flows through the capillary endothelial cell membranes through water-selective channels called **aquaporins,** a large family of intrinsic membrane proteins (28 to 30 kDa) that function as water channels. Each of these pore-forming proteins consists of six transmembrane segments that form a monomer; this structure is incorporated into membranes as homotetramers. The aquaporins are permeable to H_2O and other substances (glycerol, urea, Cl^-) having diameters of 3.4Å (0.34 nm) or less. Water also flows through apertures (pores) in the endothelial walls of the capillaries (Figures 8-5 and 8-6). Calculations based on the transcapillary movement of small molecules have led to the prediction of capillary pores with diameters of about 4 nm in skeletal and cardiac muscle. In agreement with this prediction, electron microscopy has revealed clefts between adjacent endothelial cells with gaps of about 4 nm (see Figures 8-5 and 8-6). The clefts (pores) are sparse and represent only about 0.02% of the capillary surface area. In cerebral capillaries, there is a blood-brain barrier to many small molecules.

In addition to clefts, some of the more porous capillaries (e.g., in kidney and intestine) contain **fenestrations** (see Figure 8-5) that are 20 to 100 nm wide, whereas in other sites (e.g., in the liver) **the endothelium is discontinuous** (see Figure 8-5). Fenestrations and discontinuous endothelium permit passage of molecules that are too large to pass through the intercellular clefts of the endothelium.

In pathological states such as with tissue inflammation, the enhanced permeability of the endothelium of the venules may be mainly attributed to transcellular pores that develop within the endothelial cells, and not to opening of the interendothelial cell pores.

Diffusion Is the Most Important Means of Water and Solute Transfer Across the Endothelium

Under normal conditions, only about 0.06 mL of water per minute moves back and forth across the capillary wall per 100 g of tissue. The fluid movement is a result of filtration and absorption. However, about 300 mL of water diffuses per minute per 100 g of tissue. The difference is 5000-fold.

When filtration and diffusion are related to blood flow, about 2% of the plasma passing through the capillaries is filtered. In contrast, the diffusion of water is 40 times greater than the rate at which it is brought to the capillaries by blood flow. The transcapillary exchange of solutes is also governed primarily by diffusion. *Thus, diffusion is the key factor in promoting the exchange of gases, substrates, and waste products between the capillaries and the tissue cells.* However, the *net transfer* of fluid across the capillary and venule endothelium is achieved mainly by filtration and absorption.

The process of diffusion is described by Fick's law, as follows:

$$J = -DA\, dc/dx \qquad (4)$$

where J is the quantity of a substance moved per unit time (t), D is the free diffusion coefficient for a particular molecule (the value is inversely related to the square root of the molecular weight), A is the cross-sectional area of the diffusion pathway, and dc/dx is the concentration gradient of the solute.

Fick's law is also expressed as follows:

$$J = -PS(C_0 - C_i) \qquad (5)$$

where P is the capillary permeability of the substance, S is capillary surface area, C_i is the concentration of the substance inside the capillary, and C_o is the concentration of the substance outside the capillary. Hence the PS product provides a convenient expression of available capillary surface, because permeability is rarely altered under physiologic conditions.

Diffusion of Lipid-Insoluble Molecules Is Restricted to the Pores

The mean pore size can be calculated by measurement of the diffusion rate of an uncharged molecule whose

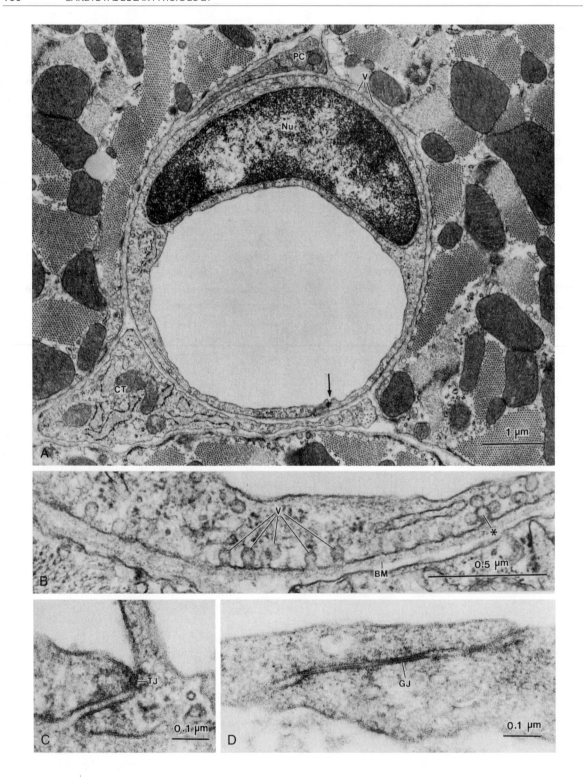

FIGURE 8-6 ■ **A,** Cross-sectioned capillary in a mouse ventricular wall. The luminal diameter is approximately 4 μm. In this thin section, the capillary wall is formed by a single endothelial cell (Nu, endothelial nucleus), which forms a functional complex (*arrow*) with itself. The thin pericapillary space is occupied by a pericyte (PC) and a connective tissue (CT) cell ("fibroblast"). Note the numerous endothelial vesicles (V). **B,** Detail of the endothelial cell in panel **A,** showing plasmalemmal vesicles (V) attached to the endothelial cell surface. These vesicles are especially prominent in vascular endothelium and are involved in transport of substances across the blood vessel wall. Note the complex alveolar vesicle (*). BM, basement membrane. **C,** Junctional complex in a capillary of mouse heart. "Tight" junctions (TJs) typically form in these small blood vessels and appear to consist of fusions between apposed endothelial cell surface membranes. **D,** Interendothelial junction in a muscular artery of monkey papillary muscle. Although tight junctions similar to those in capillaries are found in these large blood vessels, extensive junctions that resemble gap junctions in the intercalated disks between myocardial cells often appear in arterial endothelium (example shown at GJ).

free diffusion coefficient is known. Movement of solutes across the endothelium is complex. The movement involves (1) corrections for attraction between solute and solvent molecules, (2) interactions between solute molecules and pore configuration, and (3) the charge on the molecules relative to the charge on the endothelial cells. Solute movement is not simply a question of random thermal movements of molecules down a concentration gradient.

When the movement of solutes is compared with the movement of water across the intact endothelium, solutes exhibit some degree of restriction based on molecular size. Molecules larger than about 60,000 molecular weight (MW) do not penetrate the endothelium, whereas those smaller than 60,000 MW penetrate at a rate that is inversely proportional to their size. This filtering effect appears to be due to the restrictive size of the pore and to a fiber matrix within it. However, the **glycocalyx,** a 0.5-μm layer lining the luminal side of the endothelium, may also serve as a molecular filter. The glycocalyx is shown in Figure 8-7, where it appears as a clear area between the luminal endothelial membrane and the red blood cell that was moving through the capillary.

For small molecules, such as water, NaCl, urea, and glucose, the capillary pores offer little restriction to diffusion (the **reflection coefficient** is low). Diffusion

Capillary diameter   Red cell width   Endothelial cell surface   Glycocalyx

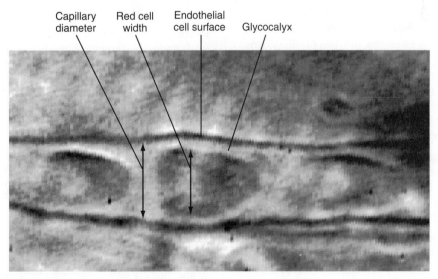

FIGURE 8-7 ■ A single capillary in a hamster cheek pouch showing the glycocalyx. Micrograph was taken during normal blood flow. *(Courtesy of Charmaine Henry.)*

is so rapid that the mean concentration gradient across the capillary endothelium is extremely small (see Figure 8-8). The only limit to the net movement of small molecules across the capillary wall is the rate at which blood flow transports the molecules to the capillaries (**flow limited**).

When transport across the capillary is flow limited, the concentration of a small solute molecule in the blood reaches equilibrium with its concentration in the interstitial fluid (ISF) near the origin of the capillary from the cognate arteriole. If an inert small molecule tracer is infused intra-arterially, its concentration falls to negligible levels near the arterial end of the capillary (Figure 8-8A). If the flow is large, the small molecule tracer will be detectable farther downstream in the capillary. A somewhat larger molecule moves farther along the capillary before it reaches an insignificant concentration in the blood. The number of still larger molecules that enter the arterial end of the capillary and that cannot pass through the capillary pores is the same as the number that leave the venous end of the capillary (Figure 8-8A).

Diffusion of large molecules across the capillaries becomes a limiting factor (**diffusion limited**). In other words, capillary permeability to a large molecule solute limits its transport across the capillary wall (Figure 8-8A). The diffusion of small, insoluble lipid molecules is so rapid that diffusion becomes limiting in blood-tissue exchange, when the distances between the capillaries and parenchymal cells are large (e.g., in the presence of tissue edema, or when capillary density is very low; see Figure 8-8B).

Lipid-Soluble Molecules Pass Directly Through the Lipid Membranes of the Endothelium and the Pores

Lipid-soluble molecules move very rapidly between blood and tissue. The degree of lipid solubility (oil-to-water partition coefficient) provides a good index of the ease of transfer of lipid molecules through the endothelium.

O_2 and CO_2 are both lipid soluble, and they pass readily through the endothelial cells. The O_2 supply of normal tissue at rest and during activity is not limited by diffusion or by the number of open capillaries, as indicated by calculations based on (1) the diffusion coefficient for O_2, (2) the capillary density and

diffusion distances, (3) the blood flow, and (4) the tissue O_2 consumption.

Measurements of Po_2 and the saturation of blood in the microvessels indicate that, in many tissues, O_2 saturation at the entrance of the capillaries has already

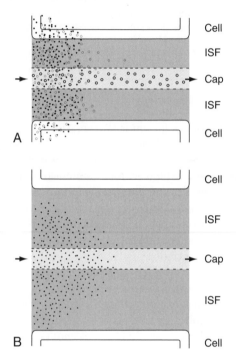

FIGURE 8-8 ■ Flow- and diffusion-limited transport from capillaries (Cap) to tissue. **A,** Flow-limited transport. The smallest water-soluble inert tracer particles (*black dots*) reach negligible concentrations after passing only a short distance down the capillary. Larger particles (*blue circles*) with similar properties travel farther along the capillary before reaching insignificant intracapillary concentrations. Both substances cross the interstitial fluid (ISF) and reach the parenchymal tissue (cell). Because of their size, more of the smaller particles are taken up by the tissue cells. The largest particles (*black circles*) cannot penetrate the capillary pores and hence do not escape from the capillary lumen except by pinocytotic vesicle transport. An increase in either the volume of blood flow or capillary density increases tissue supply for the diffusible solutes. Note that capillary permeability is greater at the venous end of the capillary (and especially in the venule, *not shown*) because of the larger number of pores in this region. **B,** Diffusion-limited transport. When the distance between the capillaries and the parenchymal tissue is large as a result of edema or low capillary density, diffusion becomes a limiting factor in the transport of solutes from capillary to tissue, even at high rates of capillary blood flow.

decreased to about 80% as a result of diffusion of O_2 from arterioles and small arteries. Also, CO_2 loading and the resultant intravascular shifts in the oxyhemoglobin dissociation curve occur in the precapillary vessels. Hence direct flux of O_2 and CO_2 occurs between adjacent arterioles, between venules, and possibly between arteries and veins (**countercurrent exchange**), in addition to gas exchange at the level of the capillaries. This countercurrent exchange of gas represents a diffusional shunt of gas around the capillaries, and at low blood flow rates the supply of O_2 to the tissue may be limited.

Capillary Filtration Is Regulated by the Hydrostatic and Osmotic Forces Across the Endothelium

The direction and magnitude of the movement of water across the capillary wall are determined by the algebraic sum of the hydrostatic and osmotic pressures that exist across the membrane. An increase in intracapillary hydrostatic pressure favors movement of fluid from the vessel to the interstitial space. Conversely, an increase in the concentration of osmotically active particles within the vessels favors movement of fluid into the vessels from the interstitial space.

Hydrostatic Forces

The hydrostatic pressure (**blood pressure**) within the capillaries is not constant, and the forces depend on the arterial pressure, the venous pressure, and the precapillary and postcapillary vessel resistances. An increase in small artery and arterial pressure or in venous pressure elevates capillary hydrostatic pressure, whereas a reduction in each of these pressures has the opposite effect. An increase in arteriolar resistance or closure of arteries reduces capillary pressure, whereas greater resistance in the venules and veins increases the capillary pressure.

Hydrostatic Pressure is the Principal Force in Capillary Filtration

Changes in the venous resistance affect capillary hydrostatic pressure more than do changes in arteriolar resistance. A given change in venous pressure produces a greater effect on the capillary hydrostatic pressure than does the same change in arterial pressure, and about 80% of an increase in venous pressure is transmitted back to the capillaries.

Despite the fact that capillary hydrostatic pressure (P_c) varies from tissue to tissue (even within the same tissue), average values, obtained from many direct measurements in human skin, are about 32 mm Hg at the arterial end of the capillaries and 15 mm Hg at the venous end of the capillaries at the level of the heart (Figure 8-9). When a person stands, the hydrostatic pressure is higher in the legs and lower in the head.

Tissue pressure, or more specifically ISF pressure (P_i) outside the capillaries, opposes capillary filtration. It is $P_c - P_i$ that constitutes the hydrostatic driving force for filtration. In the normal (nonedematous) state of the subcutaneous tissue, P_i is close to zero or slightly negative (-1 to -4 mm Hg). Hence P_c represents essentially the hydrostatic driving force.

Osmotic Forces

The key factor that restrains fluid loss from the capillaries is the osmotic pressure of the plasma proteins—usually termed colloid osmotic pressure or oncotic pressure (π_p). The total osmotic pressure of plasma is about 6000 mm Hg, whereas the oncotic pressure is only about 25 mm Hg. However, this small oncotic pressure plays an important role in fluid exchange across the capillary wall, because the plasma proteins are essentially confined to the intravascular space. Consequently, the electrolytes that are responsible for the major fraction of plasma osmotic pressure are practically equal in concentration on the two sides of the capillary endothelium. The relative permeability of solute to water influences the actual magnitude of the osmotic pressure. The **reflection coefficient** (σ) is the relative impediment to the passage of a substance through the capillary wall. The reflection coefficient of water is 0, and that of albumin, to which the endothelium is almost impermeable, is 1. Filterable solutes have reflection coefficients between 0 and 1. Also, different tissues have different reflection coefficients for the same molecule. Therefore, movement of a given solute across the endothelial wall varies with the tissue. The true oncotic pressure (π) is defined by

$$\pi = \sigma \, RT(C_i - C_0) \tag{6}$$

where σ is the reflection coefficient, R is gas constant, T is absolute temperature, and C_i and C_o are solute

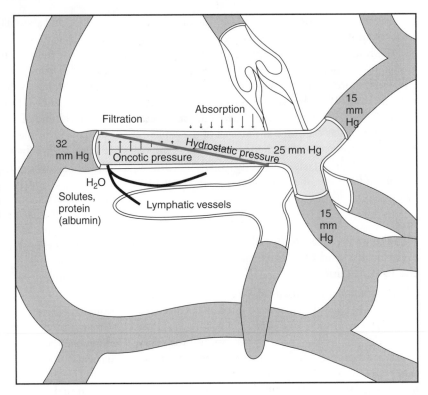

FIGURE 8-9 ▪ Schematic representation of the factors responsible for filtration and absorption across the capillary wall as well as the formation of lymph.

(**albumin**) concentrations, respectively, inside and outside the capillary.

Of the plasma proteins, albumin predominates in determining oncotic pressure. The average albumin molecule (**69,000 MW**) is approximately half the size of the average globulin molecule (**150,000 MW**). The albumin molecule is present in almost twice the concentration as the globulins (4.5 versus 2.5 g per dL of plasma). Albumin also exerts a greater osmotic force than can be accounted for solely on the basis of the number of molecules dissolved in the plasma. Therefore, it cannot be completely replaced by inert substances of appropriate molecular size, such as dextran. This additional osmotic force becomes disproportionately greater at high concentrations of albumin (**as in plasma**), and it is weak to absent in dilute solutions of albumin (**as in ISF**).

The reason for this behavior of albumin is its negative charge at normal blood pH and the attraction and retention of cations (principally Na^+) in the vascular compartment (the **Gibbs-Donnan effect**). Furthermore, albumin binds a small number of

Cl^- ions, a change that increases its negative charge and, hence, its ability to retain more Na^+ inside the capillaries. The small increase in electrolyte concentration of the plasma over that of the ISF produced by the negatively charged albumin enhances its osmotic force to that of an ideal solution containing a solute of 37,000 MW. If albumin did indeed have a molecular weight of 37,000, it would not be retained by the capillary endothelium, because of its small size. Hence, it could not function as a counterforce to capillary hydrostatic pressure. If, however, albumin did not have an enhanced osmotic force, it would require a concentration of about 12 g of albumin per dL of plasma to achieve a plasma oncotic pressure of 25 mm Hg. Such a high albumin concentration would greatly increase blood viscosity as well as the resistance to blood flow through the vascular system.

Some albumin escapes from the capillaries and enters the ISF, where it exerts an osmotic force of up to about 30% of plasma oncotic pressure. This observation of a higher ISF oncotic pressure than previously thought prompted the conclusion that filtration occurs in diminishing amounts along the entire length of the capillary in skin and skeletal muscle during steady-state conditions. Abrupt reductions in capillary hydrostatic pressure can cause transient reabsorption of fluid from the ISF compartment. However, plasma proteins continue to leak out of the capillaries, and this leakage plus the removal of water from the ISF compartment by the lymphatics concentrates the ISF proteins and changes absorption to filtration.

Balance of Hydrostatic and Osmotic Forces

The relationship between hydrostatic pressure and oncotic pressure, and the role of these forces in regulating fluid passage across the capillary endothelium, were expounded by Starling in 1896. This explanation constituted the Starling hypothesis and is expressed by the equation:

$$Q_f = k[(P_c - P_i) - \sigma(\pi_p - \pi_i)] \tag{7}$$

where Q_f is fluid movement across the capillary wall, P_c is capillary hydrostatic pressure, P_i is ISF hydrostatic pressure, π_p is plasma oncotic pressure, π_i is ISF oncotic pressure, k is the filtration constant for capillary membrane, and σ is reflection coefficient.

Filtration occurs when the algebraic sum is positive; absorption occurs when it is negative. Originally, it was proposed that filtration occurs at the arterial end of the capillary and that absorption occurs at the venous end, because of the gradient of hydrostatic pressure along the capillary. This may apply for the idealized capillary, as depicted in Figure 8-9, but direct observations have revealed that many capillaries show only filtration, whereas others show only absorption. In some vascular beds (e.g., the renal glomerulus) hydrostatic pressure in the capillary is high enough to result in filtration along the entire length of the capillary. In other vascular beds (e.g., the **intestinal mucosa**), the hydrostatic and oncotic forces allow absorption along the whole capillary.

As discussed previously, capillary pressure is variable and depends on several factors. The principal factor relates to the contractile state of the precapillary vessels. In the normal steady-state, arterial pressure, venous pressure, postcapillary resistance, ISF hydrostatic and oncotic pressures, and plasma oncotic pressure are relatively constant. A change in precapillary resistance appears to be the determining factor with respect to fluid movement across the vascular wall. The hydrostatic and osmotic forces are nearly in equilibrium along the entire capillary because water moves so quickly across the capillary endothelium. Hence, filtration and absorption in the normal state occur at very small degrees of pressure imbalance across the capillary wall. Only a small percentage (**about 2%**) of the plasma flowing through the vascular system is filtered. Some is reabsorbed and the rest is returned to the circulating blood via the lymphatic system.

In the lungs, the mean capillary hydrostatic pressure is only 8 to 10 mm Hg, and the plasma oncotic pressure is 25 mm Hg. Also, the lung ISF pressure is approximately 15 mm Hg, and the oncotic pressure of the interstitial fluid is 16 to 20 mg Hg. Thus, the net force favors reabsorption, yet pulmonary lymph is formed, and it consists of fluid that is osmotically drawn out of the capillaries by the plasma protein that escapes through the capillary endothelium.

The Capillary Filtration Coefficient Provides a Method to Estimate the Rate of Fluid Movement Across the Endothelium

The rate of fluid movement (Q_f) across the capillary membrane depends not only on the algebraic sum of the hydrostatic and osmotic forces across the endothelium (ΔP), but also on the area of the capillary wall available for filtration (A_m), the distance across the capillary wall (Δx), the viscosity of the filtrate (η), and the filtration constant of the membrane (k). These factors may be expressed by the equation:

$$Q_f = kA_m \Delta P / (\eta \Delta x) \tag{8}$$

The dimensions are units of flow per unit of pressure gradient across the capillary wall per unit of capillary surface area. This expression, which describes the flow of fluid through a porous membrane, is essentially Poiseuille's law for flow through tubes (see p. 125).

In pathological conditions such as left ventricular failure or stenosis of the mitral valve, pulmonary capillary hydrostatic pressure may exceed plasma oncotic pressure. When it does, pulmonary edema, a condition that seriously interferes with gas exchange in the lungs, may occur.

Because the thickness of the capillary wall and the viscosity of the filtrate are relatively constant, they can be included in the filtration constant, k. If the area of the capillary membrane is not known, the rate of filtration can be expressed per unit weight of tissue. Hence the equation can be simplified to:

$$Q_f = k_t \, \Delta P \tag{9}$$

where k_t is the capillary filtration coefficient for a given tissue and the units for Q_f are milliliters per minute per 100 g of tissue per millimeter of mercury pressure.

In any given tissue the filtration coefficient per unit area of capillary surface, and hence capillary permeability, is not changed by different physiological conditions, such as arteriolar dilation and capillary distention, or by such adverse conditions as hypoxia, hypercapnia, and reduced pH.

With capillary injury (toxins, severe burns), capillary permeability increases, as indicated by the filtration coefficient, and significant amounts of fluid and protein leak out of the capillaries into the interstitial space. The escaped protein enhances the oncotic pressure of the interstitial fluid, leading to additional fluid loss and dehydration. One of the important therapeutic measures in the treatment of extensive burns is replacement of fluid and plasma proteins.

The filtration coefficient can be used to determine the relative number of open capillaries (total capillary surface area available for filtration in tissue) because capillary permeability is constant under normal conditions. For example, increased metabolic activity of contracting skeletal muscle induces relaxation of precapillary resistance vessels with the opening of more capillaries (**capillary recruitment**), resulting in an increased filtering surface area.

Disturbances in Hydrostatic-Osmotic Balance

Changes in arterial pressure per se may have little effect on filtration, because the change in pressure may be countered by adjustments of the precapillary resistance vessels (**autoregulation;** see p. 179), so that hydrostatic pressure in the open capillaries remains the same.

With severe reduction in arterial pressure, as may occur in hemorrhage, there may be arteriolar constriction mediated by the sympathetic nervous system and a fall in venous pressure resulting from the blood loss. These changes lead to a decrease in capillary hydrostatic pressure. Furthermore, the low blood pressure in hemorrhage causes a decrease in blood flow (and hence O_2 supply) to the tissue, with the result that vasodilator metabolites accumulate and induce relaxation of arterioles. Precapillary vessel relaxation is also engendered by the reduced transmural pressure (autoregulation, see p. 179). As a consequence of these several factors, absorption predominates over filtration and occurs at a larger capillary surface area. This process is one of the compensatory mechanisms employed by the body to restore blood volume (p. 272).

An increase in venous pressure alone, as occurs in the feet when one changes from the lying to the standing position, would elevate capillary pressure and enhance filtration. However, the increase in transmural pressure causes precapillary vessel closure (myogenic mechanism; see p. 179) so that the capillary filtration coefficient actually decreases. This reduction in capillary surface available for filtration protects against the extravasation of large amounts of fluid into the interstitial space (edema).

With prolonged standing, particularly when associated with some elevation of venous pressure in the legs (such as that caused by pregnancy) or with sustained rises in venous pressure (as seen in congestive heart failure), filtration is greatly enhanced and exceeds the capacity of the lymphatic system to remove the capillary filtrate from the interstitial space (see also Figure 10-25).

A large amount of fluid can move across the capillary wall in a relatively short time. In a normal individual, the filtration coefficient (k_t) for the whole body is about 0.0061 mL/min/100 g of tissue/mm Hg. In a 70-kg man, a venous pressure elevation of 10 mm Hg for 10 minutes would increase filtration from capillaries by 342 mL. This would not lead to edema formation, because the fluid is returned to the vascular compartment by the lymphatic vessels. When edema develops, it usually appears in the dependent parts of the body, where the hydrostatic pressure is greatest. However, its location and magnitude are also determined by the type of tissue. Loose tissues, such as the subcutaneous tissue around the eyes or the scrotum, are more prone to collect larger quantities of interstitial fluid than are firm tissues, such as muscle, or encapsulated structures, such as the kidney.

The vascular endothelial growth factors (**VEGFs**), of which there are at least five, induce angiogenesis. They also elicit vasodilation and, as described originally, increase the endothelial permeability. By causing vasodilation, VEGF permits perfusion of more capillaries, an effect that can be misinterpreted as altered permeability. Nevertheless, in vitro and in vivo studies show VEGF increases capillary permeability. Some of the increased permeability results from opening of tight junctions between endothelial cells and from formation of fenestrations in them. These properties of the VEGFs must be considered in the evaluation of the exciting prospects of VEGFs in promoting angiogenesis in poorly perfused myocardium.

Pinocytosis Enables Large Molecules to Cross the Endothelium

Some transfer of substances across the capillary wall can occur in tiny pinocytotic vesicles (pinocytosis). These vesicles (see Figures 8-5 and 8-6) are formed by a pinching off of the surface membrane. Substances taken up on one side of the capillary wall move by thermal kinetic energy across the endothelial cell and deposit their contents at the other side. The amount of material that can be transported in this way is very small. However, pinocytosis may be responsible for the movement of large lipid-insoluble molecules (30 nm) between blood and interstitial fluid. The number of pinocytotic vesicles in endothelium varies with the tissue (muscle > lung > brain) and increases from the arterial to the venous end of the capillary.

The concentration of the plasma proteins may change in different pathological states and thus alter the osmotic force and movement of fluid across the capillary membrane. The plasma protein concentration is increased in dehydration (e.g., water deprivation, prolonged sweating, severe vomiting, and diarrhea), and water moves by osmotic forces from the tissues to the vascular compartment. In contrast, the plasma protein concentration is reduced in **nephrosis** (a renal disease in which there is loss of protein in the urine), and edema may occur.

THE LYMPHATICS RETURN THE FLUID AND SOLUTES THAT ESCAPE THROUGH THE ENDOTHELIUM TO THE CIRCULATING BLOOD

The terminal vessels of the lymphatic system consist of a widely distributed closed-end network of highly permeable lymph capillaries that resemble blood capillaries. However, they often lack tight junctions between endothelial cells, and they possess fine filaments that anchor them to the surrounding connective tissue. These fine strands distort the lymphatic vessel to open spaces between the endothelial cells and to permit the entrance of protein and large particles that are present in the interstitial fluid. The lymph capillaries drain into larger vessels that finally enter the right and left subclavian veins at their junctions with the respective internal jugular veins. Only cartilage, bone, epithelium, and tissues of the central nervous system are devoid of lymphatic vessels. The plasma capillary filtrate is returned to the circulation by virtue of tissue pressure, facilitated by intermittent skeletal muscle activity, contractions of the lymphatic vessels, and an extensive system of one-way valves. In this respect, they resemble the veins, although even the larger lymphatic vessels have thinner walls than do the corresponding veins, and they contain only a small amount of elastic tissue and smooth muscle.

When either the volume of interstitial fluid exceeds the drainage capacity of the lymphatics or the lymphatic vessels become blocked, as may occur in certain disease states such as **elephantiasis** (caused by **filariasis,** a worm infestation), interstitial fluid accumulates (edema) chiefly in the more compliant tissues (e.g., subcutaneous tissue).

The volume of fluid transported through the lymphatics in 24 hours is about equal to an animal's total plasma volume. The proteins returned by the lymphatics to the blood in a day are about one fourth to one half of the circulating plasma proteins. This is the only means by which protein (albumin) that leaves the vascular compartment can be returned to the blood, because back-diffusion into the capillaries cannot occur against the large albumin concentration gradient. If the protein was not removed by the lymph vessels, it would accumulate in the interstitial fluid. It would then act as an oncotic force to draw fluid from the blood capillaries to produce edema. In addition to returning fluid and protein to the vascular bed, the lymphatic system filters the lymph at the lymph nodes and removes foreign particles such as bacteria. The largest lymphatic vessel, the **thoracic duct,** in addition to draining the lower extremities, returns protein lost through the permeable liver capillaries. Substances absorbed from the gastrointestinal tract, principally fat in the form of chylomicrons, are delivered to the circulating blood.

Lymph flow varies considerably, being almost nil from resting skeletal muscle, and increasing during exercise in proportion to the degree of muscular activity. It is increased by any mechanism that enhances the rate of blood capillary filtration—for example, increased capillary pressure or permeability or decreased plasma oncotic pressure.

SUMMARY

- Blood flow through the capillaries is chiefly regulated by contraction and relaxation of the arterioles (resistance vessels).
- The capillaries, which consist of a single layer of endothelial cells, can withstand high transmural pressure by virtue of their small diameter. According to the law of Laplace, T (wall tension) = ΔP (transmural pressure difference) $\times$ r (radius of the capillary).
- The endothelium is the source of an endothelium-derived relaxing factor (EDRF), identified as nitric oxide (NO), and of prostacyclin, both of which relax vascular smooth muscles.
- Mechanical forces that act on the glycocalyx and on the basement membrane are transduced into signals that modify gene expression of endothelial cells whose morphology and function are changed.
- Movement of water and small solutes between the vascular and interstitial fluid compartments occurs through capillary pores mainly by diffusion but also by filtration and absorption.
- Exchange of small lipid-insoluble molecules is flow limited because the rate of diffusion is about 40 times greater than the blood flow in the tissue. The larger the molecule, the slower is its diffusion. Large lipid-insoluble molecules are diffusion limited.

Molecules larger than about 70,000 MW are essentially confined to the vascular compartment.
- Lipid-soluble substances such as CO_2 and O_2 pass directly through the lipid membranes of the capillary, and the ease of transfer is directly proportional to the degree of lipid solubility of the substance.
- Capillary filtration and absorption are described by the Starling equation:

$$\text{Fluid movement} = k[(P_c - P_i) - \sigma (\pi_p - \pi_i)]$$

where P_c is capillary hydrostatic pressure, P_i is interstitial fluid hydrostatic pressure, π_i is interstitial fluid oncotic pressure, π_p is plasma oncotic pressure, i is capillary membrane filtration constant and σ is the reflection coefficient. Filtration occurs when the algebraic sum is positive; absorption occurs when it is negative.
- Large molecules can move across the capillary wall in vesicles formed from the lipid membrane of the capillaries by a process called pinocytosis.
- Fluid and protein that have escaped from the blood capillaries enter the lymphatic capillaries and are transported via the lymphatic system back to the blood vascular compartment.

ADDITIONAL READING

Bates DO: Vascular endothelial growth factors and vascular permeability, *Cardiovasc Res* 87:262, 2010.

Bendayan M: Morphological and cytochemical aspects of capillary permeability, *Microsc Res Tech* 57:327, 2002.

Boardman KC, Swartz MA: Interstitial flow as a guide for lymphangiogenesis, *Circ Res* 92:801, 2003.

Chiu J-J, Chien S: Effects of disturbed flow on vascular endothelium: pathophysiological basis and clinical perspectives, *Physiol Rev* 91:327, 2011.

Gomes D, Agasse A, Thiébaud P, et al: Aquaporins are multifunctional water and solute transporters highly divergent in living organisms, *Biochim Biophys Acta* 1788:1213, 2009.

Michel CC: Microvascular permeability, ultrafiltration, and restricted diffusion, *Am J Physiol* 287:H1887, 2004.

Michel CC, Neal CR: Openings through endothelial cells associated with increased microvascular permeability, *Microcirculation* 6:45, 1999.

Miserocchi G, Negrini D, Passi A, De Luca G: Development of lung edema: Interstitial fluid dynamics and molecular structure, *News Physiol Sci* 16:66, 2001.

Schmid-Schonbein GW: The second valve system in lymphatics, *Lymphat Res Biol* 1:25, 2003.

Starling EH: On the absorption of fluids from the connective tissue spaces, *J Physiol* 19:312, 1896.

Swartz MA: The physiology of the lymphatic system, *Adv Drug Deliv Rev* 50:3, 2001.

Tarbell JM, Weinbaum S, Kamm RD: Cellular fluid mechanics and mechanotransduction, *Annals Biomed Eng* 33:1719, 2005.

Tzima E, Irani-Tehrani, Kiosses WB, et al: A mechanosensory complex that mediates the endothelial cell response to fluid shear stress, *Nature* 437:426, 2005.

Welsh DG, Segal SS: Endothelial and smooth muscle cell conduction in arterioles controlling blood flow, *Am J Physiol* 274:H178, 1998.

Xia J, Duling BR: Patterns of excitation-contraction coupling in arterioles: Dependence on time and concentration, *Am J Physiol* 274:H323, 1998.

CASE 8-1

HISTORY

A 45-year-old man with a long history of alcoholism (averaging a liter of whiskey per day) was admitted to the hospital as an emergency because of vomiting of blood and fainting. In the past few months, he noted progressive anorexia, fatigue, jaundice, generalized itching, and abdominal swelling. Physical examination showed a semicomatose man with pallor, jaundice, and ascites. Blood pressure was 90 mm Hg systolic/40 mm Hg diastolic, heart rate was 100 beats/min, and hematocrit

was 35%. Liver function tests indicated severe liver damage. The diagnosis was advanced cirrhosis of the liver. Immediate treatment was transfusion with three units of blood. The following pressures were noted:

Mesenteric capillary hydrostatic pressure: 44 mm Hg
Plasma oncotic pressure: 23 mm Hg
Pressure in peritoneal cavity: 8 mm Hg
Peritoneal fluid oncotic pressure: 3 mm Hg

QUESTIONS

1. The transcapillary pressure responsible for the ascites was (assume the filtration coefficient is 1.0 and the reflection coefficient is 0.7):
   a. 5 mm Hg.
   b. 15 mm Hg.
   c. 19 mm Hg.
   d. 22 mm Hg.
   e. 36 mm Hg.
2. After lost blood was replaced by transfusion, the treatment for the patient's condition was:
   a. dialysis.
   b. high-fat diet.
   c. portal-caval shunt.
   d. cholecystectomy.
   e. erythromycin.
3. The substance mainly responsible for the oncotic pressure of the patient's plasma was:
   a. sodium.
   b. albumin.
   c. chloride.
   d. globulin.
   e. potassium.

CASE 8-2

HISTORY

A 25-year-old man suffered third-degree burns over the upper three quarters of his body in a fire in his home. Several hours elapsed before he reached the hospital. On admission, he was in a shocklike state. Blood pressure was 90 mm Hg systolic/70 mm Hg diastolic, heart rate was 110 mm Hg, and hematocrit was 55%. Blood analysis revealed a sodium level of 145 mEq/L, a potassium level of 4 mEq/L, a chloride level of 105 mEq/L, and an albumin level of 3.5 g/dL.

QUESTIONS

1. The most effective treatment is an intravenous infusion of:
   a. saline.
   b. whole blood.
   c. 5% glucose.
   d. dextran.
   e. plasma.

2. After several months of treatment with extensive artificial skin grafts, the patient was able to walk and to resume an almost normal life. After prolonged standing, he noted slight ankle swelling but no ecchymoses in his feet. Capillaries in his feet did not rupture when he stood because:
   a. arterioles reflexively constrict and prevent exposure of the capillaries to high pressure.
   b. tissue pressure rises and opposes an increase in capillary pressure.
   c. total capillary cross-sectional area is large enough to distribute the pressure and thereby compensate for the high intracapillary pressure.
   d. capillary diameter is so small that the capillary wall tension is low.
   e. capillaries constrict via a myogenic mechanism.

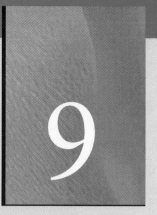

9

THE PERIPHERAL CIRCULATION AND ITS CONTROL

OBJECTIVES

1. Indicate the intrinsic and extrinsic (neural and humoral) factors that regulate peripheral blood flow.

2. Explain autoregulation of blood flow and the myogenic mechanism for local adjustments of blood flow.

3. Elucidate metabolic regulation of blood flow.

4. Explain the role of the sympathetic nerves in blood flow regulation.

5. Describe vascular reflexes in the control of blood flow.

6. Describe the role of humoral agents in the regulation of blood flow.

THE FUNCTIONS OF THE HEART AND LARGE BLOOD VESSELS

The principal function of the heart is to pump blood to the tissues of the body. However, the distribution of blood to the crucial regions of the body depends on the large and small arteries and arterioles. *The regulation of peripheral blood flow is essentially under dual control: centrally, by the nervous system, and locally, in the tissues by the conditions in the immediate vicinity of the blood vessels.* The relative importance of the central and local control mechanisms varies among tissues. In some areas of the body, such as the skin and the splanchnic regions, neural regulation of blood flow predominates; in other regions, such as the heart and the brain, local factors are dominant.

The small arteries and arterioles that regulate the blood flow throughout the body are called the **resistance vessels.** These vessels offer the greatest resistance to the flow of blood pumped to the tissues by the heart. As such, they are important in the maintenance of arterial blood pressure. Smooth muscle fibers are the main component of the walls of the resistance vessels (see Figure 1-2). Hence, the vessel lumen can vary from complete obliteration by strong contraction of the smooth muscle with infolding of the endothelial lining, to maximal dilation by full relaxation of the smooth muscle. At any given time, some resistance vessels are closed by partial contraction (**tone**) of the arteriolar smooth muscle. If all the resistance vessels in the body dilated simultaneously, blood pressure would fall precipitously. Passive stretch of the microvessels by an increase in intravascular pressure decreases vascular resistance, whereas a decrease in intravascular pressure increases vascular resistance by recoil of the stretched vascular muscle.

CONTRACTION AND RELAXATION OF ARTERIOLAR VASCULAR SMOOTH MUSCLE REGULATE PERIPHERAL BLOOD FLOW

Vascular smooth muscle is responsible for the control of total peripheral resistance, arterial and venous tone, and the distribution of blood flow throughout the body. The smooth muscle cells are small, mononucleate, and spindle shaped. They are usually arranged in helical or circular layers around the large blood vessels and in a single circular layer around arterioles (Figure 9-1A and B). Also, parts of endothelial cells project into the vascular smooth muscle layer (**myoendothelial junctions**) at various points along the arterioles (Figure 9-1C). These projections suggest a functional interaction between endothelium and adjacent vascular smooth muscle.

In general, the close association between action potentials and contraction observed in skeletal and cardiac muscle cells cannot be demonstrated in vascular smooth muscle. Also, vascular smooth muscle lacks transverse tubules. Graded changes in membrane potential are often associated with changes in force. Contractile activity is generally elicited by neural or humoral stimuli, and the activity of smooth muscle varies in different vessels. For example, some vessels, particularly in the portal or mesenteric circulation, contain longitudinally oriented smooth muscle. This muscle is spontaneously active, and it displays action potentials that are correlated with the contractions and the electrical coupling between cells.

Vascular smooth muscle cells contain large numbers of thin actin filaments and small numbers of thick myosin filaments. These filaments are aligned in the long axis of the cell, but they do not form visible sarcomeres with striations. Nevertheless, the sliding filament mechanism is believed to operate in this tissue, and phosphorylation of crossbridges regulates their rate of cycling. Compared with skeletal muscle, the smooth muscle contracts very slowly, develops high forces, and maintains force for long periods. The adenosine triphosphate (ATP) utilization is diminished, and it operates over a considerable range of lengths under physiological conditions. Cell-to-cell conduction occurs via gap junctions, as it does in cardiac muscle (see p. 57).

In smooth muscle, the interaction between myosin and actin, which leads to contraction, is controlled by the myoplasmic Ca^{++} concentration, as it is in cardiac and skeletal muscle. The molecular mechanism by which Ca^{++} regulates contraction in smooth muscle (Figure 9-2) is fundamentally different, however, because smooth muscle does not utilize the Ca^{++}-binding regulatory protein troponin. For smooth muscle crossbridges to be activated to cycle, the 20-kDa regulatory light chain of myosin (MLC_{20}, a protein subunit of myosin) must be phosphorylated. MLC_{20} is phosphorylated by myosin light-chain kinase (MLCK) and de-phosphorylated by myosin light-chain phosphatase (MLCP). This requirement for phosphorylation provides a means to regulate contraction in smooth muscle in addition to that in cardiac and skeletal muscles, because both MLCK and MLCP are themselves regulated by other kinases.

FIGURE 9-1 ■ **A,** Low-magnification electron micrograph of an arteriole in cross section (inner diameter of approximately 40 μm) in cat ventricle. The wall of the blood vessel is composed largely of vascular smooth muscle cells (SM) whose long axes are directed approximately circularly around the vessel. A single layer of endothelial cells (E) forms the innermost portion of the blood vessel. Connective tissue elements (CT), such as fibroblasts and collagen, make up the adventitial layer at the periphery of the vessel; nerve bundles also appear in this layer (N). EN, endothelial cell nucleus. **B,** Detail of the wall of the blood vessel in **A.** This field contains a single endothelial layer (E), the medial smooth muscle layer (with three smooth muscle cell profiles: SM_1, SM_2, and SM_3), and the adventitial layer, containing nerves (N) and connective tissue (CT). SMN, smooth muscle nucleus. **C,** Another region of the arteriole, showing the area in which the endothelial (E) and smooth muscle (SM) layers are apposed. A projection of an endothelial cell (between *arrows*) is closely applied to the surface of the overlying smooth muscle, forming a "myoendothelial junction." Plasmalemmal vesicles (V) are prominent in both the endothelium and the smooth muscle cell (where such vesicles are known as "caveolae" [C]).

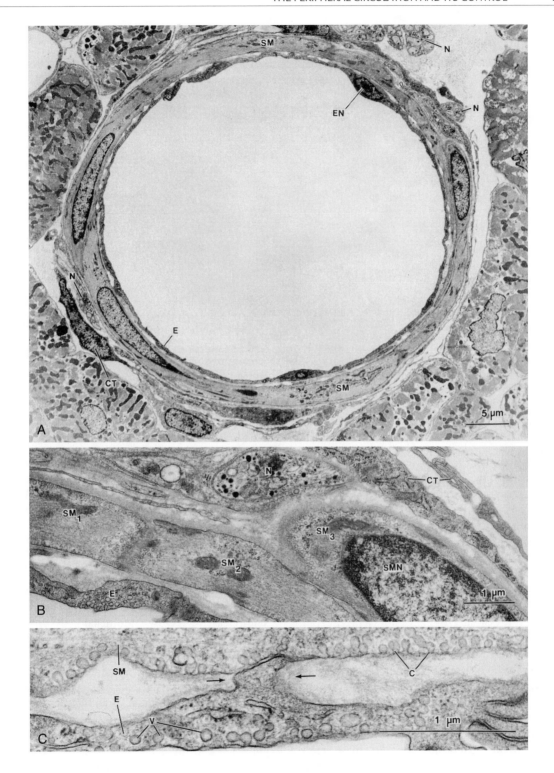

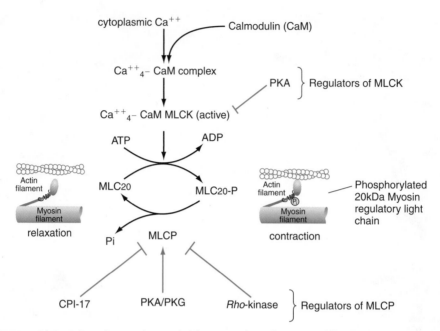

FIGURE 9-2 ■ For smooth muscle actin-myosin crossbridges to cycle and generate force or shortening, the 20-kDa myosin regulatory light-chain subunit (MLC_{20}) of myosin must be phosphorylated. Phosphorylation of MLC_{20} is controlled by myosin light-chain kinase (MLCK) and myosin light-chain phosphatase (MLCP). MLCK activity is inhibited by protein kinase A (PKA). MLCP activity is inhibited by *Rho*-kinase and CPI-17 (17-kDa C-kinase potentiated protein phosphatase-1 inhibitor). P_i, inorganic phosphate, released from MLC_{20}-P by the phosphatase action of MLCP; PKA, cyclic adenosine monophosphate (AMP)–dependent protein kinase; PKG, cyclic guanosine monophosphate (GMP)–dependent protein kinase.

MLCK is activated by a complex between 4 Ca^{++} and the Ca^{++}-binding messenger protein **calmodulin (CaM)**, which is present in high abundance in smooth muscle cells. The concentration of Ca^{++}/calmodulin, and thus the activation of MLCK, is driven by the cytoplasmic Ca^{++} concentration (i.e., "'Ca^{++}'activation" of contraction). However, the level of phosphorylation of the MLC_{20} is also determined by MLCP. Inhibiting the activity of MLCP has the effect of increasing contraction, even when cytoplasmic Ca^{++} (and MLCK activity) does not change, because inhibition of MLCP results in increased phosphorylation of MLC_{20}. Inhibition of MLCP activity thus increases the "'Ca^{++}'sensitivity" of contraction. Conversely, stimulation of MLCP activity decreases MLC_{20} phosphorylation and contraction, even at a constant Ca^{++}, and thus decreases Ca^{++} sensitivity of contraction.

MLCP is inhibited primarily by *rho*-kinase (a regulator of the cytoskeleton in many types of cells).

Rho-kinase is activated in a signaling cascade that begins with activation of certain G-protein–coupled receptors (GPCRs) on the surface membrane. Another protein, CPI-17 (17-kDa C-protein–potentiated inhibitor of protein phosphatase), which is activated by protein kinase C (PKC), also inhibits MLCP. Activity of MLCP may also be increased, particularly by nitric oxide (NO), through cyclic GMP and protein kinase G (PKG), and by cyclic adenosine monophosphate (AMP), acting through protein kinase A (PKA). The release of NO by endothelial cells, and subsequent stimulation of smooth muscle MLCP, constitutes a major mechanism by which endothelium may cause smooth muscle relaxation and arterial or venous dilation. In summary, regulation of smooth muscle contraction by neurotransmitters, circulating hormones, and autocoids often involves both changes in "'Ca^{++}'activation" of contraction (MLCK) and in Ca^{++} sensitivity of contraction (MLCP) (see later). The contractile state of smooth

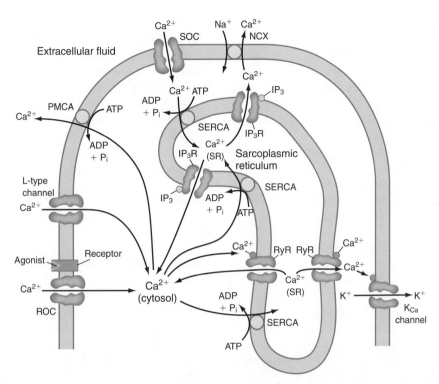

FIGURE 9-3 ▪ Control of cytoplasmic calcium ion ($[Ca^{++}]$, shown as Ca^{2+} here) in vascular smooth muscle. Calcium can enter the cell via electrically activated channels (e.g., voltage-operated Ca^{++} channel, L-type Ca^{++} channel), via receptor-operated channels (ROCs) in the sarcolemma, or via store-operated channels (SOCs). SOCs open when the sarcoplasmic reticulum (SR) becomes depleted of Ca^{++}. Calcium is also released from the sarcoplasmic reticulum through ryanodine receptor channels (RyRs) and through inositol triphosphate receptors (IP_3Rs) in response to inositol triphosphate (IP_3) stimulation and is taken back into the SR by a calcium pump (SERCA). Calcium is extruded from the cell by a plasma membrane calcium pump (PMCA) and by the Na-Ca exchanger (NCX). Membrane potential is determined by K_{Ca} channels, which may be activated by local Ca^{++}, and by ROCs, which are permeable to both Na^+ and Ca^{++}. ADP, adenosine diphosphate; ATP, adenosine triphosphate; MLCK, myosin light-chain kinase; MLCP, myosin light-chain phosphatase; P_i, inorganic phosphate. *(Modified from Blaustein MP, Kao JPY, Matteson DR:* Cellular Physiology, *Philadelphia, 2004, Mosby.)*

muscle is thus governed finally by the *ratio* of Ca^{++}-activated MLCK activity to MLCP activity, because this ratio determines the level of phosphorylation of MLC_{20}.

Cytoplasmic Ca^{++} is Regulated to Control Contraction, via MLCK

The cytoplasmic Ca^{++} concentration, and thus MLCK activity, is determined by the summation of the Ca^{++} that enters the cytosol (influx) and that leaving the cytosol (efflux) (Figure 9-3). Ca^{++} enters the cytosol in two ways: (1) from the extracellular space, via influx through voltage-operated calcium channels (typically

L-type, activated by depolarization), receptor-operated calcium channels (ROCs, activated after the action of agonists on membrane receptors), and store-operated calcium channels (activated after depletion of sarcoplasmic reticulum Ca^{++} stores), and (2) from the sarcoplasmic reticulum (SR) via activation of either ryanodine receptor channels, RyRs or inositol-1,4,5 triphosphate (IP_3) receptor channels (IP_3-stimulated) located on the SR. Ca^{++} ions leave the cytosol via ATP-driven calcium transporters (i.e., Ca^{++} pumps) located on both the SR (termed SERCAs) and plasma membrane (termed PMCAs) as well as activation of the Na/Ca exchangers on the plasma membrane as in cardiac muscle (see Figure 4-8).

Contraction is Controlled By Excitation-Contraction Coupling and/or Pharmacomechanical Coupling

Cellular responses to agonist vary among different blood vessels as well as smooth muscle types. This diversity arises partly from differences in ion channels that may be present (such as potassium and calcium channels important in excitation-contraction [E-C] coupling) and in agonist-specific receptors (such as those that bind angiotensin II, norepinephrine, serotonin, histamine, and acetylcholine) expressed on the plasma membrane of vascular smooth muscle.

Excitation-Contraction Coupling in Vascular Smooth Muscle

The potential across the plasma membrane of vascular smooth muscle is an important determinant of cytoplasmic Ca^{++}, and thus of contractile state of vascular smooth muscle. The reason is that both entry of Ca^{++} into the cell and extrusion of Ca^{++} from the cell are voltage-dependent (involving voltage-dependent Ca^{++} channels and sodium/calcium exchange [NCX]). Depolarization increases Ca^{++} influx and decreases Ca^{++} efflux. In many types of arteries, membrane potential is strongly influenced by the transmural pressure (i.e., the blood pressure) through the "'myogenic'" mechanism (discussed later in this chapter), with increases in pressure tending to cause depolarization and consequent entry of Ca^{++} through voltage-dependent Ca^{++} channels. Membrane potential is, however, always strongly influenced by K^+ channels, with activation of K^+ channels tending to hyperpolarize the membrane and inhibition of K^+ channels tending to depolarize it. Some types of vascular smooth muscle produce action potentials in which the depolarizing current is carried by voltage-dependent (L-type) Ca^{++} channels. The resting membrane potential of vascular smooth muscle is determined primarily by K^+ permeability because of the relative abundant expression of K^+ channels. Stimuli that open K^+ channels can alter membrane potential by altering K^+ efflux across the plasma membrane (since resting potassium concentration inside the cell, $[K^+]_i$, is greater than that outside the cell, $[K^+]_o$). Opening of K^+ channels causes hyperpolarization (due to increased K^+ efflux) of the membrane potential, whereas closure of K^+ channels causes depolarization (due to decreased K^+ efflux). L-type calcium channels are voltage-sensitive and are activated (i.e., opened) by membrane depolarization, resulting in influx of extracellular Ca^{++} and elevating intracellular Ca^{++} concentration. If the increase in Ca^{++} levels is sufficient, then the Ca^{++}/calmodulin complex activates MLCK, promoting actin-myosin interaction and contraction. Thus, changes in membrane potential alter extracellular Ca^{++} influx and efflux, modulate intracellular cytoplasmic Ca^{++}, and affect vascular smooth muscle contraction, artery diameter, and vascular resistance.

Pharmacomechanical Coupling

Contraction of arteries and veins is very importantly modulated by hormones, neurotransmitters, and autocoids acting on receptors located in the plasma membrane (Figure 9-4). Most of these receptors are GPCRs. Pharmacomechanical (PM) coupling is a mechanism of contractile activation that causes little or no change in membrane potential (making it distinct from E-C coupling). Pharmacomechanical coupling can result either in contraction (Figure 9-4A) or relaxation (Figure 9-4B). The three major components of PM coupling are (1) the GPCR itself, (2) the coupling complex, and (3) the second messenger (e.g., cyclic AMP or IP$_3$). G-protein coupled receptors are characterized by the ligands they bind (e.g., adrenergic [catecholamines], serotinergic [serotonin], cholinergic [acetylcholine]) and by the particular heterotrimeric G-proteins to which they are coupled. Important G-proteins coupled to GPCRs on vascular smooth muscle cells include $G\alpha_{q/11}$, $G\alpha_{12/13}$, $G\alpha_s$, and $G\alpha_{i/o}$. The G-protein α subunits, and sometimes the G-protein $\beta\gamma$ subunits, activate specific effector molecules, such as kinases. In many cases, second messenger molecules are ultimately generated that stimulate downstream cellular mechanisms (ion influx, Ca^{++} release, enzyme activation or inhibition). G-protein–coupled receptors are important regulators of cardiovascular function, with many drugs acting on them. (It has been estimated that, overall, about 40% of currently used drugs act on GPCRs in the cardiovascular system and elsewhere in the body).

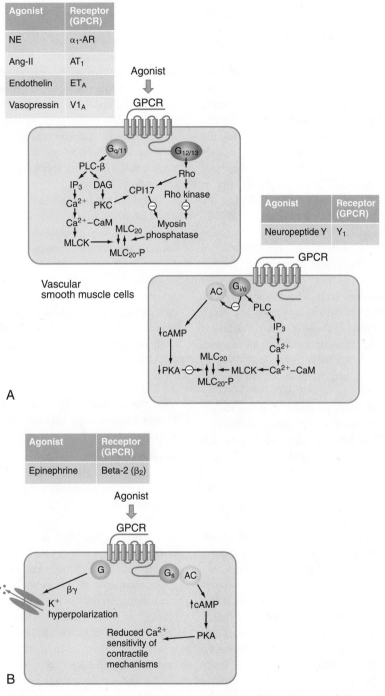

FIGURE 9-4 Key physiological neurotransmitters and hormones that control vascular tone, their receptors and intracellular mechanisms. **A,** Physiological agonists bind to G-protein–coupled receptors (GPCRs) that are coupled to different G proteins and to different effector molecules and second messengers. These pathways all result in vasoconstriction. The α subunits of the G-proteins are: $G\alpha_{q/11}$, $G\alpha_{12/13}$, and $G\alpha_{i/o}$. AC, adenyl cyclase; CaM, calmodulin; CPI-17, 17-kDa C-protein–potentiated inhibitor of protein phosphatase; DAG, diacylglycerol; IP$_3$, inositol triphosphate; MLC$_{20}$, 20-kDa myosin regulatory light chain; MLCK, myosin light-chain kinase; MLCP, myosin light-chain phosphatase (also known as protein phosphatase); PKC, protein kinase C; PLC-β, phospholipase C-β. **B,** Epinephrine binds to the GPCR β$_2$-AR (β$_2$-adrenoceptor, AR) to promote vasodilation through increased cyclic adenosine monophosphate (cAMP) and activation of K$^+$ channels. β$_2$-AR is coupled to the G-protein Gα$_S$, which inhibits MLCK via phosphorylation by its effector, cAMP-dependent protein kinase A (PKA).

Control of Vascular Tone by Catecholamines

The catecholamines norepinephrine (NE) and epinephrine are key controllers of cardiovascular function. Norepinephrine is released from sympathetic nerve endings in the heart and blood vessels and acts locally, whereas epinephrine is released from the adrenal medulla and circulates in the blood to act widely throughout the body. In general, the GPCRs that bind catecholamines are known as "'adrenoceptors'," a term deriving from the fact that these receptors all bind the adrenal medullary hormones, epinephrine and NE, although with varying affinities. The adrenoceptors are large and diverse family of GPCRs, consisting of five major types (α_1, α_2, β_1, β_2, β_3) and several subtypes, and a full discussion of their function and pharmacology is reserved for pharmacology texts. In arteries and veins, NE binds most strongly to α_1-adrenoceptors (α_1-ARs), which are GPCRs located in the sympathetic neuroeffector junctions, on the smooth muscle cell membrane. These receptors couple to both $G\alpha_{q/11}$ and $G\alpha_{12/13}$ (see Figure 9-4A), and their activation results in contraction (PM coupling). $G\alpha_{q/11}$ activates phospholipase C (PLC), which catalyzes the production of diacylglycerol (DAG) and IP_3 from PIP_2 (phosphatidylinositol 4,5-bisphosphate). Diacylglycerol activates PKC, which in turn activates CPI-17, which inhibits MLCP. IP_3 activates IP_3 receptors (IP_3Rs) on the SR membrane to release Ca^{++}, which binds to CaM and activates MLCK. Thus, phosphorylation of MLC_{20} is increased as a result of increased "Ca^{++} activation" of contraction, and as a result of increased "Ca^{++} sensitivity" of contraction. Release of NE from sympathetic nerve endings, and the subsequent contraction of vascular smooth muscle, is a major way in which vascular resistance and vascular capacitance (through contraction of small veins) are regulated. (Note that heart tissue contains few α_1-ARs, and there NE acts primarily on β_1 receptors, which are coupled to Ga_s, increasing cAMP and strengthening cardiac contraction (see Figures 5-23 and 5-28). Many vascular tissues contain few or no β_1-ARs). Most of the arteries and veins of the body are innervated solely by fibers of the sympathetic nervous system, and thus neurally released NE plays a major role in controlling vascular function, through sympathetic nerve activity directed by the central nervous system. The sympathetic nerve fibers release NE to exert a tonic vasoconstrictor effect on the blood vessels, as evidenced by the fact that cutting or freezing the sympathetic nerves to a vascular bed (such as muscle) increases the blood flow. Activation of the sympathetic nerves either directly or reflexly (see pp. 184 and 185) enhances vascular resistance. (In contrast to the sympathetic nerves, the parasympathetic nerves tend to decrease vascular resistance. However, these nerves innervate only a small fraction of the blood vessels in the body, mainly in certain viscera and pelvic organs.)

Epinephrine is released from the adrenal medulla and circulates in the blood. Epinephrine acts most potently on β_2-ARs on vascular smooth muscle and causes vasodilation, through increases in cAMP (see Figure 9-4B) and reduced "Ca^{++} sensitivity" of contraction. At very high concentrations in the plasma, however, epinephrine also binds to a_1-ARs to cause contraction and vasoconstriction, overriding its effects mediated by the vascular β_2-ARs. In the heart, both epinephrine and NE bind equally well to β_1-ARs.

Control of Vascular Contraction by Other Hormones, Other Neurotransmitters, and Autocoids

Angiotensin II has many actions, most acting to increase arterial blood pressure. It is a direct vasoconstrictor, acting primarily on AT_1 receptors, which are coupled to both both $G\alpha_{q/11}$ and $G\alpha_{12/13}$ (see Figure 9-4A). Endothelin, a 21–amino acid peptide, acts primarily on ET_A receptors on vascular smooth muscle to cause vasoconstriction (see Figure 9-4A). Endothelin is synthesized and released from endothelial cells. Vasopressin, or antidiuretic hormone (ADH), is a neurohypophysial hormone that is a potent constrictor that is called into play to elevate blood pressure (and conserve fluid volume) particularly as a compensatory mechanism in hemorrhage. Vasopressin binds primarily to the $V1_A$ receptor, which is coupled to $G\alpha_{q/11}$ and $G\alpha_{12/13}$. Neuropeptide Y is a sympathetic neurotransmitter that is co-released with NE from sympathetic nerve endings on vascular smooth muscle and binds primarily to the Y_1 receptor, which is coupled to $G\alpha_{i/o}$. Activation of Y_1 thus can decrease cAMP and enhance contraction by decreasing the PKA-mediated inhibition of MLCP.

INTRINSIC CONTROL OF PERIPHERAL BLOOD FLOW

Autoregulation and the Myogenic Mechanism Tend to Keep Blood Flow Constant

Blood flow is adjusted to the existing metabolic activity of the tissue. Furthermore, imposed changes in the arterial perfusion pressure at constant levels of tissue metabolism are met with vascular resistance changes that maintain a constant blood flow. This mechanism is commonly referred to as the **autoregulation** of blood flow, which is illustrated in Figure 9-5. In the skeletal muscle preparation from which these data were derived, the muscle was completely isolated from the rest of the animal and was in a resting state. From a control pressure of 100 mm Hg, the pressure was abruptly increased or decreased, and the blood flows observed immediately after changing the perfusion pressure are represented by the *closed circles* in the figure. Maintenance of the altered pressure at each new level was followed within 30 to 60 seconds by a return of flow toward the control levels; the *open circles* represent these steady-state flows. Over the pressure range of 20 to 120 mm Hg, the steady-state flow is relatively constant. Calculation of resistance across the vascular

bed (**pressure/flow**) during steady-state conditions indicates that, with elevation of perfusion pressure, the resistance vessels have constricted, whereas with reduction of perfusion pressure, they have dilated.

The reason for this constancy of blood flow in the presence of an altered perfusion pressure is not known. It is explained best by the **myogenic mechanism.** *According to this mechanism, the vascular smooth muscle contracts in response to an increase in transmural pressure, and it relaxes in response to a decrease in transmural pressure.* Therefore, the initial flow increment is produced by an abrupt increase in perfusion pressure. This increase passively distends the blood vessels. The distention is followed by a return of flow to the previous control level by contraction of the vascular smooth muscles.

An example of a myogenic response is shown in Figure 9-6. Arterioles isolated from the hearts of young pigs were cannulated at each end, and the transmural pressure (**intravascular pressure minus extravascular pressure**) and flow through the arteriole could be adjusted to desired levels. With no flow through the arteriole, successive increases in transmural pressure elicited progressive decreases in the vessel diameter (Figure 9-6A). This effect was independent of the endothelium, because the responses were identical in intact vessels and in vessels that were denuded of endothelium (Figure 9-6B). Arterioles that were relaxed by direct action of **nitroprusside** on the vascular smooth muscle showed only a passive increase in diameter when transmural pressure was increased. In vascular smooth muscle having spontaneous action potentials (arterioles, portal vein), the action potential frequency increases with stretch to cause greater Ca^{++} influx via electromechanical coupling. In vascular smooth muscle lacking spontaneous action potentials, stretch activates plasma membrane Ca^{++} channels to elevate intracellular Ca^{++}. The nature of the Ca^{++} sensor that allows this process is not completely understood, but it allows an increase in transmural pressure to activate membrane calcium channels. Indeed, membrane depolarization itself has been shown to activate phospholipase C and thereby generate second messengers.

It would be expected that operation of a myogenic mechanism would be minimized, because blood pressure is reflexly maintained at a fairly constant level under normal conditions. However, when a person

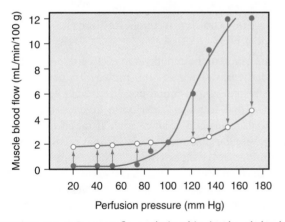

FIGURE 9-5 ■ Pressure-flow relationship in the skeletal muscle vascular bed of the dog. *Closed circles* represent the flows obtained immediately after abrupt changes in perfusion pressure from the control level (point where *lines* cross). *Open circles* represent the steady-state flows obtained at the new perfusion pressure. *(Redrawn from Jones RD, Berne RM: Intrinsic regulation of skeletal muscle blood flow. Circ Res 14:126, 1964.)*

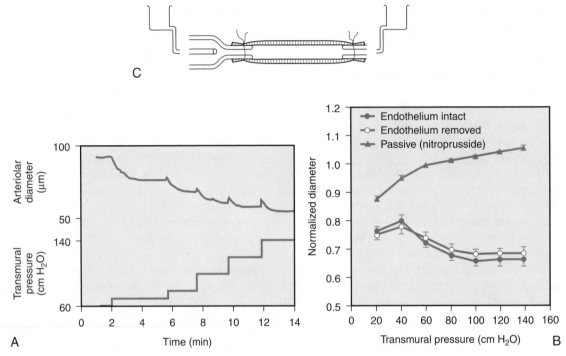

FIGURE 9-6 ■ A, Constriction of an isolated cardiac arteriole in response to increases in transmural pressure without flow through the blood vessel. **B,** Constrictor response of the arteriole to an increase in transmural pressure is unaffected by removal of its endothelium. **C,** Diagram of cannulated arteriole. When the smooth muscle is relaxed by nitroprusside, the arteriole is passively distended by the increase in transmural pressure. *(Redrawn from Kuo L, Davis MJ, Chilian WM: Endothelium-dependent, flow-induced dilation of isolated coronary arterioles. Am J Physiol 259:H1063, 1990.)*

changes position (e.g., from lying to standing), a large change in transmural pressure occurs in the lower extremities. The precapillary vessels constrict in response to this imposed stretch. Consequently, flow ceases in most capillaries. After flow stops, capillary filtration diminishes until the increase in plasma oncotic pressure and the increase in interstitial fluid pressure balance the elevated capillary hydrostatic pressure that is produced by changing from a horizontal to a vertical position (see Chapters 8 and 10).

> If arteriolar resistance did not increase with standing, the hydrostatic pressure in the lower parts of the legs would reach such high levels that large volumes of fluid would pass from the capillaries into the interstitial fluid compartment and produce edema.

The Endothelium Actively Regulates Blood Flow

Stimulation of the endothelium elicits a response of the underlying vascular smooth muscle. To demonstrate this response, transmural pressure is kept constant in an isolated arteriole. A perfusion fluid reservoir connected to one end of an arteriole is raised to increase intravascular pressure. A reservoir that is connected to the other end of the arteriole is lowered simultaneously by an equal distance. This maneuver increases the longitudinal pressure gradient along the vessel, and flow-mediated vasodilation occurs (Figure 9-7A). If the arteriole is denuded of endothelium, the dilation of the vessel in response to increased flow is abolished (Figure 9-7B). The mechanism of flow-mediated vasodilation is ascribed to endothelial-derived hyperpolarization factor (EDHF), which comprises several soluble components released from endothelial cells in response to shear stress secondary to the increase in velocity of flow.

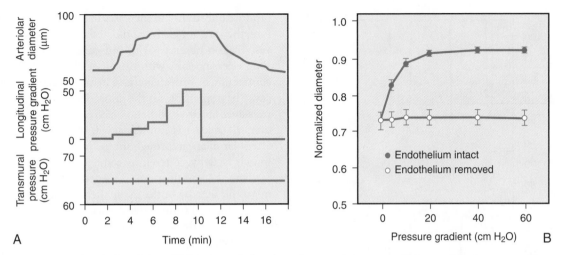

FIGURE 9-7 ■ **A,** Flow-induced vasodilation in an isolated cardiac arteriole at constant transmural pressure. Flow was increased progressively by increasing the pressure gradient in the long axis of the arteriole (longitudinal pressure gradient). **B,** Flow-induced vasodilation is abolished by removal of the endothelium of the arteriole. *(Redrawn from Kuo L, Davis MJ, Chilian WM: Endothelium-dependent, flow-induced dilation of isolated coronary arterioles.* Am J Physiol *259:H1063, 1990.)*

The mechanism of EDHF's action includes a hyperpolarization of the endothelial cell itself as well as of adjacent vascular smooth muscle. Hyperpolarization of the endothelial cell is initiated by activation of small (K_{Ca} 2.3) and intermediate (K_{Ca} 3.1) conductance K^+ channels from which K^+ leaves the cell. The rise of extracellular K^+ also stimulates the Na^+,K^+-ATPase, an action that contributes to endothelial cell hyperpolarization. The hyperpolarization is transmitted to adjacent vascular smooth muscle cells via myoendothelial cell gap junctions. The endothelial cell also releases soluble factors (NO, prostacyclin, H_2O_2, and epoxyeicosatrienoic acid) that cause hyperpolarization of vascular smooth muscle by activation of large conductance K_{Ca} channels (BK_{Ca}). This action moves the membrane potential farther from the threshold at which Ca^{++} entry occurs. EDHF becomes an increasingly important as a vasodilator in the microcirculation as vessel radius decreases.

Tissue Metabolic Activity Is the Main Factor in the Local Regulation of Blood Flow

According to the metabolic mechanism, any intervention that results in an O2 supply that is inadequate for the requirements of the tissue gives rise to the formation of vasodilator metabolites. These metabolites are released from the tissue, and they act locally to dilate the resistance vessels. When the metabolic rate of the tissue increases or the O_2 delivery to the tissue decreases, more vasodilator substance is released and the metabolite concentration in the tissue increases.

Many substances have been proposed as mediators of metabolic vasodilation. Some of the earliest substances suggested are lactic acid, CO_2, and hydrogen ions. However, the decrease in vascular resistance induced by supernormal concentrations of these dilator agents falls considerably short of the dilation observed under conditions of increased metabolic activity.

Changes in O_2 tension can evoke changes in the contractile state of vascular smooth muscle; an increase in Po_2 elicits contraction, whereas a decrease in Po_2 evokes relaxation. If significant reductions in the intravascular Po_2 occur before the arterial blood reaches the resistance vessels (diffusion through the arterial and arteriolar walls; see p. 157), small changes in O_2 supply or in consumption could elicit contraction or relaxation of the resistance vessels. However, direct measurements of Po_2 at the resistance vessels indicate that over a wide range of Po_2 (11 to 343 mm Hg), there is no correlation between O_2 tension and arteriolar diameter. Furthermore, if Po_2 were directly

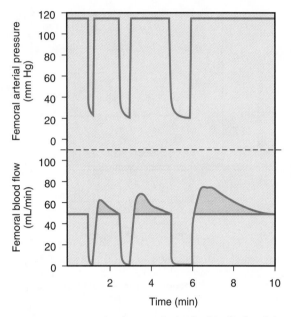

FIGURE 9-8 ■ Reactive hyperemia in the hindlimb of the dog after 15-, 30-, and 60-second occlusions of the femoral artery. *(From Berne RM: Unpublished observations.)*

responsible for vascular smooth muscle tension, one would not expect to find a parallelism between the duration of arterial occlusion and the duration of the reactive hyperemia (Figure 9-8). In response to either short occlusions (5 to 10 seconds) or long occlusions (1 to 3 minutes), the venous blood becomes bright red (well-oxygenated) within 1 or 2 seconds after release of the arterial occlusion. Hence the smooth muscle of the resistance vessels must be exposed to a high Po_2 in each instance. Nevertheless, the longer occlusions result in longer periods of reactive hyperemia. These observations are more compatible with the release of a vasodilator metabolite from the tissue than with a direct effect of Po_2 on the vascular smooth muscle.

Potassium ions, inorganic phosphate, and interstitial fluid osmolarity can also induce vasodilation. Because K^+ and phosphate are released and osmolarity is increased during skeletal muscle contraction, these factors may contribute to **active hyperemia** (i.e., increased blood flow caused by enhanced tissue activity). However, significant increases of phosphate concentration and osmolarity are not consistently observed during muscle contraction, and they may

produce only transient increases in blood flow. Therefore, they are not likely candidates as mediators of the vasodilation observed with muscular activity. Potassium release occurs with the onset of skeletal muscle contraction or with an increase in cardiac activity. This could be responsible for the initial decrease in vascular resistance observed with increased cardiac work. However, K^+ release is not sustained, despite continued arteriolar dilation throughout the period of enhanced muscle activity. Therefore some other agent must mediate the vasodilation associated with the greater metabolic activity of the tissue. Reoxygenated venous blood obtained from active cardiac and skeletal muscles under steady-state conditions of exercise does not elicit vasodilation when infused into a test vascular bed. It is difficult to see how oxygenation of the venous blood could alter its K^+ or phosphate content or its osmolarity and thereby destroy its vasodilator effect.

Adenosine, which is involved in coronary blood flow regulation, may also participate in the control of the resistance vessels in skeletal muscle. Furthermore, nitric oxide (NO) and prostaglandins have a role in flow-induced dilation of isolated perfused arterioles. In one study, wild-type (WT) mice and knockout (KO) mice (mice with deletion of the gene for encoding endothelial NO synthase) showed the same degree of arteriolar dilation to enhanced flow. In another, N^G-nitro-L-arginine methyl ester, an inhibitor of NO synthase, partially reduced the increased flow response in WT mice, but it had no effect on the response in the KO mice. Indomethacin, an inhibitor of prostaglandin synthesis, elicited partial reduction of flow-induced dilation in WT mice, but it abolished the response in KO mice. Combined administration of L-arginine and indomethacin abolished flow-induced dilation in the WT and in the KO mice.

Thus, a number of candidates exist for the role of mediator of metabolic vasodilation. The relative contribution of each of the various factors remains the subject for future investigation. Several factors may be involved in any given vascular bed, and different factors predominate in different tissues.

Metabolic control of vascular resistance by the release of a vasodilator substance is predicated on the existence of basal vessel tone. This tonic activity, or **basal tone,** of the vascular smooth muscle is readily demonstrable. However, in contrast to tone in skeletal muscle, it is independent of the nervous system. The factors responsible for basal tone in blood vessels are not known, but one or more of the following factors may be involved: (1) an expression of myogenic activity in response to the stretch imposed by the blood pressure, (2) the high O_2 tension of arterial blood, (3) the presence of Ca^{++}, or (4) some unknown factor in plasma, because addition of plasma to the bathing solution of isolated vessel segments evokes partial contraction of the smooth muscle.

If arterial inflow to a vascular bed is discontinued briefly, the blood flow, on release of the occlusion, immediately exceeds the flow before occlusion. The period of **reactive hyperemia** only gradually returns to the control level. This response is illustrated in Figure 9-8: Blood flow to the leg was stopped by clamping the femoral artery for 15, 30, and 60 seconds. Release of the 60-second occlusion resulted in a peak blood flow that was 70% greater than the control flow, and the flow returned to the control level within about 110 seconds. When this same experiment is performed in humans by inflating a blood pressure cuff on the upper arm, dilation of the resistance vessels of the hand and forearm, immediately after release of the cuff, is evident from the bright red color of the skin and the fullness of the veins. Within limits, the peak flow and particularly the duration of the reactive hyperemia are proportional to the duration of the occlusion (see Figure 9-8). If the extremity is exercised during the occlusion period, reactive hyperemia increases. These observations, and the close relationship that exists between metabolic activity and blood flow in the unoccluded limb, are consonant with a metabolic mechanism in the local regulation of tissue blood flow.

When the vascular smooth muscle of the arterioles relaxes in response to vasodilator metabolites released by a decrease in the O_2 supply/O_2 demand ratio of the tissue, resistance may diminish in the arteries that feed these arterioles. This results in a greater blood flow than is produced by arteriolar dilation alone. Two possible mechanisms can account for this coordination of arterial and arteriolar dilation. First, vasodilation in the microvessels is propagated, and when initiated in the arterioles, it can propagate from arterioles back to arteries. Second, the metabolite-mediated dilation of the arterioles accelerates blood flow in the feeder arteries.

This increases the shear stress on the arterial endothelium and thereby induces vasodilation.

EXTRINSIC CONTROL OF PERIPHERAL BLOOD FLOW IS MEDIATED MAINLY BY THE SYMPATHETIC NERVOUS SYSTEM

Impulses that Arise in the Medulla Descend in the Sympathetic Nerves to Increase Vascular Resistance

Several regions in the medulla influence cardiovascular activity. Some of the effects of stimulation of the dorsal lateral medulla (**pressor region**) are vasoconstriction, cardiac acceleration, and enhanced myocardial contractility. Caudal and ventromedial to the pressor region is a zone whose stimulation decreases the blood pressure. This **depressor area** exerts its effect by direct spinal inhibition and also by inhibition of the medullary pressor region. These areas constitute a center—not in an anatomic sense in that a discrete group of cells is discernible, but, in a physiologic sense, in that the stimulation of the pressor region produces the responses described previously. From the vasoconstrictor regions, fibers descend in the spinal cord and synapse at different levels of the thoracolumbar region (T1 to L2 or L3). Fibers from the intermediolateral gray matter of the cord emerge with the ventral roots, but they leave the motor fibers to join the paravertebral sympathetic chains through the white communicating branches. These preganglionic white (**myelinated**) fibers may pass up or down the sympathetic chains to synapse in the various ganglia. Postganglionic gray branches (**unmyelinated**) then join the corresponding segmental spinal nerves and accompany them to the periphery to innervate the arteries and veins. Postganglionic sympathetic fibers from the various ganglia join the large arteries and accompany them as an investing network of fibers to the resistance vessels (**small arteries and arterioles**) and capacitance vessels (**veins**).

The vasoconstrictor regions are tonically active, and reflexes or humoral stimuli that enhance this activity increase the frequency of impulses that reach the terminal branches to the vessels. At this location, a constrictor neurotransmitter (**norepinephrine**) is released and elicits constriction (α-adrenergic effect) of the resistance vessels. Inhibition of the vasoconstrictor areas reduces their tonic activity. Hence the frequency of impulses in the efferent nerve fibers diminishes, resulting in vasodilation. In this manner, neural regulation of the peripheral circulation is accomplished primarily by alteration of the frequency of impulses that pass down the vasoconstrictor fibers of the sympathetic nerves to the blood vessels. The vasomotor regions may show rhythmic changes in tonic activity that are manifested as oscillations of arterial pressure. Some oscillations occur at the frequency of respiration (**Traube-Hering waves**), and they are caused by an increase in sympathetic impulses to the resistance vessels coincident with inspiration. Other oscillations occur at a lower frequency than that of respiration (**Mayer waves**).

Sympathetic Nerves Regulate the Contractile State of the Resistance and Capacitance Vessels

The vasoconstrictor fibers of the sympathetic nervous system supply the arteries, arterioles, and veins. However, neural influence on the larger vessels is far less important than it is on the arterioles and small arteries. Capacitance vessels are more responsive to sympathetic nerve stimulation than are resistance vessels; they reach the maximal constriction at a lower frequency of stimulation than do the resistance vessels. However, capacitance vessels respond less to vasodilator metabolites. NE is the neurotransmitter released at the sympathetic nerve terminals in the blood vessels. Many factors, such as circulating hormones and in particular locally released substances, modify the liberation of norepinephrine from the vesicles of the nerve terminals.

The response of the resistance and capacitance vessels to stimulation of the sympathetic fibers is illustrated in Figure 9-9. At constant arterial pressure, sympathetic fiber stimulation reduces blood flow (**constriction of the resistance vessels**) and decreases blood volume of the tissues (**constriction of the capacitance vessels**). The abrupt decrease in tissue volume shown in the figure was caused by the movement of blood out of the capacitance vessels and out of the hindquarters of the cat, whereas the late, slow,

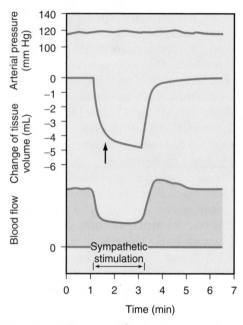

FIGURE 9-9 ■ Effect of sympathetic nerve stimulation (2 Hz) on blood flow and tissue volume in the hindquarters of the cat. The *arrow* denotes the change in slope of the tissue volume curve where the volume decrease caused by emptying of capacitance vessels ceases and loss of extravascular fluid becomes evident. *(Redrawn from Mellander S: Comparative studies on the adrenergic neuro-hormonal control of resistance and capacitance blood vessels in the cat. Acta Physiol Scand 50[Suppl 176]:1, 1960.)*

progressive decline in volume (to the right of the *arrow*) was caused by the movement of extravascular fluid into the capillaries and, hence, away from the tissue. The loss of tissue fluid is a consequence of the lowered capillary hydrostatic pressure brought about by constriction of the resistance vessels. A new equilibrium of the forces responsible for filtration and absorption was established across the capillary wall (see p. 165).

Section of the sympathetic nerves to an extremity, as might occur during peripheral arterial surgery, abolishes sympathetic vascular tone, thereby increasing limb flow. With time, vascular tone is regained by an increase in basal (intrinsic) tone.

Approximately one third of the blood volume of a tissue can be mobilized on stimulation of the sympathetic nerves at basal physiological frequencies. The basal tone is very low in capacitance vessels. When the veins are denervated, only small increases in volume are obtained with maximal doses of acetylcholine. Therefore, the blood volume at basal tone is close to the maximal blood volume of the tissue. More blood can be mobilized from the skin than from the muscle capacitance vessels. This action depends in part on the greater sensitivity of the skin vessels to sympathetic stimulation, but also because basal tone is lower in skin vessels than in muscle vessels. Therefore in the absence of neural influence, the skin capacitance vessels contain more blood than do the muscle capacitance vessels.

Blood is mobilized from capacitance vessels in response to physiological stimuli. In exercise, activation of the sympathetic nerve fibers constricts the veins and hence augments the cardiac filling pressure. In **arterial hypotension,** as induced by hemorrhage, the capacitance vessels constrict and thereby aid in overcoming the associated decrease in central venous pressure. Furthermore, the resistance vessels constrict in **hemorrhage shock,** and thereby help to restore the arterial pressure (see Chapter 13). Also, extravascular fluid is mobilized by a greater reabsorption of fluid from the tissues into the capillaries in response to the lowered capillary hydrostatic pressure that is caused by the lower arterial pressure.

Neural and humoral stimuli can exert similar or dissimilar effects on different segments of the vascular tree. In so doing, they can alter blood flow, tissue blood volume, and extravascular volume to meet the physiological requirements of the organism.

The Parasympathetic Nervous System Innervates Blood Vessels Only in the Cranial and Sacral Regions of the Body

The efferent fibers of the cranial division of the parasympathetic nervous system supply blood vessels of the head and viscera, whereas fibers of the sacral division supply blood vessels of the genitalia, bladder, and large bowel. Skeletal muscle and skin do not receive parasympathetic innervation. Because only a small proportion of the resistance vessels of the body receive parasympathetic fibers, the effect of these cholinergic fibers on total vascular resistance is small.

Epinephrine and Norepinephrine Are the Main Humoral Factors That Affect Vascular Resistance

Epinephrine and norepinephrine exert a profound effect on the peripheral blood vessels. In skeletal muscle, epinephrine in low concentrations dilates resistance vessels (**β-adrenergic effect**), and in high concentrations, it produces constriction (**α-adrenergic effect**). In skin, only vasoconstriction is obtained with epinephrine, whereas in all vascular beds the primary effect of norepinephrine is vasoconstriction. When stimulated, the adrenal gland can release epinephrine and norepinephrine into the systemic circulation. However, under physiologic conditions, the effect of catecholamine release from the adrenal medulla is less important than the norepinephrine released by sympathetic nerve activation.

The Vascular Reflexes Are Responsible for Rapid Adjustments of Blood Pressure

Areas of the medulla that mediate sympathetic and vagal effects are under the influence of neural impulses that arise in the baroreceptors, chemoreceptors, hypothalamus, cerebral cortex, and skin. These areas of the medulla are also affected by changes in the blood concentrations of CO_2 and O_2.

Arterial Baroreceptors

The **baroreceptors** (or **pressoreceptors**) are stretch receptors located in the **carotid sinuses** (slightly widened areas of the internal carotid arteries at their points of origin from the common carotid arteries) and in the **aortic arch** (Figure 9-10). Impulses that arise in the carotid sinus travel up the sinus nerve to the glossopharyngeal nerve and, via the latter, to the **nucleus of the tractus solitarius** (**NTS**) in the medulla. The NTS is the site of central projection of the chemoreceptors and baroreceptors. Stimulation of the NTS inhibits sympathetic nerve impulses to the peripheral blood vessels (**depressor effect**), whereas lesions of the NTS produce vasoconstriction (**pressor effect**). Impulses arising in the pressoreceptors of the aortic

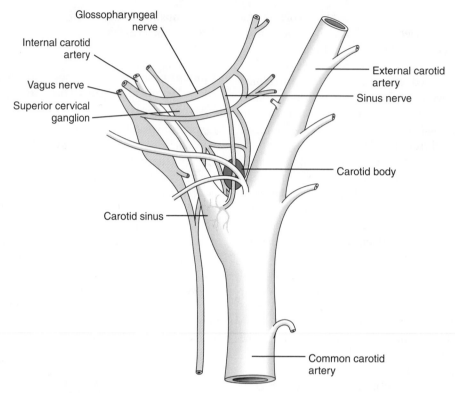

FIGURE 9-10 ■ Diagrammatic representation of the carotid sinus and carotid body and their innervation in the dog. *(Redrawn from Adams WE:* The comparative morphology of the carotid body and carotid sinus, *Springfield, Ill, 1958, Charles C Thomas.)*

arch reach the NTS via afferent fibers in the vagus nerves. *The pressoreceptor nerve terminals in the walls of the carotid sinus and aortic arch respond to the stretch and deformation of the vessel induced by the arterial pressure. The frequency of firing is enhanced by an increase in blood pressure and diminished by a reduction in blood pressure.* An increase in impulse frequency, as occurs with a rise in arterial pressure, inhibits the vasoconstrictor regions. This inhibition results in peripheral vasodilation and a lowering of blood pressure. Bradycardia, elicited by stimulation of the vagal nuclei in the medulla, contributes to a lowering of the blood pressure.

The carotid sinus and aortic baroreceptors are not equipotent in their effects on peripheral resistance in response to nonpulsatile alterations in blood pressure. Baroreceptors in the carotid sinus are more sensitive than are those in the aortic arch. Changes in pressure in the carotid sinus evoke greater alterations in systemic arterial pressure than do equivalent changes in

aortic arch pressure. However, with pulsatile changes in blood pressure, the two sets of baroreceptors respond similarly.

The carotid sinus, with the sinus nerve intact, can be isolated from the rest of the circulation and perfused by either a donor animal or an artificial perfusion system. Under these conditions, changes in the pressure within the carotid sinus are associated with reciprocal changes in the blood pressure of the experimental animal. The receptors in the walls of the carotid sinus display adaptation. Therefore, they respond more to constantly changing pressures than to sustained constant pressures. This is illustrated in Figure 9-11, which shows that at normal levels of mean blood pressure (about 100 mm Hg) a barrage of impulses from a single fiber of the sinus nerve is initiated in early systole by the pressure rise. Only a few spikes are observed during late systole and early diastole. At lower pressures, these phasic changes are even more evident, and the overall frequency of discharge is

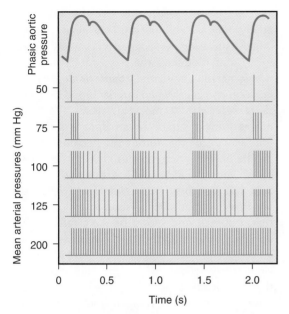

FIGURE 9-11 ▦ Relationship of phasic aortic blood pressure in the firing of a single afferent nerve fiber from the carotid sinus at different levels of mean arterial pressure.

reduced. The blood pressure threshold for eliciting sinus nerve impulses is about 50 mm Hg. A maximal, sustained firing is reached at around 200 mm Hg.

Because the pressoreceptors show some degree of adaptation, their response at any level of mean arterial pressure is greater with a large than with a small pulse pressure. This is illustrated in Figure 9-12, which shows the effects of damping pulsations in the carotid sinus on the frequency of firing in a the sinus nerve fiber and on the systemic arterial pressure. When the pulse pressure in the carotid sinuses is reduced with an air chamber, but mean pressure remains constant, the rate of electrical impulses recorded from a sinus nerve fiber decreases and the systemic arterial pressure increases. Restoration of the pulse pressure in the carotid sinus restores the frequency of sinus nerve discharge and systemic arterial pressure to control levels (see Figure 9-12).

The increases in resistance that occur in the peripheral vascular beds in response to reduced pressure in the carotid sinus vary from one vascular bed to another and thereby produce a redistribution of blood flow. For example, in the dog the resistance changes elicited by altering carotid sinus pressure around the normal operating sinus pressure are greatest in the femoral vessels, less in the renal, and least in the mesenteric and

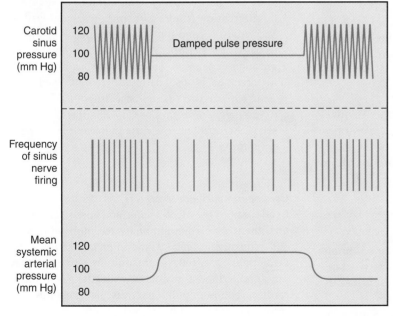

FIGURE 9-12 ▦ Effect of reducing pulse pressure in the vascularly isolated perfused carotid sinuses *(top record)* on impulses recorded from a fiber of a sinus nerve *(middle record)* and on mean systemic arterial pressure *(bottom record)*. Mean pressure in the carotid sinuses *(horizontal line, top record)* is held constant when pulse pressure is damped.

celiac vessels. Furthermore, the sensitivity of the carotid sinus reflex can be altered. Local application of norepinephrine, or stimulation of sympathetic nerve fibers to the carotid sinuses, enhances the sensitivity of the receptors in the sinus. Hence, a given increase in intrasinus pressure produces a greater depressor response. A decrease in baroreceptor sensitivity occurs in hypertension, when the carotid sinus becomes stiffer and less deformable as a result of the high intra-arterial pressure. Under these conditions, a given increase in carotid sinus pressure elicits a smaller decrement in systemic arterial pressure than it does at normal levels of blood pressure. In other words, the set-point of the baroreceptors is raised in hypertension, such that the threshold is increased and the receptors are less sensitive to change in transmural pressure.

As would be expected, denervation of the carotid sinuses can produce temporary, and in some instances prolonged, hypertension. *The arterial baroreceptors play a key role in short-term adjustments of blood pressure,* when relatively abrupt changes in blood volume, cardiac output, or peripheral resistance occur (as in exercise). However, *long-term control of blood pressure—that is, over days, weeks, and longer—is determined by the fluid balance of the individual, namely, the balance between fluid intake and fluid output.* By far the single most important organ in the control of body fluid volume, and hence of blood pressure, is the kidney. With overhydration, excessive fluid intake is excreted, whereas with dehydration, there is a marked reduction in urine output.

In some individuals the carotid sinus is quite sensitive to pressure. Hence tight collars or other forms of external pressure over the region of the carotid sinus may elicit marked hypotension and fainting.

CLINICAL BOX

Arterial blood pressure is maintained upon assuming an upright position because the tendency for blood to pool in peripheral vessels is opposed by the myogenic mechanism in arterioles (see Figure 9-6), by compression of veins by

contracting skeletal muscle (see Figure 12-2), and by baroreceptor-mediated reflexes (see Figure 9-10) that modulate the output of the autonomic nervous system. **Orthostatic** or **postural hypotension** occurs when arterial blood pressure decreases (>10-20 mm Hg) when a subject moves from a supine to an upright position. Malfunction of the autonomic nervous system can be one of several various causes of this disorder. Thus, the increased heart rate (see Figure 5-9) and vasoconstriction (see Figure 9-9) arising from sympathetic nervous activity are less than optimal, and blood pressure falls in the upright position. Orthostatic hypotension can arise from primary autonomic failure in which either preganglionic or postganglionic sympathetic neurons degenerate. The reduction of transmitter release at the ganglionic synapse or at the neuroeffector junction impairs the reflex adjustments needed to sustain arterial pressure. Medical management of orthostatic hypotension due to primary autonomic failure includes increased salt and fluid consumption, physical exercises before rising, and elastic support stockings. In more severe cases, drugs that activate α-adrenergic receptors (midodrine) or cause fluid retention (fludrocortisone) are employed. Secondary autonomic failure can occur in subjects having peripheral neuropathies involving autonomic neurons, as in diabetes. Orthostatic hypotension is also caused by drugs used to treat hypertension (diuretics, drugs that block α-adrenergic receptors or Ca^{++} channels on vessels). Adjustment of dose can alleviate the condition.

Cardiopulmonary Baroreceptors

In addition to the carotid sinus and aortic baroreceptors, there are cardiopulmonary receptors with vagal and sympathetic afferent and efferent nerves. These cardiopulmonary reflexes are tonically active, and they can alter peripheral resistance with changes in intracardiac, venous, or pulmonary vascular pressures. The receptors are located in the atria, ventricles, and pulmonary vessels.

The atria contain two types of receptors: those activated by the tension developed during atrial contraction (**A receptors**) and those activated by the stretch of the atria during atrial filling (**B receptors**). Stimulation of these atrial receptors sends impulses up vagal fibers to the vagal center in the medulla. Consequently, the sympathetic activity is decreased to the kidney and increased to the sinoatrial (SA) node. These changes in sympathetic activity increase renal blood flow, urine flow, and heart rate.

Activation of the cardiopulmonary receptors can also lower blood pressure reflexly by inhibiting the vasoconstrictor center in the medulla. Stimulation of the receptors inhibits angiotensin, aldosterone, and vasopressin (ADH) release; and interruption of the reflex pathway has the opposite effects. Changes in urine volume elicited by changes in cardiopulmonary baroreceptor activation are important in the regulation of blood volume. For example, a decrease in blood volume (hypovolemia), as occurs in hemorrhage, enhances sympathetic vasoconstriction in the kidney and increases secretion of renin, angiotensin, aldosterone, and ADH. The renal vasoconstriction (primarily afferent arteriolar) reduces glomerular filtration and increases **renin** release from the kidney. Renin acts on a plasma substrate to form **angiotensin I**, a decapeptide. In turn, angiotensin I is metabolized to **angiotensin II** by angiotensin-converting enzyme. Angiotensin II increases aldosterone release from the adrenal cortex, which in turn enhances retention of NaCl. The enhanced release of ADH increases water reabsorption. The net result is retention of salt and water by the kidney and a sensation of thirst. Angiotensin II also causes vasoconstriction to raise systemic arteriolar tone.

The Peripheral Chemoreceptors Are Stimulated by Decreases in Blood Oxygen Tension and pH and by Increases in Carbon Dioxide Tension

The peripheral chemoreceptors consist of small, highly vascular bodies in the region of the aortic arch (**aortic bodies**) and in the carotid bodies just medial to the carotid sinuses (see Figure 9-10). Although they are primarily concerned with the regulation of respiration, the chemoreceptors reflexly influence the vasomotor

regions to a minor degree. A reduction in arterial blood O_2 tension (Pao_2) stimulates the chemoreceptors. The consequent increase in the number of impulses in the afferent nerve fibers from the carotid and aortic bodies stimulates the vasoconstrictor regions. This action increases the tone of the resistance and capacitance vessels.

Stimulation of the peripheral chemoreceptors by increased arterial blood CO_2 tension ($Paco_2$) and reduced pH elicit a reflex response that is minimal compared with the direct effect of **hypercapnia** (high $Paco_2$) and of H^+ on the vasomotor regions in the medulla. When hypoxia and hypercapnia coexist (asphyxia), the stimulation of the chemoreceptors is greater than the sum of the two gas stimuli when each acts alone. The effects of asphyxia on blood pressure, heart rate, and respiration are shown in Figure 9-13 (see also Figures 5-14 and 5-15).

When the chemoreceptors are stimulated simultaneously with a pressure reduction in the baroreceptors, the chemoreceptors potentiate the vasoconstriction observed in the peripheral vessels. However, when the baroreceptors and chemoreceptors are stimulated together (e.g., high carotid sinus pressure and low $Paco_2$), the effects of the baroreceptors predominate.

Chemoreceptors with sympathetic afferent fibers are present in the heart. These cardiac chemoreceptors are activated by ischemia and transmit the precordial pain (**angina pectoris**) associated with an inadequate blood supply to the myocardium.

The Central Chemoreceptors Are Sensitive to Changes in $Paco_2$

Increases of $Paco_2$ stimulate chemosensitive regions of the medulla, thereby eliciting vasoconstriction and increased peripheral resistance. Reduction in $Paco_2$ below normal levels (as with hyperventilation) decreases the degree of tonic activity of these areas in the medulla, thereby reducing peripheral resistance. The chemosensitive regions are also affected by changes in pH. A lowering of blood pH stimulates, and a rise in blood pH inhibits, these areas. These effects of

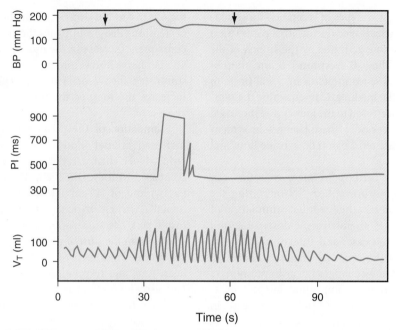

FIGURE 9-13 ▪ Effects of stimulation of the isolated perfused carotid body chemoreceptors at constant carotid sinus perfusion pressure, through substitution of hypoxic hypercapnic blood (P_{O_2}, 31.1 mm Hg; P_{CO_2}, 84.9 mm Hg; pH, 7.242) for arterial blood (P_{O_2}, 140.4 mm Hg; P_{CO_2}, 42.1 mm Hg; pH, 7.33) between *arrows*. Note that the bradycardia was transient. The increase in pulse interval (PI) indicates a decrease in heart rate. The enhanced respiratory response *(bottom record)* abolishes bradycardia and can produce tachycardia, especially with sustained stimulation of the carotid body receptors (see Figures 5-16 and 5-17). BP, mean arterial blood pressure; V_T, tidal volume. *(Redrawn from de Burgh Daly M, Korner PI, Angell-James JE, et al: Cardiovascular and respiratory effects of carotid body stimulation in the monkey. Clin Exp Pharmacol Physiol 5:511, 1978.)*

changes in Pa_{CO_2} and blood pH possibly operate through changes in cerebrospinal fluid pH, as appears to apply to the respiratory center.

Oxygen tension has relatively little direct effect on the medullary vasomotor region. The primary effect of hypoxia is reflexly mediated via the carotid and aortic chemoreceptors. Moderate reduction of Pa_{CO_2} stimulates the vasomotor region, but severe reduction depresses vasomotor activity, in the same manner that other areas of the brain are depressed by very low O_2 tensions.

At high altitudes, the low Pa_{O_2} stimulates the peripheral chemoreceptors to increase the rate and depth of respiration. This is the main mechanism involved in an attempt to restore the oxygen supply to the body.

Other Vascular Reflexes

Hypothalamus

Optimal function of the cardiovascular reflexes requires the integrity of the pontine and hypothalamic structures. Furthermore, these structures are responsible for behavioral and emotional control of the cardiovascular system. Stimulation of the anterior hypothalamus decreases the blood pressure and heart rate, whereas stimulation of the posterolateral region of the hypothalamus increases the blood pressure and heart rate. The hypothalamus also contains a temperature-regulating center that affects the skin vessels. Stimulation by cold applications to the skin or by cooling of the blood perfusing the hypothalamus results in constriction of the skin vessels and heat conservation, whereas warm stimuli result in cutaneous vasodilation and enhanced heat loss (see Chapter 12).

Cerebrum

The cerebral cortex can also exert a significant effect on blood flow distribution in the body. Stimulation of the motor and premotor areas can affect blood pressure; usually a pressor response is obtained. However, vasodilation and depressor responses may be evoked (e.g., blushing or fainting) in response to an emotional stimulus.

> Cerebral ischemia, which may occur because of excessive pressure exerted by an expanding intracranial tumor, results in a marked increase in peripheral vasoconstriction. The stimulation is probably caused by a local accumulation of CO_2 and reduction of O_2, and possibly by excitation of intracranial baroreceptors. With prolonged, severe ischemia, central depression eventually supervenes and blood pressure falls.

Skin and Viscera

Painful stimuli can elicit either pressor or depressor responses, depending on the magnitude and location of the stimulus. Distention of the viscera often evokes a depressor response, whereas painful stimuli on the body surface usually evoke a pressor response.

Pulmonary Reflexes

Inflation of the lungs reflexly induces systemic vasodilation and a decrease in arterial blood pressure. Conversely, collapse of the lungs evokes systemic vasoconstriction. Afferent fibers that mediate this reflex are carried by the vagus nerves. Their stimulation, by stretch of the lungs, inhibits the vasomotor areas. The magnitude of the depressor response to lung inflation is directly related to the degree of inflation and to the existing level of vasoconstrictor tone; the greater the vascular tone, the greater the hypotension produced by lung inflation.

BALANCE BETWEEN EXTRINSIC AND INTRINSIC FACTORS IN REGULATION OF PERIPHERAL BLOOD FLOW

Dual control of the peripheral vessels by intrinsic and extrinsic mechanisms makes possible a number of vascular adjustments. Such regulations enable the body to direct blood flow to areas where the need is greater and

away from areas where the need is less. The relative potency of extrinsic and intrinsic mechanisms is constant in some tissues, whereas in other tissues the ratio is changeable, depending on the state of activity of that tissue.

In the brain and the heart, both vital structures with very limited tolerance for a reduced blood supply, intrinsic flow-regulating mechanisms are dominant.

> Massive discharge of the vasoconstrictor region over the sympathetic nerves, which might occur in severe, acute hemorrhage, has negligible effects on the cerebral and cardiac resistance vessels, whereas skin, renal, and splanchnic blood vessels become greatly constricted.

In the skin the extrinsic vascular control is dominant. The cutaneous vessels not only participate strongly in a general vasoconstrictor discharge but also respond selectively through hypothalamic pathways to subserve the heat loss and heat conservation function required in body temperature regulation. However, intrinsic control can be demonstrated by local changes of temperature that can modify or override the central influence on resistance and capacitance vessels.

In skeletal muscle the interplay and changing balance between extrinsic and intrinsic mechanisms can be clearly seen. In resting skeletal muscle, neural control (**vasoconstrictor tone**) is dominant, as can be demonstrated by the large increment in blood flow that occurs immediately after section of the sympathetic nerves to the tissue. In anticipation of exercise, and at the start of exercise, blood flow increases in the leg muscles. After the onset of exercise, the intrinsic flow-regulating mechanisms elicit vasodilation in the active muscles because of the local increase in metabolites. Vasoconstriction occurs in the inactive muscles as a manifestation of the general sympathetic discharge associated with exercise. However, the constrictor impulses that reach the resistance vessels of the active muscles are overridden by the local metabolic effects that dilate them. Hence, operation of this dual-control mechanism provides increased blood flow where it is required and shunts it away from inactive areas.

Similar effects may be achieved with an increase in Pa_{CO_2}. Normally, the hyperventilation associated with

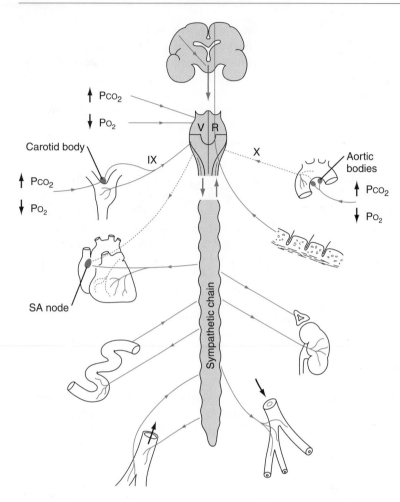

FIGURE 9-14 ■ Schematic diagram illustrating the neural input and output of the vasomotor region (VR). IX, glossopharyngeal nerve; X, vagus nerve.

exercise keeps $Paco_2$ at normal levels. However, were $Paco_2$ to increase, a generalized vasoconstriction would occur, because of stimulation of the medullary vasoconstrictor region by CO_2. In the active muscles, where the CO_2 concentration is highest, the smooth muscle of the arterioles would relax in response to the local Pco_2. Factors affecting and affected by the vasomotor region are summarized in Figure 9-14.

SUMMARY

- The arterioles, often referred to as the resistance vessels, are important in the regulation of blood flow through their cognate capillaries. The smooth muscle, which makes up a major fraction of the walls of the arterioles, contracts and relaxes in response to neural and humoral stimuli.
- Most tissues show autoregulation of blood flow, a phenomenon characterized by a constant blood flow in the face of a change in perfusion pressure. A logical explanation of autoregulation is the myogenic mechanism whereby an increase in transmural pressure elicits a contractile response, whereas a decrease in transmural pressure elicits relaxation.
- The striking parallelism between tissue blood flow and tissue O_2 consumption indicates that blood flow is largely regulated by a metabolic mechanism.

A decrease in the O_2 supply/O_2 demand ratio of a tissue releases one or more vasodilator metabolites that dilate arterioles and thereby enhance the oxygen supply.

- Neural regulation of blood flow is accomplished mainly by the sympathetic nervous system. Sympathetic nerves to blood vessels are tonically active; inhibition of the vasoconstrictor center in the medulla reduces peripheral vascular resistance. Stimulation of the sympathetic nerves constricts resistance and capacitance (veins) vessels.

- Blood vessels in the head, viscera, and genitalia are supplied by the cranial and sacral divisions of the parasympathetic nervous system as well as by the sympathetic nervous system. Parasympathetic activity usually induces vasodilation, but the effect is generally weak.

- The baroreceptors (pressoreceptors) in the internal carotid arteries and aorta are tonically active and regulate blood pressure on a moment-to-moment basis. Stretch of these receptors by an increase in arterial pressure reflexly inhibits the vasoconstrictor center in the medulla and induces vasodilation, whereas a decrease in arterial pressure disinhibits the vasoconstrictor center and induces vasoconstriction.

- The carotid baroreceptors predominate over baroreceptors in the aorta and both respond more vigorously to pulsatile (stretch) than they do to steady (nonpulsatile) pressure; they adapt to an imposed constant pressure.

- Baroreceptors are also present in the cardiac chambers and large pulmonary vessels (cardiopulmonary baroreceptors); they have less influence on blood pressure but they participate in blood volume regulation.

- Peripheral chemoreceptors (carotid and aortic bodies) and central chemoreceptors in the medulla oblongata are stimulated by a decrease in blood oxygen tension (Pao_2) and an increase in blood carbon dioxide tension ($Paco_2$). Stimulation of these chemoreceptors increases the rate and depth of respiration but also produces peripheral vasoconstriction.

- Peripheral resistance, and hence blood pressure, can be affected by stimuli arising in the skin, viscera, lungs, and brain.

- The combined effect of neural and local metabolic factors is to distribute blood to active tissues and divert it from inactive tissues. In vital structures such as the heart and brain and in contracting skeletal muscle, the metabolic factors predominate over the neural factors.

ADDITIONAL READING

Bellien JM, Iacob M, Gutierres L, et al: Crucial role of NO and endothelium-derived hyperpolarizing factor in the radial artery in humans, *Am J Physiol* 290:H1347, 2006.

Berg BR, Cohen KD, Sarelius IH: Direct coupling between blood flow and metabolism at the capillary level in striated muscle, *Am J Physiol* 272:H2693, 1997.

Bolton TB, Prestwich SA, Zholos AV, Gordienko DV: Excitation-contraction coupling in gastrointestinal and other smooth muscles, *Annu Rev Physiol* 61:85, 1999.

Dampney RA, Horiuchi J, Tagawa T, et al: Medullary and supra-medullary mechanisms regulating sympathetic vasomotor tone, *Acta Physiol Scand* 177:209, 2003.

Edwards G, Félétou M, Weston AH: Endothelium-derived hyperpolarizing factors and associated pathways: a synopsis, *Pflügers Arch* 459:863, 2010.

Kara T, Narkiewicz K, Somers VK: Chemoreflexes—physiology and clinical implications, *Acta Physiol Scand* 177:377, 2003.

Kohan DE, Rossi NF, Inscho EW, Pollock DM: Regulation of blood pressure and salt homeostasis by endothelin, *Physiol Rev* 91:1, 2011.

Liu Y, Bubolz AH, Mendoza S, et al: H_2O_2 is the transferrable factor mediating flow-induced dilation in human coronary arterioles, *Circ Res* 108:566, 2011.

Maguire JJ, Davenport AP: Regulation of vascular reactivity by established and emerging GPCRs, *Trends Pharmacol Sci* 26:448, 2005.

Mifflin SW: What does the brain know about blood pressure? *News Physiol Sci* 16:266, 2001.

Monos E, Berczi V, Nadasy G: Local control of veins: Biomechanical, metabolic, and humoral aspects, *Physiol Rev* 75:611, 1995.

Moore A, Mangoni AA, Lyons D, Jackson SH: The cardiovascular system, *Br J Clin Pharmacol* 56:254, 2003.

Osborn JW, Jacob F, Guzman P: A neural set point for the long-term control of arterial pressure: Beyond the arterial baroreceptor reflex, *Am J Physiol* 288:R846, 2005.

Persson PB: Modulation of cardiovascular control mechanisms and their interaction, *Physiol Rev* 76:193, 1996.

Shamsuzzaman AS, Somers VK: Cardiorespiratory interactions in neural circulatory control in humans, *Ann N Y Acad Sci* 940:488, 2001.

Somlyo AP, Somlyo AV: Ca^{2+} sensitivity of smooth muscle and non-muscle myosin II: modulated by G proteins, kinases, and myosin phosphatase, *Physiol Rev.* 83:1325, 2003.

Sun D, Huang A, Smith CJ, et al: Enhanced release of prostaglandins to flow-induced arteriolar dilation in eNOs knockout mice, *Circ Res* 85:288, 1999.

Thrasher TN: Baroreceptors, baroreceptor unloading, and the long-term control of blood pressure, *Am J Physiol* 288:R819, 2005.

Timmers HJ, Wieling W, Karemaker JM, Lenders JW: Cardiovascular responses to stress after carotid baroreceptor denervation in humans, *Ann N Y Acad Sci* 1018:515, 2004.

CASE 9-1

HISTORY

A 40-year-old man sees his physician because of pain in the calves of both legs when he walks moderate distances; the pain is especially noticeable when he walks uphill or when he climbs stairs. The onset of the pain was insidious and has progressively increased in frequency and severity. He has had no other symptoms. He eats a normal diet, has two cocktails before dinner, and has smoked two packs of cigarettes per day for the past 22 years. Physical examination was essentially normal except for the presence of borderline hypertension with a brachial pressure of 140/90 mm Hg and for weak pulses in the dorsalis pedis and posterior tibial arteries in both legs. Measurement of blood pressure in the dorsalis pedis artery gave a systolic pressure of 112 mm Hg. Arteriography revealed a narrowing of the major arteries of both lower legs. He was diagnosed as having thromboangiitis obliterans, a severe progressive obstructive disease of large arteries.

QUESTIONS

1. At rest the arterioles in the lower legs show:
   a. myogenic constriction.
   b. metabolic dilation.
   c. autoregulation.
   d. myogenic dilation.
   e. metabolic constriction.

2. From the blood pressure measurements you obtain an ankle-brachial index of (see Chapter 7) of:
   a. 1.24.
   b. 1.04.
   c. 0.96.
   d. 0.80.
   e. 0.64.

3. His physician would probably recommend:
   a. that he stops smoking.
   b. a vasodilator drug.
   c. bilateral sympathectomy of the lower extremities.
   d. application of heat to the lower legs 3 to 4 times daily.
   e. a vasoconstrictor drug.

10

CONTROL OF CARDIAC OUTPUT: COUPLING OF HEART AND BLOOD VESSELS

OBJECTIVES

1. Describe the principal determinants of cardiac output.

2. Describe the principal determinants of cardiac preload and afterload.

3. Explain the mechanical coupling between the heart and blood vessels.

4. Explain the effects of gravity on venous function and on arterial pressure.

Cardiac output (CO) is defined as the total flow of blood out of the left ventricle. It could be measured in the aorta, except for that portion of the total output that flows to the heart itself via the coronary circulation. Cardiac output is thus the total flow that is available to perfuse all the tissues of the body. In order to meet the metabolic demands of the body, and maintain arterial pressure, cardiac output must be able to increase substantially. During severe exercise (see Chapter 13), cardiac output can increase 4- to 5-fold. In general, this is accomplished by increases in heart rate (up to 3-fold, in young adults) and increases in stroke volume (up to about 1.5-fold). In such exercise, this increase in cardiac output enables an increase in overall O_2 consumption of approximately 12 times (untrained young male). Because total peripheral resistance during exercise decreases to a little as one-third the resting value, the increase in cardiac output is essential to maintain the mean arterial pressure.

Changes in both the heart and the systemic vasculature are required to produce the increased cardiac output.

FACTORS CONTROLLING CARDIAC OUTPUT

Four factors that control cardiac output are heart rate, myocardial contractility, preload, and afterload (Figure 10-1). Heart rate and myocardial contractility are strictly cardiac factors. They are characteristics of the cardiac tissues, although they are modulated by various neural and humoral mechanisms. Preload and afterload, however, depend on the characteristics of both the heart and the vascular system. *On the one hand, preload and afterload are important determinants of cardiac output. On the other hand, preload and afterload are themselves determined by the cardiac output and by certain vascular*

195

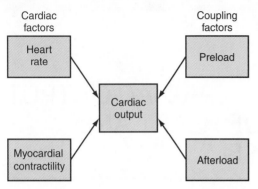

FIGURE 10-1 ▓ The four factors that determine cardiac output.

characteristics. Preload and afterload may be designated as coupling factors because they constitute a functional coupling between the heart and blood vessels.

To understand the regulation of cardiac output, one must appreciate the nature of the coupling between the heart and the vascular system. Graphic techniques have been developed to analyze the interactions between the cardiac and vascular components of the circulatory system. The graphic analysis involves two simultaneous functional relationships between **cardiac output** and **central venous pressure** (i.e., the pressure in the right atrium and thoracic venae cavae).

The **cardiac function curve** (**CFC**) defines one of these relationships. It is an expression of the well-known Frank-Starling relationship (see Chapters 4 and 5), and it reflects the dependence of cardiac output on preload (i.e., on central venous, or right atrial, pressure). *The cardiac function curve is a characteristic of the heart itself,* and it has been studied in hearts that have been completely isolated from the rest of the circulatory system.

The **vascular function curve** defines the dependence of the central venous pressure on the cardiac output. This relationship depends only on certain vascular system characteristics, namely peripheral resistance, arterial and venous compliances, and blood volume. *The vascular function curve is entirely independent of the characteristics of the heart,* and it can be evaluated even if the heart was replaced by a mechanical pump.

THE CARDIAC FUNCTION CURVE RELATES CENTRAL VENOUS PRESSURE (PRELOAD) TO CARDIAC OUTPUT

Preload or Filling Pressure of the heart

The greater the preload of the heart, the greater the cardiac output. In the intact circulation, it will be the pressure in the great veins (i.e., the central venous pressure [CVP]) that constitutes the preload of the heart. In the whole heart, the stretch of the ventricles prior to systole will determine the strength of the subsequent contraction, by the cellular mechanisms discussed earlier (see Chapter 4). The cardiac output is the output of the left ventricle, but it is the preload of the right ventricle that ultimately actually determines the cardiac output. The reason is that, during periods when cardiac output is constant, and within limits, the left ventricle will pump whatever volume of blood comes to it, from the right side of the heart. Thus, it is the filling pressure on the right side of the heart that ultimately determines the output on the left. The filling pressure on the right side of the heart is functionally equal to the central venous pressure. In the intact circulation, the preload is considered to be the CVP, which is approximately equal to the mean right atrial pressure ($\overline{P}_{ra}$), which, when the tricuspid valve is open, is approximately equal to the right ventricular pressure. The relationship between preload or filling pressure and stroke volume (or cardiac output) is shown in the cardiac function curve. Cardiac function curves are also known as "Starling curves" or ventricular function curves. Partial curves can be obtained in human subjects, through the use of intracardiac pressure and volume transducers. The cardiac function curve is a manifestation of the Frank-Starling relationship or length-dependence of cardiac contraction.

Cardiac Function Curve

The CFC will be derived by using left ventricular pressure-volume (P-V) loops to illustrate the effect that varying preload has on the stroke volume (SV). In the CFC, stroke volume (or the proportional quantity, CO) is plotted as a function of filling pressure, or preload. For the left ventricle, a measure of preload is the

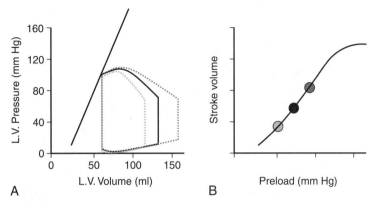

FIGURE 10-2 ■ The cardiac function curve (CFC) shows the relationship between preload and cardiac output (or stroke volume). A single CFC (panel **B**) can be obtained by varying preload to produce different stroke volumes of the left ventricle (LV), as shown in the pressure-volume loops (panel **A**). The *straight line* represents the end-systolic pressure-volume relationship (ESPVR). Three individual P-V loops are illustrated, and each is characterized by a different stroke volume. The three different stroke volumes are plotted in **B** vs. the preload at which they were obtained. When stroke volume is measured at many different preloads, the continuous curve in **B** is obtained, which is the complete cardiac function curve.

left ventricular end-diastolic pressure (LVEDP). In an experimental situation in which an isolated animal heart is used, the preload of the left ventricle may be varied by changing the height of a reservoir of blood that is connected to the left ventricle (see Chapter 5). Raising or lowering the reservoir increases or decreases the pressure in the left ventricle and is one way in which preload can be changed in an experimental setting. The effect of changing preload on the left ventricular P-V loop is shown in Figure 10-2A. Decreased preload is associated with decreased end-diastolic volume, and increased preload with increased end-diastolic volume. However, the contractility of the ventricle has not changed in this example, and thus the end-systolic pressure-volume relationship (the *straight line* that indicates the maximum pressure the ventricle can produce at a given volume) has not changed and therefore the end-systolic volume does not change when preload changes. The result is that increased preload results in an increased stroke volume and decreased preload results in a decreased stroke volume. When the different stroke volumes are then plotted against the preload pressures at which they occurred (Figure 10-2B), the entire relationship yields the CFC. A CFC obtained from measurements in 75 patients in whom left ventricular end-diastolic pressure was varied (by various means) (Figure 10-3)

verifies that the CFC is a feature of cardiac function in humans.

Factors that Change the Cardiac Function Curve

Contractility
Increases in cardiac contractility, as produced by the actions of norepinephrine or epinephrine on the heart, are a primary way in which cardiac output is increased physiologically. These substances, acting to increase contractility by the cellular mechanisms already presented (see Chapters 4 and 5), have the effect of raising the peak pressure that can be developed at a given left ventricular volume. Increases in contractility are reflected in an end-systolic pressure-volume relationship that is shifted upward and to the left (increased slope), and vice versa for decreases in contractility, as might occur with cardiac damage. Increases in contractility thus increase stroke volume by decreasing end-systolic volume (Figure 10-4A). At each preload, stroke volume is increased with increased contractility, and thus the entire cardiac function curve is increased upwardly (Figure 10-4B). Decreased contractility results in a decreased stroke volume at all preloads. With a change in contractility, the heart will be characterized by a completely new cardiac function curve, which still,

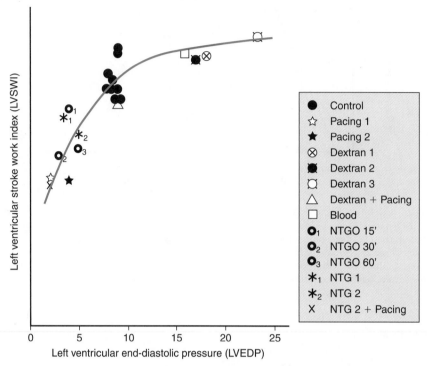

FIGURE 10-3 ■ Cardiac function curve in humans. Preload of the left ventricle (measured as left ventricular end-diastolic pressure) was varied by various interventions in 75 patients. A composite graph for 75 patients in whom left ventricular end-diastolic pressure (LVEDP) was modified as shown. Each *point* represents the mean value for a particular intervention and includes from 4 to 21 patients, with a total of 102 interventions. Left ventricular stroke work index (LVSWI) is positively related to LVEDP up to 10 mm Hg (LVSWI = 24.4 + 2.70 LVEDP); thereafter, there is little increase in LVSWI as LVEDP increases further. NTG, sublingual nitroglycerin; NTGO, nitroglycerin ointment with observations made after 15, 30, and 60 minutes. *(Modified from Parker JO, Case RB: Normal left ventricular function.* Circulation *60:4, 1979.)*

however, reflects the Frank-Starling relationship or the length-dependence of cardiac contraction.

Afterload

Afterload is the load experienced by the left ventricle after the aortic valve opens (ending the isovolumic contraction phase). Afterload is thus related to the arterial blood pressure as well as to the hemodynamic properties of the arterial system (which will influence the dynamics of the arterial blood pressure during ejection of the stroke volume into the arterial system; see Chapter 7). Increases in afterload are represented on the left ventricular P-V loop as a higher pressure throughout the ejection phase (Figure 10-5A). When the diastolic arterial blood pressure is elevated, the isovolumic contraction must then develop a higher pressure in the left ventricle (compared with normal basal

state) before the aortic valve can be forced open. If ventricular contractility is constant, the end-systolic P-V relationship is not altered, and therefore the stroke volume is reduced, because the heart is not able to achieve a lower end-systolic volume (it does not have an increased ability to "squeeze down" against the elevated pressure). Conversely, decreases in afterload result in increased stroke volume, because the heart is able to squeeze down more, achieving a lower end-systolic volume. A change in afterload places the left ventricle on a completely new function curve (Figure 10-5B), which still displays the length-dependence of cardiac contraction.

Myocardial Compliance

Damaged or ischemic heart muscle is less compliant ("stiffer") than normal heart muscle. In the absence of

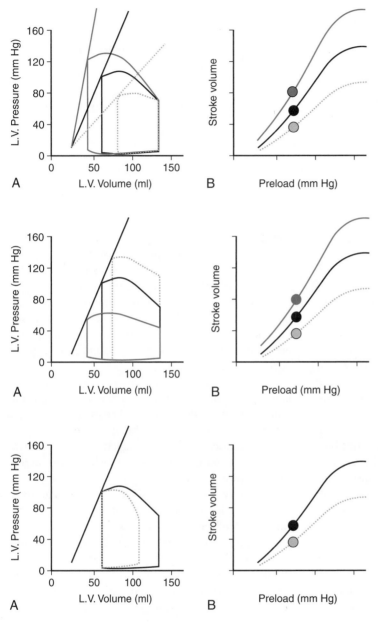

FIGURE 10-4 ■ Effect of altered contractility on left ventricular (L.V.) pressure-volume loops (**A**) and cardiac function curves (**B**). Increasing left ventricular contractility increases the slope of the end-systolic pressure volume relation, decreases end-systolic volume, and increases stroke volume. Solid black lines represent the normal, basal state; dotted blue lines, decreased contractility; and solid blue lines, increased contractility. Filled circles in (**B**) represent the stroke volumes of the correspondingly colored pressure-volume loops in (**A**).

FIGURE 10-5 ■ Effect of altered afterload on left ventricular (L.V.) pressure-volume loops (**A**) and cardiac function curves (**B**). Increasing afterload results in decreased stroke volume, because of increased end-systolic volume. Black solid lines represent normal basal state; blue dotted lines, increased afterload; and solid blue lines, decreased afterload. Filled circles in (**B**) represent the stroke volumes of the correspondingly colored pressure-volume loops in (**A**).

FIGURE 10-6 ■ Effect of decreasing ventricular compliance on the left ventricular (L.V.) pressure-volume loop (**A**) and the cardiac function curve (**B**). Decreased myocardial compliance results in reduced filling during diastole, hence decreased end-diastolic volume and stroke volume. Black solid lines represent normal basal state; and dotted blue line, decreased ventricular compliance. Filled circles in (**B**) represent the stroke volumes of the correspondingly colored pressure-volume loops in (**A**).

any other changes, the result is less filling during diastole and a reduced end-diastolic volume (Figure 10-6A). If contractility is not changed, then the stroke volume will be markedly reduced and the left ventricle will operate on a new cardiac function curve (Figure 10-6B) that is depressed compared with the normal basal state.

Cardiac Function Curves and Physiological Function

Heart rate is a major physiological determinant of cardiac output, because CO = HR × SV. Thus, it is useful to plot cardiac output, rather than stroke volume, as a function of preload (Figure 10-7). Increased heart rate, increased contractility, and decreased afterload are all

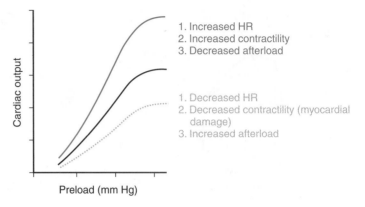

1. Increased HR
2. Increased contractility
3. Decreased afterload

1. Decreased HR
2. Decreased contractility (myocardial damage)
3. Increased afterload

FIGURE 10-7 ▌ Summary of factors that change the cardiac function curve and can thus affect cardiac output. HR, heart rate.

factors that increase cardiac output at a given preload. Conversely, decreased heart rate, decreased contractility, increased afterload, and decreased compliance all decrease cardiac output at a given preload. Physiologically, the changes in cardiac function are rarely (if ever) as simple as can be achieved in isolated heart preparations, as illustrated in the simple schemes shown in Figures 10-2, and 10-4 through 10-6). For example, an increase in contractility produced by increased sympathetic drive to the heart (increased release of norepinephrine) tends to raise stroke volume as shown (see Figure 10-4), but heart rate also increases, with a resultant greater cardiac output. Because mean arterial pressure is the arithmetic product of cardiac output and total peripheral resistance, there is an increase in mean arterial pressure, which constitutes an increase in afterload, an effect that tends to decrease stroke volume. Thus, it is important to remember that physiologically, multiple changes usually occur simultaneously. Most importantly, the filling pressure of the heart is greatly influenced by conditions in the systemic blood vessels. The effect that factors in the systemic vasculature have on the filling pressure of the heart, and hence on cardiac output, are quantified with the **vascular function curve, or VFC**, as discussed next.

THE VASCULAR FUNCTION CURVE RELATES CENTRAL VENOUS PRESSURE TO CARDIAC OUTPUT

The vascular function curve is independent of the Frank-Starling relationship, length-dependence of cardiac contraction. *The vascular function curve defines the changes in central venous pressure evoked by changes in cardiac output;* that is, central venous pressure is the **dependent variable** (or **response**), and cardiac output is the **independent variable** (or **stimulus**). This situation contrasts with that in the cardiac function curve, in which central venous pressure (or preload) is the independent variable and cardiac output is the dependent variable.

A simplified model of the circulation helps explain how cardiac output determines the level of central venous pressure (Figure 10-8). The essential components of the cardiovascular system have been lumped into four elements. The right and left sides of the heart, as well as the pulmonary vascular bed, are considered simply a **pump,** much as that employed during open heart surgery. The high-resistance microcirculation is designated the **peripheral resistance.** Finally, the compliance of the system is subdivided into two components, the **arterial compliance, C_a,** and the **venous compliance, C_v.** As defined in Chapter 7, compliance (C) is the increment of volume (ΔV) accommodated per unit change of pressure (ΔP); that is:

$$C = \Delta V / \Delta P \qquad (1)$$

The venous compliance is about 20 times as great as the arterial compliance. In the example that follows, the ratio of C_v to C_a is set at 19:1 to simplify certain calculations. Thus, if it was necessary to add x mL of blood to the arterial system to produce a 1–mm Hg increment in arterial pressure, it would be necessary to add 19x mL of blood to the venous system to raise venous pressure by the same amount.

A Control state

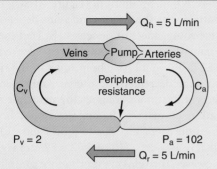

$Q_h = 5$ L/min

Veins Pump Arteries

C_v

Peripheral resistance

C_a

$P_v = 2$ $P_a = 102$

$Q_r = 5$ L/min

R = (102 − 2) / 5 = 20 mm Hg/L/min

Control state. The flow (Q_r) across the peripheral resistance is equal to the flow (Q_h) generated by the heart. The mean arterial pressure (P_a) is 102 mm Hg, the central venous pressure (P_v) is 2 mm Hg, and the peripheral resistance is 20 mm Hg/L/min.

B Beginning of cardiac arrest

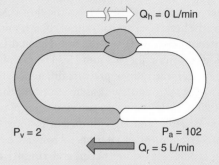

$Q_h = 0$ L/min

$P_v = 2$ $P_a = 102$

$Q_r = 5$ L/min

At the very beginning of cardiac arrest (i.e., $Q_h = 0$ L/min), P_a and P_v have not yet changed. Hence, Q_r is still 5 L/min through a resistance of 20 mm Hg/L/min. Because of the disparity between Q_h and Q_r, P_a will begin to decrease rapidly, and P_v will begin to rise rapidly.

C Cardiac arrest: steady-state

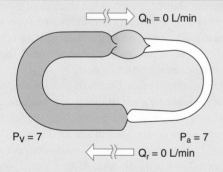

$Q_h = 0$ L/min

$P_v = 7$ $P_a = 7$

$Q_r = 0$ L/min

When the effects of cardiac arrest have attained the steady-state, P_a will have fallen to 7 mm Hg and P_v will have risen to the same value. Because $P_a − P_v = 0$, flow across the resistance will cease (i.e., $Q_r = 0$).

D Beginning of cardiac resuscitation

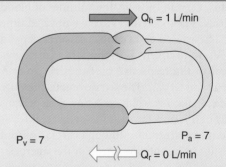

$Q_h = 1$ L/min

$P_v = 7$ $P_a = 7$

$Q_r = 0$ L/min

The heart is resuscitated, and it begins to pump at a constant value of $Q_h = 1$ L/min. At the very beginning of resuscitation, P_a and P_v have not had time to change, and therefore Q_r is still 0 L/min. Because Q_h exceeds Q_r by 1 L/min, P_a will rise rapidly and P_v will fall rapidly. A new equilibrium will be attained when P_a increases to 26 mm Hg and P_v falls to 6 mm Hg. When $P_a − P_v = 20$ mm Hg, the flow (Q_r) through the resistance will be 1 L/min, which equals the cardiac output (Q_h).

FIGURE 10-8 ■ Simplified model of the cardiovascular system, consisting of a pump, arterial compliance (C_a), peripheral resistance, and venous compliance (C_v).

To illustrate how central venous pressure varies inversely with cardiac output, let us first give our model certain characteristics that resemble those of an average adult person (see Figure 10-8A). Let the flow (Q_h) generated by the heart (i.e., cardiac output) be 5 L/min; let mean arterial pressure, P_a, be 102 mm Hg; and let central venous pressure, P_v, be 2 mm Hg. The peripheral resistance, R, is the ratio of pressure difference ($P_a - P_v$) to flow (Q_r) through the resistance vessels; this ratio equals 20 mm Hg/L/min. An arteriovenous pressure difference of 100 mm Hg is sufficient to force a flow (Q_r) of 5 L/min through a peripheral resistance of 20 mm Hg/L/min. This flow (**peripheral runoff**) is precisely equal to the flow (Q_h) generated by the heart. From heartbeat to heartbeat, the volume of blood in the arteries (V_a) and the volume of blood in the veins (V_v) remain constant, because the volume of blood transferred from the veins to the arteries by the heart equals the volume of blood that flows from the arteries through the resistance vessels and into the veins.

Figure 10-8B illustrates the status of the circulation at the very beginning of an episode of cardiac arrest, that is, $Q_h = 0$. Initially, the volumes of blood in the arteries (V_a) and veins (V_v) have not had time to change. The arterial and venous pressures depend on V_a and V_v, respectively. Therefore these pressures are identical to the respective pressures in panel A (i.e., $P_a = 102$ and $P_v = 2$). The arteriovenous pressure gradient of 100 mm Hg will force a flow (the peripheral runoff) of 5 L/min through the peripheral resistance of 20 mm Hg/L/min. Although cardiac output now equals 0 L/min, the flow through the microcirculation *transiently* equals 5 L/min. In other words, the potential energy stored in the arteries by the previous pumping action of the heart causes blood to be transferred from arteries to veins. This transfer occurs initially at the control rate, even though the heart can no longer transfer blood from the veins into the arteries.

As time passes, the blood volume in the arteries progressively decreases, and the blood volume in the veins progressively increases. Because the vessels are elastic structures, arterial pressure falls gradually and venous pressure rises gradually. This process continues until the arterial and venous pressures become equal (Figure 10-8C). Once this condition is reached, the flow (Q_r) from the arteries to the veins through the resistance vessels is zero, as is the cardiac output (Q_h).

At zero flow equilibrium (Figure 10-8C), the pressure attained in the arteries and veins depends on the relative compliances of these vessels. Had the arterial (C_a) and venous (C_v) compliances been equal, the decline in P_a would have been equal to the rise in P_v, because the decrement in arterial volume equals the increment in venous volume (**the principle of "conservation of mass"**). P_a and P_v would both have attained the average of P_a and P_v in Figure 10-8A and B—that is, $P_a = P_v = (102 + 2)/2 = 52$ mm Hg.

However, the veins are much more compliant than are the arteries; the compliance ratio is approximately equal to the ratio ($C_v:C_a = 19$) that we have assumed for the model. Hence, the transfer of blood from arteries to veins at equilibrium would induce a fall in arterial pressure that is 19 times as great as the concomitant rise in venous pressure. As shown in Figure 10-8C, P_v would increase by 5 mm Hg (from 2 to 7 mm Hg), whereas P_a would fall by $19 \times 5 = 95$ mm Hg (from 102 to 7 mm Hg). This equilibrium pressure that prevails in the circulatory system in the absence of flow is often referred to as the **mean circulatory pressure,** or **static pressure.** The pressure in the static system reflects the total volume of blood in the system and the overall compliance of the entire system.

The example of cardiac arrest in Figure 10-8 provides the basis for understanding the vascular function curves. Two important points on the curve have already been derived, as shown in Figure 10-9. One point (A) represents the normal operating status (depicted in Figure 10-8A). At that point, when cardiac output was 5 L/min, P_v was 2 mm Hg. Then, when flow stopped (cardiac output = 0), P_v became 7 mm Hg at equilibrium; this pressure is the mean circulatory pressure, P_{mc}.

The inverse relationship between central venous pressure and cardiac output (see Figure 10-9) simply denotes that when cardiac output is suddenly decreased, the peripheral runoff from arteries to veins is temporarily greater than the rate at which the heart pumps the blood from the veins back into the arteries. During that transient period, a net volume of blood is translocated from arteries to veins; hence P_a falls and P_v rises.

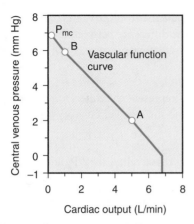

FIGURE 10-9 ■ Changes in central venous pressure produced by changes in cardiac output. The mean circulatory pressure (or static pressure), P_{mc}, is the equilibrium pressure throughout the cardiovascular system when cardiac output is 0. Points B and A represent the values of venous pressure at cardiac outputs of 1 and 5 L/min, respectively.

An example of a sudden increase in cardiac output, but with peripheral resistance remaining constant, illustrates how a third point, B, on the vascular function curve is derived. Consider that the arrested heart is suddenly restarted and that it immediately begins pumping blood from the veins into the arteries at a rate of 1 L/min (Figure 10-8D). When the heart first begins to beat, the arteriovenous pressure gradient is zero, and hence no blood flows from the arteries into the veins. When beating has just resumed, blood is being depleted from the veins at the rate of 1 L/min, and the arterial volume is being repleted at the same rate. Hence P_v begins to fall and P_a begins to rise. Because of the difference in compliances, P_a will rise 19 times more rapidly than P_v will fall.

The resulting pressure gradient causes blood to flow through the resistance. If the heart maintains a constant output of 1 L/min, P_a continues to rise and P_v continues to fall until the pressure gradient becomes 20 mm Hg. This gradient forces a flow of 1 L/min through a resistance of 20 mm Hg/L/min. This gradient is achieved by a 19–mm Hg rise (to 26 mm Hg) in P_a and a 1–mm Hg fall (to 6 mm Hg) in P_v. This equilibrium value of $P_v = 6$ mm Hg for a cardiac output of 1 L/min also appears (point B in Figure 10-9) on the

vascular function curve. The curve reflects a net transfer of blood from the venous to the arterial side of the circuit after the heart has been restarted, and consequently, P_v is reduced.

The reduction of P_v that can be achieved by an increase in cardiac output is limited. At some critical maximal value of cardiac output, sufficient fluid is translocated from the venous to the arterial side of the circuit to reduce P_v below the ambient pressure. In a system of very distensible vessels, such as the venous system, the vessels collapse when the intravascular pressure falls below the extravascular pressure. This venous collapse constitutes an impediment to venous return to the heart. Hence, in the example in Figure 10-9, it limits the maximal value of cardiac output to 7 L/min, regardless of the capabilities of the pump. For readers interested in the mathematical derivation of these results, the basic equations are presented in the next section.

Mathematical Analysis of the Vascular Function Curve

From the definition of peripheral resistance (see Chapter 6):

$$R = (P_a - P_v)/Q_r \qquad (2)$$

where R is resistance, P_a is arterial pressure, P_v is venous pressure, and Q_r is blood flow through the resistance vessels. At equilibrium, Q_r equals cardiac output, Q_h. Assume that $R = 20$ and that Q_h had been 0 but that it had then been increased to a constant value of 1 L/min (Figure 10-10, *arrow 1*). If we solve Equation 2 for P_a when the system is in equilibrium (i.e., $Q_r = Q_h$), then:

$$P_a = P_v + Q_r R = P_v + (1 \times 20) \qquad (3)$$

Thus P_a increases to a value 20 mm Hg greater than P_v. It continues to be 20 mm Hg above P_v, as long as the pump output is maintained at 1 L/min and the peripheral resistance remains at 20 mm Hg/L/min. We can calculate what the actual changes in P_a and P_v will be when Q_r attains a constant value of 1 L/min. The arterial volume increment needed to achieve the required level of P_a depends entirely on the arterial compliance, C_a. For a rigid arterial system (**low compliance**), this

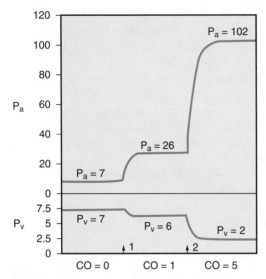

FIGURE 10-10 ▓ Changes in arterial (P_a) and venous (P_v) pressures in the circulatory model shown in Figure 10-8. The total peripheral resistance is 20 mm Hg/l/min, and the ratio of C_v to C_a is 19:1. The cardiac output (CO) is 0 to the left of *arrow 1*. It is increased to 1 L/min at *arrow* i, and to 5 L/min at *arrow 2*.

volume is small; for a distensible system, the volume is large. Whatever the magnitude, however, the change in volume represents the translocation of some quantity of blood from the venous to the arterial side of the circuit.

For a given total blood volume, any increment in arterial volume (ΔV_a) must equal the decrement in venous volume (ΔV_v); that is:

$$\Delta V_a = -\Delta V_v \qquad (4)$$

From the definition of compliance:

$$C_a = \Delta V_a / \Delta P_a \qquad (5)$$

and

$$C_v = \Delta V_v / \Delta P_v \qquad (6)$$

By substitution into equation 4:

$$\Delta P_v / \Delta P_a = -C_a / C_v \qquad (7)$$

Given that C_v is 19 times as great as C_a, the increment in P_a is 19 times as great as the decrement in P_v; that is:

$$\Delta P_a = -19 \Delta P_v \qquad (8)$$

To calculate the absolute values of P_a and P_v, let ΔP_a represent the difference between the prevailing P_a and the mean circulatory pressure (P_{mc}); that is, let:

$$\Delta P_a = P_a - P_{mc} \qquad (9)$$

and let ΔP_v represent the difference between the prevailing P_v and the mean circulatory pressure. Then:

$$\Delta P_v = P_v - P_{mc} \qquad (10)$$

Substituting these values for ΔP_a and ΔP_v into Equation 8:

$$P_a - P_{mc} = -19(P_v - P_{mc}) \qquad (11)$$

By solving equations 3 and 11 simultaneously:

$$P_a = P_{mc} + 19 \qquad (12)$$

and

$$P_v = P_{mc} - 1 \qquad (13)$$

Hence, for a mean circulatory pressure of 7 mm Hg, P_a increases to 26 mm Hg and P_v decreases to 6 mm Hg when Q_h increases from 0 to 1 L/min (see Figure 10-10). These pressure changes provide the required arteriovenous pressure gradient of 20 mm Hg.

If the pump output is abruptly increased to a constant level of 5 L/min (Figure 10-10, *arrow 2*) and peripheral resistance remains constant at 20 mm Hg/L/min, an additional volume of blood is translocated from the venous to the arterial side of the circuit. The blood progressively accumulates in the arteries until P_a reaches a level of 100 mm Hg above P_v, as shown by substitution into Equation 3:

$$P_a = P_v + Q_r R = P_v + (5 \times 20) \qquad (14)$$

By solving equations 11 and 14 simultaneously, we find that P_a rises to a value of 95 mm Hg above P_{mc}, and P_v falls to a value 5 mm Hg below P_{mc}. In Figure 10-10, therefore, P_v declines to 2 mm Hg and P_a rises to 102 mm Hg. The resulting pressure gradient of 100 mm Hg will force a cardiac output of 5 L/min through a constant peripheral resistance of 20 mm Hg/L/min.

The following equation for P_v as a function of Q_r in the model is derived from equations 2, 7, 9, and 10:

$$P_v = -(RC_a/C_a + C_v)Q_r + P_{mc} \qquad (15)$$

Equation 15 has the form of a straight line and satisfies the relation y = mx + b. Note that the slope (m)

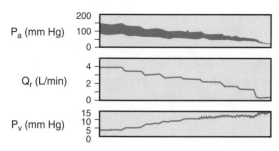

FIGURE 10-11 ■ Changes in arterial (P_a) and central venous (P_v) pressures produced by changes in systemic blood flow (Q_r) in a canine right-heart bypass preparation. Stepwise changes in Q_r were produced by altering the rate of a mechanical pump. *(From Levy MN: The cardiac and vascular factors that determine systemic blood flow. Circ Res 44:739, 1979.)*

depends only on R, C_a and C_v. Note also that when $Q_r = 0$, then $P_v = P_{mc}$; that is, at zero flow, P_v equals the mean circulatory pressure.

Venous Pressure Depends on Cardiac Output

Experimental and clinical observations have shown that changes in cardiac output do indeed evoke the alterations in P_a and P_v that have been predicted previously for our simplified model. In an experiment on an anesthetized dog, for example, a mechanical pump was substituted for the right ventricle (Figure 10-11). As the cardiac output, Q, was diminished in a series of small steps, P_a fell and P_v rose.

CLINICAL BOX

Similarly, a major coronary artery may suddenly become occluded in a human patient. The resultant acute **myocardial infarction** (**death of myocardial tissue**) often diminishes cardiac output, which is attended by a fall in arterial pressure and a rise in central venous pressure.

Blood Volume

The vascular function curve is affected by variations in total blood volume. During circulatory standstill (i.e., **zero cardiac output**), the mean circulatory pressure depends only on total vascular compliance and blood volume, as stated previously. Thus, for a given vascular

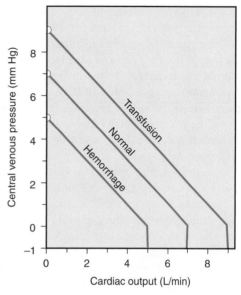

FIGURE 10-12 ■ Effects of increased blood volume (Transfusion curve) and of decreased blood volume (Hemorrhage curve) on the vascular function curve. Similar shifts in the vascular function curve are produced by increases and decreases, respectively, in venomotor tone.

compliance, the mean circulatory pressure will increase when the blood volume is expanded (**hypervolemia**), and it will decrease when the blood volume is diminished (**hypovolemia**). This is illustrated by the y-axis intercepts in Figure 10-12, in which the mean circulatory pressure is 5 mm Hg after hemorrhage and is 9 mm Hg after transfusion. These values compare with that of 7 mm Hg when the blood volume is normal (**normovolemia**).

Figure 10-12 shows that the cardiac output at which $P_v = 0$ varies directly with the blood volume. Therefore, the maximal value of cardiac output becomes progressively more limited as the total blood volume is reduced. However, the pressure ($P_v = 0$) at which the veins collapse (denoted by the sharp change in slope of the vascular function curve) is not altered appreciably by changes in blood volume. This pressure depends only on the pressure surrounding the central veins.

Furthermore, the differences in P_v during hypervolemia, normovolemia, and hypovolemia in the static system are preserved at each level of cardiac output, such that the vascular function curves parallel one another (see Figure 10-12). To illustrate, consider the example of hypervolemia, in which the mean circulatory pressure is 9 mm Hg. In Figure 10-12, both P_a and P_v would be 9 mm Hg, instead of 7 mm Hg, when the cardiac output is zero. With a sudden increase in cardiac output to 1 L/min (at *arrow 1* in Figure 10-10), if the peripheral resistance were still 20 mm Hg/L/min, an arteriovenous pressure gradient of 20 mm Hg would still be necessary for 1 L/min to flow through the resistance vessels. This does not differ from the example for normovolemia. If we assume the same C_v:C_a ratio of 19:1, the pressure gradient would be achieved by a 1–mm Hg decline in P_v and a 19–mm Hg rise in P_a. Hence a change in cardiac output from 0 to 1 L/min would evoke the same 1–mm Hg reduction in P_v. This change in P_v would apply, irrespective of the blood volume, as long as C_a, C_v, and the peripheral resistance were independent of the blood volume. Equation 15 also discloses that the slope of the vascular function curve remains constant as long as R, C_v, and C_a do not change.

Venomotor Tone

The effects of changes in venomotor tone on the vascular function curve closely resemble those of changes in blood volume. In Figure 10-12, for example, the transfusion curve could just as well represent increased venomotor tone, whereas the hemorrhage curve could represent decreased tone. During circulatory standstill, for a given blood volume, the pressure within the vascular system will rise as the tension exerted by the smooth muscle within the vascular walls increases. It is principally the arteriolar and venous smooth muscles that are mainly under nervous or humoral control. The fraction of the blood volume located within the arterioles is very small, whereas the blood volume in the veins is large (see Table 1-1). Therefore, if the blood volume remains constant, only changes in venous tone can alter the mean circulatory pressure appreciably. Hence, mean circulatory pressure rises with increased venomotor tone and falls with diminished tone.

Experimentally, the pressure attained shortly after abrupt circulatory standstill is usually above 7 mm Hg, even when blood volume is normal. The pressure change is attributable to the generalized venoconstriction elicited by cerebral ischemia, activation of the arterial and central chemoreceptors, and reduced excitation of the arterial baroreceptors. If resuscitation is not successful, this reflex response subsides as central nervous activity ceases. When blood volume is normal, the mean circulatory pressure usually approaches a value close to 7 mm Hg.

Blood Reservoirs

Venoconstriction is considerably greater in certain regions of the body than in others. Large vascular beds that undergo appreciable venoconstriction constitute blood reservoirs. The vascular bed of the skin is one of the major blood reservoirs in humans. Blood loss evokes profound subcutaneous venoconstriction, which is responsible for the characteristic pale appearance of the skin in people who have lost a substantial amount of blood. The resulting diversion of blood away from the skin liberates several hundred milliliters of blood, to be perfused through more vital regions. The vascular beds of the liver, lungs, and spleen are also important blood reservoirs. In the dog, the spleen is packed with red blood cells, and it can constrict to a small fraction of its normal size. During hemorrhage, this mechanism autotransfuses blood of high erythrocyte content into the general circulation. However, in humans the volume changes of the spleen are considerably smaller (see also Chapter 13).

Peripheral Resistance

The changes in the vascular function curve induced by changes in arteriolar tone are shown in Figure 10-13. The arterioles contain only about 3% of the total blood volume (see Table 1-1). Changes in the contractile state of these vessels do not significantly alter the mean circulatory pressure, as stated previously. Thus, the family of vascular function curves that represent different peripheral resistances converges at a common point on the ordinate.

At any given cardiac output, P_v varies inversely with the arteriolar tone, all other factors remaining constant. Arteriolar constriction sufficient to double the peripheral resistance causes a twofold rise in P_a (see Chapter 7). In the example shown in Figure 10-10, a change in the cardiac output from 0 to 1 L/min (*arrow 1*) caused P_a to rise from 7 to 26 mm Hg, an increment

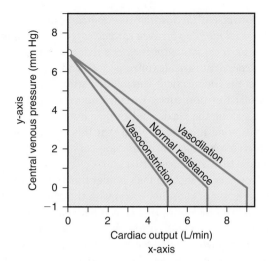

FIGURE 10-13 ■ Effects of arteriolar vasodilation and vasoconstriction on the vascular function curve.

of 19 mm Hg. If peripheral resistance had been twice as great, the same change in cardiac output would have evoked twice as great an increment in P_a.

To achieve this greater rise in P_a, twice as great an increment in blood volume would be required on the arterial side of the circulation, if the arterial compliance remained constant. Given a constant total blood volume, this larger arterial volume signifies a corresponding reduction in venous volume. Hence, the decrement in venous volume would be twice as great when the peripheral resistance was doubled.

If venous compliance remained constant, a twofold reduction in venous volume would be reflected by a twofold decline in P_v. Therefore, an increase in cardiac output from 0 L/min to 1 L/min (Figure 10-10, *arrow 1*) would have caused a 2–mm Hg decrement in P_v, to a level of 5 mm Hg. Similarly, greater increases in cardiac output would have evoked proportionately greater decrements in P_v under conditions of increased peripheral resistance than when the levels of resistance were normal.

This relationship between the peripheral resistance and the decrement in P_v, together with the failure of peripheral resistance to affect the mean circulatory pressure, accounts for the clockwise rotation of the vascular function curves with increased peripheral resistance (see Figure 10-13). Conversely, arteriolar vasodilation is associated with a counterclockwise

rotation from the same vertical axis intercept. A higher maximal level of cardiac output is attainable when the resistance vessels are dilated than when they are constricted.

CARDIAC OUTPUT AND VENOUS RETURN ARE CLOSELY ASSOCIATED

Except for small, transient disparities, the heart is unable to pump any more blood than is delivered to it through the venous system. Similarly, because the circulatory system is a closed circuit, the venous return must equal the cardiac output over any appreciable time interval. The flow around the entire closed circuit depends on the capability of the pump, the characteristics of the circuit, and the total volume of fluid in the system. "Cardiac output" and "venous return" are simply two terms for the flow around the closed circuit. Cardiac output is the volume of blood being pumped by the heart per unit time; venous return is the volume of blood returning to the heart per unit time. At equilibrium, these two flows are equal.

The techniques of circuit analysis are applied here in an effort to gain some insight into the control of flow around the vascular circuit. Acute changes in cardiac contractility, peripheral resistance, or blood volume may transiently affect cardiac output and venous return disparately. Except for such brief disparities, however, such factors simply alter flow around the entire circuit. Whether one thinks of that flow as **cardiac output** or as **venous return** is irrelevant. Many writers have ascribed a reduction in cardiac output during some intervention, such as hemorrhage, to a decrease in venous return. Such an explanation, however, may be an example of circular reasoning. Hemorrhage reduces flow around the entire circuit, for reasons to be elucidated. To attribute the reduction in cardiac output to a curtailment of venous return is equivalent to ascribing the decrease in total blood flow to a decrease in total blood flow!

THE HEART AND VASCULATURE ARE COUPLED FUNCTIONALLY

In accordance with Starling law of the heart, cardiac output depends intimately on the right atrial (or central venous) pressure. Furthermore, right atrial pressure is approximately equal to right ventricular end-diastolic pressure, because the normal tricuspid valve constitutes a low-resistance junction between the right atrium and right ventricle. In the discussion that follows, graphs of cardiac output as a function of central venous pressure (P_v) are called **cardiac function curves.** Extrinsic regulatory influences may be expressed as shifts in such curves, as indicated previously (see Figure 5-23).

A typical cardiac function curve is plotted on the same coordinates as a normal vascular function curve in Figure 10-14. *The cardiac function curve is plotted according to the usual convention; that is, the variable (P_v) plotted along the abscissa is the **independent variable (stimulus)**, and the variable (**cardiac output**) that is plotted along the ordinate is the **dependent variable (response)**.* In accordance with the Frank-Starling mechanism, *the cardiac function curve reveals that a rise in P_v causes an increase in cardiac output.*

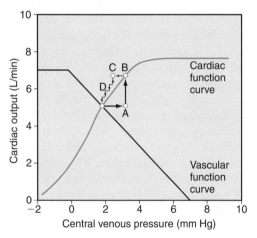

FIGURE 10-14 ■ Typical vascular and cardiac function curves plotted on the same coordinate axes. Note that to plot both curves on the same graph, it is necessary to reverse the x and y axes for the vascular function curves shown in Figures 10-9, 10-12 and 10-13. The coordinates of the equilibrium point, at the intersection of the cardiac and vascular function curves, represent the stable values of cardiac output and central venous pressure at which the system tends to operate. Any perturbation (e.g., when venous pressure is suddenly increased to point A) institutes a sequence of changes in cardiac output and venous pressure that restore these variables to their equilibrium values (points B through D; see text for explanation).

Conversely, *the vascular function curve describes an inverse relationship between cardiac output and P_v; that is, a rise in cardiac output causes a reduction in P_v.* P_v is the dependent variable (or response), and cardiac output is the independent variable (or stimulus) for the vascular function curve. By convention, P_v should be scaled along the y-axis, and cardiac output should be scaled along the x-axis. Note that this convention is observed for the vascular function curves displayed in Figures 10-9, 10-12, and 10-13.

However, to include the vascular function curve on the same set of coordinate axes with the cardiac function curve (see Figure 10-14), it is necessary to violate the plotting convention for one of these curves. *We have arbitrarily violated the convention for the vascular function curve. Note that the vascular function curve in Figure 10-14 reflects how P_v (scaled along the x-axis) varies in response to a change of cardiac output (scaled along the y-axis).*

The **equilibrium point** of a system represented by a given pair of cardiac and vascular function curves is defined by the intersection of these two curves. The coordinates of this equilibrium point represent the values of cardiac output and P_v at which such a system tends to operate. Only transient deviations from such values for cardiac output and P_v are possible, as long as the given cardiac and vascular function curves accurately describe the system.

The tendency for the cardiovascular system to operate around such an equilibrium point may best be illustrated by examining its response to a sudden perturbation. Consider the changes elicited by a sudden rise in P_v from the equilibrium point to point A in Figure 10-14. Such a change might be induced by rapid injection, during ventricular diastole, of a given volume of blood on the venous side of the circuit. The injection of the volume of blood would be accompanied by the withdrawal of an equal volume from the arterial side, so that the total blood volume would remain constant.

As defined by the cardiac function curve in Figure 10-14, this elevated P_v would increase cardiac output (A to B) during the very next ventricular systole. The increased cardiac output, in turn, would result in the net transfer of blood from the venous to the arterial side of the circuit, with a consequent reduction in P_v. In one heartbeat, the reduction in P_v would be small (B to C) because the heart would transfer only a tiny fraction of the total venous blood volume over to the arterial side. Because of this reduction in P_v, the cardiac output during the very next beat diminishes (C to D) by an amount dictated by the function curve. Because point D is still above the intersection point, the heart will pump blood from the veins to the arteries at a rate greater than that at which the blood will flow across the peripheral resistance from arteries to veins. Hence P_v will continue to fall. This process will continue, in diminishing steps, until the point of intersection is reached. Only one specific combination of cardiac output and venous pressure (denoted by the coordinates of the point of intersection) will simultaneously satisfy the requirements of the cardiac and vascular function curves.

Myocardial Contractility

Combinations of cardiac and vascular function curves help explain the effects of alterations in ventricular contractility. In Figure 10-15, the lower cardiac function curve represents the control state, whereas the upper curve reflects an increased contractility. This pair of curves is analogous to the family of ventricular

function curves shown in Figure 5-23. The enhancement of ventricular contractility might be achieved by electrical stimulation of the cardiac sympathetic nerves. If the effects of such stimulation were restricted to the heart, the vascular function curve would be unaffected. Therefore one vascular function curve would suffice, as shown in Figure 10-15.

During the control state, the equilibrium values for cardiac output and P_v are designated by point A. Cardiac sympathetic nerve stimulation would abruptly raise cardiac output to point B, because of the enhanced contractility, before P_v would change appreciably. However, this high cardiac output would increase the net transfer of blood from the venous to the arterial side of the circuit. Consequently, P_v would begin to fall (point C). Cardiac output would continue to fall until a new equilibrium point (D) was reached. This point is located at the intersection of the vascular function curve with the new cardiac function curve. The new equilibrium point (D) lies above and to the left of the control equilibrium point (A). This shift reveals that sympathetic stimulation evokes a greater cardiac output at a lower level of P_v.

Such a change accurately describes the true response. In the experiment depicted in Figure 10-16, the left stellate ganglion was stimulated between the two *arrows*. During stimulation, aortic flow (**cardiac output**) rose quickly to a peak value. The flow then fell gradually to a steady-state value, which was significantly greater than the control level. The increased aortic flow was accompanied by reductions in right and left atrial pressures (P_{RA} and P_{LA}). The initial, abrupt rise in cardiac output in this experiment represents the shift from A to B in Figure 10-15, whereas the subsequent, more gradual reductions in cardiac output and atrial pressure in the experiment represent the progressive shift from B to D.

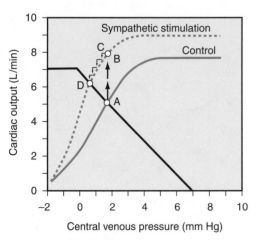

FIGURE 10-15 ■ Enhancement of myocardial contractility, as by cardiac sympathetic nerve stimulation, causes the equilibrium values of cardiac output and venous pressure (P_v) to shift from the intersection (point A) of the control vascular and cardiac function curves *(solid lines)* to the intersection (point D) of the same vascular function curve with the cardiac function curve *(dashed line)* that represents enhanced myocardial contractility. See text for explanation of points B and C.

Blood Volume

Changes in blood volume affect the vascular function curve in the manner shown in Figure 10-12. To understand the circulatory alterations evoked by a given change in blood volume, the appropriate cardiac function curve should be plotted along with the vascular function curves that represent the control and experimental states.

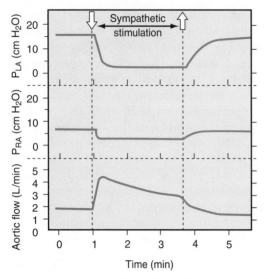

FIGURE 10-16 ▓ During electrical stimulation of the left stellate ganglion (containing cardiac sympathetic nerve fibers), aortic blood flow increased while pressures in the left atrium (P_{LA}) and right atrium (P_{RA}) diminished. These data conform to the conclusions derived from Figure 10-15, in which the equilibrium values of cardiac output and venous pressure are observed to shift from point A to point D during cardiac sympathetic nerve stimulation. *(Redrawn from Sarnoff SJ, Brockman SK, Gilmore JP, et al: Regulation of ventricular contraction. Influence of cardiac sympathetic and vagal nerve stimulation on atrial and ventricular dynamics. Circ Res 8:1108, 1960.)*

Figure 10-17 illustrates the response to a blood transfusion. Equilibrium point B, which denotes the values for cardiac output and P_v after transfusion, lies above and to the right of the control equilibrium point, A. Thus the transfusion increases both cardiac output and P_v. Hemorrhage has the opposite effect. Mechanistically, the change in ventricular filling pressure (**central venous pressure**), evoked by a given change in blood volume, alters cardiac output. This is accomplished by changing the sensitivity of the contractile proteins to the prevailing level of intracellular Ca^{++}, as explained in Chapters 4 and 5. Pure increases or decreases in venomotor tone elicit responses analogous to those evoked by augmentations or reductions, respectively, of the total blood volume, for reasons discussed later.

Peripheral Resistance

Predictions concerning the effects of changes in peripheral vascular resistance are complex because both the cardiac and vascular function curves shift. With increased peripheral resistance (Figure 10-18), the vascular function curve is rotated counterclockwise. However, it converges to the same P_v-axis intercept as does the control curve (see Figure 10-13); the directions of rotation differ in Figures 10-13 and 10-18

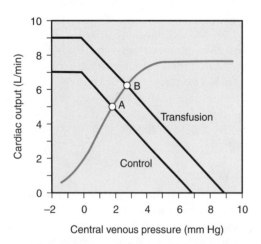

FIGURE 10-17 ▓ After a blood transfusion, the vascular function curve is shifted to the right. Therefore, cardiac output and venous pressure are both increased, as denoted by the translocation of the equilibrium point from A to B.

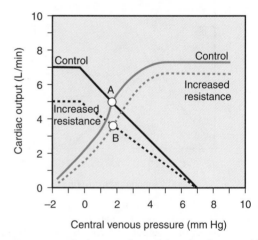

FIGURE 10-18 ▓ An increase in peripheral resistance shifts the cardiac and vascular function curves downward. At equilibrium the cardiac output is less (point B) when the peripheral resistance is high than when it is normal (point A).

because the axes were switched for the vascular function curves in the two figures. The cardiac function curve is also shifted downward because (1) as peripheral resistance increases, arterial pressure (afterload) tends to rise and (2) at any given P_v, the heart is able to pump less blood against a greater afterload. Because the cardiac and vascular function curves are both displaced downward, the new equilibrium point, B, falls below the control point, A.

Whether point B falls directly below point A or lies to the right or left of it depends on the magnitude of the shift in each curve. For example, if a given increase in peripheral resistance shifts the vascular function curve more than it does the cardiac function curve, the equilibrium point B will fall below and to the left of A; that is, both cardiac output and P_v will diminish. Conversely, if the cardiac function curve is displaced more than the vascular function curve, point B will fall below and to the right of point A; that is, cardiac output will decrease but P_v will rise somewhat.

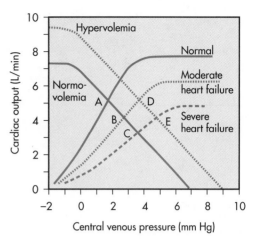

FIGURE 10-19 ■ With moderate or severe heart failure, the cardiac function curves are shifted to the right. Before any change in blood volume, cardiac output decreases and central venous pressure rises (from control equilibrium point A to point B or C). After the increase in blood volume that usually occurs in heart failure, the vascular function curve is shifted to the right. Hence, central venous pressure may be elevated with no reduction in cardiac output (point D) or (in severe heart failure) with some diminution in cardiac output (point E).

CLINICAL BOX

"Heart failure" is the general term that refers to those conditions in which the heart is not able to provide adequate blood flow to the tissues of the body. Heart failure may be acute or chronic. Acute heart failure may be caused by toxic quantities of drugs and anesthetics or by certain pathological conditions, such as a sudden coronary artery occlusion. Chronic heart failure may occur in such conditions as essential hypertension and ischemic heart disease. In these various forms of heart failure, myocardial contractility is impaired. Consequently, the cardiac function curve is shifted downward and to the right, as shown in Figure 10-19.

In **acute heart failure,** blood volume does not change immediately. Therefore, the equilibrium point of the cardiac and vascular function curves will shift from the intersection of the normal curves (Figure 10-19, point A) to the intersection of the normal vascular function curve, with a cardiac function curve that denotes impaired contractility (point B or C).

In **chronic heart failure,** both the cardiac function and vascular function curves shift. The vascular function curve shifts because of an increase in blood volume caused in part by fluid retention by the kidneys. The fluid retention is related to the concomitant reduction in glomerular filtration rate and to the

greater secretion of aldosterone by the adrenal cortex. The resulting hypervolemia is reflected by a rightward shift of the vascular function curve, as shown in Figure 10-19. Hence, with moderate degrees of heart failure, P_v is elevated, but cardiac output is approximately normal (point D). With more severe degrees of heart failure, P_v will be still higher but cardiac output will be subnormal (point E).

THE RIGHT VENTRICLE REGULATES NOT ONLY PULMONARY BLOOD FLOW BUT ALSO CENTRAL VENOUS PRESSURE

The interrelations between cardiac output and central venous pressure are complicated and perplexing. The simplified circulation model includes just one pump and only the systemic circulation. The interrelations are much more complex when the systemic and pulmonary circulations and the left and right ventricles are included in the analysis. However, the systemic and pulmonary vascular systems are

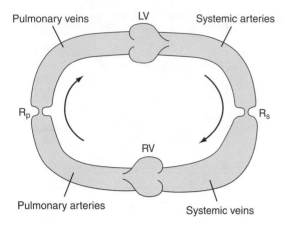

FIGURE 10-20 ■ Simplified cardiovascular system model that consists of left (LV) and right (RV) ventricles, systemic (R_s) and pulmonary (R_p) vascular resistances, systemic arterial and venous compliances, and pulmonary arterial and venous compliances. Arrows indicate direction of blood flow.

important components of the cardiovascular systems in mammals, and therefore the more complete model does merit analysis.

Figure 10-20 shows a more complete, but still oversimplified, cardiovascular system model that contains two pumps in series (**the left and right ventricles**) and two vascular beds in series (**the systemic and pulmonary vasculatures**). The series arrangement requires that the flows pumped by the two ventricles be virtually equal to each other over any substantial period. Otherwise, the blood would ultimately accumulate in one or the other of the vascular systems. Because the cardiac function curves for the two ventricles differ substantially, the filling (**atrial**) pressures for the two ventricles must differ appropriately to ensure equal stroke volumes (see Figure 5-21).

Two basic tenets about ventricular function are (1) the left ventricle is the pump that forces blood through the systemic vasculature and (2) the right ventricle is the pump that forces blood through the pulmonary vasculature. Although these assertions are essentially correct, it is instructive to examine right ventricular function in more detail.

Consider the effect on the circulatory system model shown in Figure 10-20 if the right ventricle suddenly ceases to function as a pump and instead serves as a passive, low-resistance conduit between the systemic veins and the pulmonary arteries. In such a circulatory

system, the only pump would then be the left ventricle. The left ventricle would now be required to pump blood through two vascular resistances in series, namely the systemic and pulmonary resistances. We shall consider the resistance of the right ventricle itself to be negligible.

Normally, pulmonary resistance is about 10% as great as systemic resistance. The total resistance would be 10% greater than the systemic resistance alone (see Chapter 6) because the two resistances are in series with each other. In a normal cardiovascular system, a 10% increase in systemic vascular resistance would increase mean arterial pressure (and hence **left ventricular afterload**) by approximately 10%. This would not affect left ventricular function drastically. However, when the 10% increase in total resistance is achieved by adding a small resistance (i.e., **the pulmonary resistance**) downstream of the systemic resistance, and that resistance is separated from the systemic resistance by a large compliance (**the combined systemic venous and pulmonary arterial compliance**), the 10% increase in total resistance then affects the cardiovascular system drastically.

The simulated effects of inactivating the pumping action of the right ventricle in a hydraulic analog of the circulatory system are shown in Figure 10-21. In the model, the right and left ventricles generate cardiac outputs that vary directly with their respective filling pressures. Under control conditions, the output of the right ventricle (5 L/min) is equal to that of the left ventricle. The right ventricular pumping action causes the pressure in the pulmonary artery to exceed the pressure in the pulmonary veins by an amount that will force fluid through the pulmonary vascular resistance at a rate of 5 L/min.

When the right ventricle ceases pumping (*arrow 1*), the systemic venous and pulmonary arterial systems become a common passive conduit with a large compliance. Pulmonary arterial pressure decreases (not shown), and systemic venous pressure rises to a common value (5 mm Hg in Figure 10-21). At this low pressure, however, fluid flows from the pulmonary arteries to the pulmonary veins at a greatly reduced rate. At the same time, the left ventricle initially pumps fluid from the pulmonary veins to the systemic arteries at the control rate of 5 L/min. Hence pulmonary venous pressure drops precipitously. Left ventricular

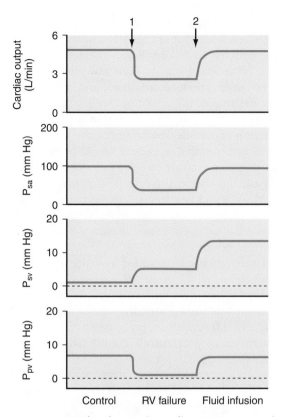

FIGURE 10-21 ■ The changes in cardiac output, systemic arterial pressure (P_{sa}), systemic venous pressure (P_{sv}), and pulmonary venous pressure (P_{pv}) evoked by simulated right ventricular failure and by simulated fluid infusion in the circulatory model shown in Figure 10-20. At *arrow 1*, the pumping action of the right ventricle was discontinued (simulated right ventricular [RV] failure), and the right ventricle served only as a low-resistance conduit. At *arrow 2*, fluid volume was expanded, and the right ventricle continued to serve only as a conduit. *(Modified from Furey SA, Zieske HA, Levy MN: The essential function of the right ventricle. Am Heart J 107:404, 1984.)*

(cardiac) output also drops abruptly because pulmonary venous pressure is the preload for the left ventricle. This effect, in turn, results in a rapid reduction in systemic arterial pressure. In summary, cessation of right ventricular pumping causes marked reductions in cardiac output, in systemic arterial pressure, and in pulmonary venous pressure as well as a modest rise in systemic venous pressure (Figure 10-21).

Most of the hemodynamic problems induced by inactivating the right ventricle can be reversed by

increasing the fluid (blood) volume of the system (*arrow 2*, Figure 10-21). If fluid is added until pulmonary venous pressure (**left ventricular preload**) is raised to its control value, cardiac output and systemic arterial pressure are restored to normal, but systemic venous pressure is abnormally elevated. In a human subject, such a rise in systemic venous pressure may lead to the accumulation of fluid (edema) in the dependent regions of the body; such edema is characteristic of **right heart failure.**

Severe contractile failure of the right ventricle is the equivalent of overstressing the left ventricle by adding in series a relatively small (10%) hydraulic resistance (pulmonary vascular resistance) to the normal systemic vascular resistance. Ordinarily, increasing the systemic vascular resistance itself by 10% does not seriously stress the cardiovascular system. However, when the 10% additional resistance is downstream of the systemic venous bed (which has a very large compliance), it may diminish cardiac output drastically. The main compensatory response of the body is to increase blood volume, in part by renal retention of fluid and electrolytes. However, this compensatory response may lead to severe peripheral edema.

With these findings in mind, we might reassess the principal function of the right ventricle as follows: From the viewpoint of providing sufficient flow of blood to all the tissues in the body, the left ventricle alone is adequate to carry out this function. The operation of two ventricles in series is not essential to provide adequate blood flow to the tissues. *The crucial function of the right ventricle is therefore to prevent the rise in systemic venous (and pulmonary arterial) pressure that would be required to force the normal cardiac output through the pulmonary vascular resistance.* Preventing the abnormal rise in systemic venous pressure also prevents extensive dependent edema.

CLINICAL BOX

Any change in contractility that affects the two ventricles disparately alters the distribution of blood volume in the two vascular systems. For example, if a coronary artery to the left ventricle becomes occluded suddenly, left ventricular contractility is impaired and **left ventricular failure** ensues. Instantaneously, left atrial pressure does not change perceptibly and the left ventricle begins to pump a diminished flow. If the right ventricle is not affected by the acute coronary artery occlusion, the right ventricle initially continues to pump the normal flow. The disparate right and left ventricular outputs result in a progressive increase in left atrial pressure and a progressive decrease in right atrial pressure. Therefore left ventricular output increases toward the normal value and the right ventricular output falls below the normal value. This process continues until the outputs of the two ventricles become equal again. At this new equilibrium, the outputs of the two ventricles are subnormal. The elevated left atrial pressure is accompanied by an equally elevated pulmonary venous pressure, which can have serious clinical consequences. The high pulmonary venous pressure can increase lung stiffness and lead to respiratory distress by increasing the mechanical work of pulmonary ventilation. Furthermore, the high pulmonary venous pressure elevates the hydrostatic pressure in the pulmonary capillaries, and hence may lead to transudation of fluid from the pulmonary capillaries to the pulmonary interstitium or into the alveoli themselves (**pulmonary edema**). The last of these consequences may be lethal.

CLINICAL BOX

In humans, **right heart failure** may be caused by occlusive disease predominantly of the coronary vessels to the right ventricle; these vessels are affected much less commonly than are the vessels to the left ventricle. The major hemodynamic effects of acute right heart failure are pronounced reductions in cardiac output and in arterial blood pressure, and the principal treatment consists of infusion of blood or plasma. Bypass of the right ventricle is not infrequently implemented surgically for patients with certain **congenital cardiac defects,** such as severe narrowing of the tricuspid valve and maldevelopment of the right ventricle. The effects of acute right heart failure or of right ventricular bypass are directionally similar to those predicted by the model study (see Figure 10-21).

HEART RATE HAS AMBIVALENT EFFECTS ON CARDIAC OUTPUT

Cardiac output is the product of stroke volume and heart rate. The preceding analysis of the control of cardiac output was, in reality, restricted to the control

of stroke volume, and the role of heart rate was neglected. The effect of changes in heart rate on cardiac output are now considered. The analysis is complex, because a change in heart rate alters the other three factors (**preload, afterload, and contractility**) that determine stroke volume (see Figure 10-1). An increase in heart rate, for example, would decrease the duration of diastole. Hence, ventricular filling would be diminished; that is, preload would be reduced. If the proposed increase in heart rate did alter cardiac output, the arterial pressure would change; that is, afterload would be changed. Finally, the rise in heart rate would increase the net rate of Ca^{++} influx into the myocardial cells, enhancing myocardial contractility (see Chapter 4).

Heart rate has been varied by artificial pacing in many types of experimental preparations and in humans. The effects on cardiac output have usually resembled the experimental results shown in Figure 10-22. In this experiment on an anesthetized dog, the stroke volume progressively diminished as the atrial

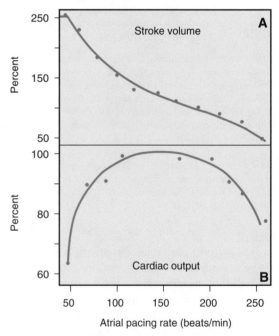

FIGURE 10-22 ■ The changes in stroke volume (**A**) and cardiac output (**B**) induced by changing the rate of atrial pacing in an anesthetized dog. *(Redrawn from Kumada M, Azuma T, Matsuda K: The cardiac output-heart rate relationship under different conditions. Jpn J Physiol 17:538, 1967.)*

pacing frequency was gradually increased (Figure 10-22A). Presumably, the curtailment of stroke volume was induced by the abridged time for ventricular filling.

The change in cardiac output induced by a change in heart rate is influenced markedly by the actual level of the heart rate. In the experiment shown in Figure 10-22, for example, as the pacing frequency was increased within the range of 50 to 100 beats per minute (beats/min), an increase in heart rate augmented the cardiac output (Q_h). Over this lower frequency range, the reduction in stroke volume evoked by a given increase in heart rate (HR) was proportionately less than the increase in heart rate itself. Consequently, because $Q_h = SV \times HR$, a given increment in HR would exceed the induced decrement in SV. Hence the induced Q_h would exceed the initial Q_h.

Over the frequency range from about 100 to 200 beats/min, however, cardiac output was not affected appreciably by changes in pacing frequency (Figure 10-22B). As the pacing frequency was increased, the stroke volume decreased in proportion to the increase in heart rate. Finally, at excessively high pacing frequencies (above 200 beats/min), increments in heart rate decreased the cardiac output. Therefore the induced decrement in SV must have exceeded the increment in HR over this high range of pacing frequencies. Although the relationship of Q_h to HR is characteristically that of an inverted U, the relationship varies quantitatively among subjects and among physiological states in any given subject.

The reason for the observed correlations between cardiac output and heart rate should be interpreted very cautiously. During physical exercise, for example, cardiac output and heart rate often rise proportionately, and stroke volume may change very little (see Chapter 13). One is tempted to conclude that the increase in cardiac output must be caused by the observed increase in heart rate, because the correlation between cardiac output and heart rate is striking. However, Figure 10-22 emphasizes that, over a wide range of heart rates, a change in heart rate has little influence on cardiac output. Several studies on exercising subjects have confirmed that, even during exercise, changes in pacing frequency over a substantial frequency range do not alter cardiac output very much.

CLINICAL BOX

The characteristic relationship between cardiac output and heart rate explains the urgent need for treatment of patients who have excessively slow or excessively fast heart rates. Profound **bradycardias** (slow rates) may occur as the result of a very slow sinus rhythm in patients with **sick sinus syndrome** or as the result of a slow idioventricular rhythm in patients with **complete atrioventricular block.** In either rhythm disturbance, the capacity of the ventricles to fill during a prolonged diastole is limited (often by the noncompliant pericardium). Hence, cardiac output usually decreases substantially because the very slow heart rate cannot be overcome by a sufficiently great stroke volume. Consequently, these rhythm disturbances often require installation of an artificial pacemaker.

At the other end of the heart rate spectrum, excessively high heart rates in patients with **supraventricular** or **ventricular tachycardias** often require emergency treatment because their cardiac outputs may be critically low. In such patients, the filling time is so restricted at very high heart rates that small additional reductions in filling time elicit disproportionately severe reductions in filling volume. Reversion of the tachycardia to a more normal rhythm can usually be accomplished pharmacologically. However, **cardioversion,** which delivers a strong electric current across the thorax or directly to the heart through an implanted device, may be required in emergencies.

The principal increase in cardiac output during exercise must therefore, be ascribed to (1) the pronounced reduction in peripheral vascular resistance, (2) the positive inotropic effect of the increased sympathetic neural activity on the ventricular myocardium, and (3) the auxiliary pumping action of the contracting skeletal muscles. These factors are combined with the directional effects on blood flow brought about by the venous valves (as explained later in this chapter). The attendant changes in heart rate are not inconsequential, however. If the heart rate cannot increase normally during exercise, the augmentation of cardiac output and the capacity for exercise may be severely limited. The increase in heart rate plays a *permissive role* in augmenting cardiac output, even if it is not proper to assign HR to a primary, causative role. The mechanisms responsible for raising heart rate in precise proportion to the increase in cardiac output are undoubtedly neural in origin, but the specific components of the reflex arcs have not yet been elucidated.

ANCILLARY FACTORS AFFECT THE VENOUS SYSTEM AND CARDIAC OUTPUT

The interrelationships between central venous pressure and cardiac output have been explained in an oversimplified fashion, and the described effects have been evoked by changes in isolated variables. However, because many feedback control loops regulate the cardiovascular system, an isolated change in a single variable rarely occurs. A change in blood volume, for example, reflexly alters cardiac function, peripheral resistance, and venomotor tone. Several auxiliary factors also regulate cardiac output. Such ancillary factors may be considered to modulate the more basic factors that we have considered here.

Gravity

Gravitational forces may affect cardiac output profoundly. It is not unusual for some soldiers standing at attention to faint because cardiac output is reduced. Gravitational effects are exaggerated in airplane pilots during pullouts from dives. The centrifugal force in the footward direction may be several times greater than the force of gravity. Such individuals characteristically black out momentarily during the maneuver, as blood is drained from the cephalic regions and pooled in the lower parts of the body.

The explanation for the reduction in cardiac output under such conditions is often specious. It is frequently argued that when an individual is standing, the forces of gravity impede venous return from the dependent regions of the body. This statement is incomplete, however, because it ignores the facilitative counterforce on the arterial side of the same circuit.

In this sense the vascular system resembles a **U tube.** To comprehend the action of gravity on flow through such a system, the models depicted in Figures 10-23 and 10-24 are analyzed. In Figure 10-23, for example, all the U tubes represent rigid cylinders of constant diameter. With both limbs of the U tube

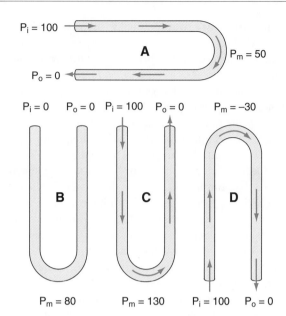

FIGURE 10-23 ■ Pressure distributions in rigid U tubes with constant internal diameters, all with the same dimensions. For a given inflow pressure ($P_i = 100$) and outflow pressure ($P_o = 0$), the pressure at the midpoint (P_m) depends on the orientation of the U tube, but the flow through the tube is independent of the orientation.

oriented horizontally (Figure 10-23A), the flow depends only on the pressures at the inflow and outflow ends of the tube (P_i and P_o, respectively), the viscosity of the fluid, and the length and radius of the tube, in accordance with **Poiseuille's equation** (see Chapter 6). With a constant cross section, the pressure gradient is uniform; hence, the pressure midway down the tube (P_m) equals the average of the inflow and outflow pressures.

When the U tube is oriented vertically (Figure 10-23B to D), hydrostatic forces must be taken into consideration. In tube B, both limbs are open to atmospheric pressure, and both ends are located at the same hydrostatic level; hence, there is no flow. The pressure at the midpoint of the tube is simply ρhg. The pressure depends on the density of the fluid, ρ; the height of the U tube, h; and the acceleration of gravity, g. In the example in Figure 10-23, the length of the U tube is such that the midpoint pressure is 80 mm Hg.

Now consider tube C, which is oriented the same as is tube B but in which a 100–mm Hg pressure difference is applied across the two ends. The flow precisely

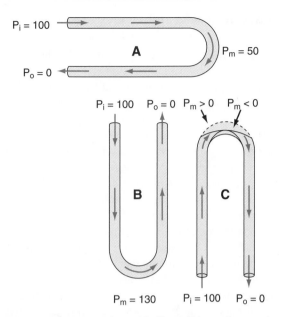

$P_i = 100$ $P_o = 0$ $P_m > 0$ $P_m < 0$

B   C

$P_m = 130$ $P_i = 100$ $P_o = 0$

FIGURE 10-24 ■ In U tubes with distensible sections at the bends, even when inflow (P_i) and outflow (P_o) pressures are the same, the resistance to flow, and the fluid volume contained within each tube, varies with the orientation of the tube. P_m, pressure at the midpoint of the tube.

equals that in tube A, because the pressure gradient, tube dimensions, and fluid viscosity are all the same. Gravitational forces are precisely equal in magnitude, but opposite in direction, in the two limbs of the U tube. Because the flow is the same as that in A, there is a pressure drop of 50 mm Hg at the midpoint as a result of the viscous losses that result from flow. Furthermore, gravity tends to increase pressure by 80 mm Hg at the midpoint, just as in tube B. The actual pressure at the midpoint of tube C is the result of the viscous loss and hydrostatic gain, or 130 mm Hg in this example.

In tube D, a pressure gradient of 100 mm Hg is applied to the same U tube, but the tube is oriented in the opposite direction. Gravitational forces are so directed that the pressure at the midpoint tends to be 80 mm Hg less than that at the end of the U tube. Viscous losses still produce a 50–mm Hg pressure drop at the midpoint, relative to P_i. With this orientation, pressure at the midpoint of the U tube is 30 mm Hg below ambient pressure. Flow is the same as in tubes A and C, for the reasons stated in relation to C.

In a system of rigid U tubes, gravitational effects do not alter the rate of fluid flow. However, experience shows that gravity does affect the cardiovascular system. The reason is that the vessels are distensible rather than rigid. To explain the gravitational effects, the pressures in a set of U tubes with distensible components (at the bends in the tubes of Figure 10-24) are examined. In tubes A and B in Figure 10-24, the pressure distributions resemble those in tubes A and C, respectively, in Figure 10-23. In Figure 10-24, because the pressure is higher at the bend of tube B than at the bend of tube A, and because the segments are distensible in this region, the distention at the bend in tube B exceeds that at the bend in tube A. The extent of the distention depends on the compliance of these tube segments. Because flow varies directly with the tube diameter, the flow through tube B exceeds the flow through tube A for a given pressure difference applied at the ends.

Orienting a U tube with its bend downward actually increases, rather than diminishes, the flow. How then is the observed impairment of cardiovascular function explained when the body is similarly oriented? The explanation is that the cardiovascular system is a closed circuit of constant fluid (blood) volume, whereas the U tube is an open conduit that is supplied by a fluid source of unlimited volume. In the dependent regions of the cardiovascular system, the distention occurs more on the venous than on the arterial side of the circuit, because the venous compliance is so much greater than the arterial compliance. Such venous distention is readily observed on the back of the hands when the arms are allowed to hang down. The hemodynamic effects of such venous distention (**venous pooling**) resemble those caused by the hemorrhage of an equivalent volume of blood from the body. When an adult person shifts from a supine position to a relaxed standing position, 300 to 800 mL of blood is pooled in the legs. This change may reduce cardiac output by about 2 L/min.

The compensatory adjustments to the erect position are similar to the adjustments to blood loss. For example, the diminished baroreceptor excitation reflexly speeds the heart, strengthens the cardiac contraction, and constricts the arterioles and veins. The baroreceptor reflex has a greater effect on the resistance vessels than on the capacitance vessels. Warm, ambient temperatures interfere with the compensatory vasomotor reactions, and the absence of muscular activity exaggerates the effects.

When the U tube is rotated so that the bend is directed upward (Figure 10-24, tube C), the effects are opposite to those that take place in tube B. The pressure at the bend of tube C would tend to be −30 mm Hg, just as in tube D in Figure 10-23. However, the distensible segment of tube C collapses because the ambient pressure exceeds the internal pressure. Flow then ceases, and therefore the pressure decrease associated with viscous flow does not occur. In U tube C, when flow stops, the pressure at the top of each limb is 80 mm Hg less than at the bottom (**the hydrostatic pressure difference**). Hence, in the left (or inflow) limb, the pressure begins to rise rapidly from a negative value. If the tube remained collapsed at the bend, the pressure to the left of the collapsed segment would rapidly approach 20 mm Hg. However, as soon as this pressure exceeds the ambient pressure (0 mm Hg), the collapsed tubing is forced open, and flow begins. With the onset of flow, however, pressure at the bend again drops below the ambient pressure. Thus, the tubing at the bend flutters; that is, it fluctuates between the open and closed states.

When an arm is raised, the cutaneous veins in the hand and forearm collapse, for the reasons described previously. Fluttering does not occur, because the deeper veins are protected from collapse by being tethered to surrounding structures. This protection allows these deeper veins to accommodate the flow that is ordinarily carried by the collapsed superficial veins. The analogy would be to add a rigid tube (which represents the deeper veins) in parallel with the collapsible tube (which represents the superficial veins) at the bend of tube C in Figure 10-24. The collapsible tube would no longer flutter but it would remain closed. All flow would occur through the rigid tube, just as in tube D in Figure 10-23.

CLINICAL BOX

Many of the drugs used to treat **hypertension** also interfere with the reflex adaptation to standing. Similarly, astronauts exposed to weightlessness lose their adaptations after a few days in space and experience difficulties when they first return to earth. When individuals with impaired reflex adaptation stand, their blood pressure may drop substantially. This response, called **orthostatic hypotension**, may cause lightheadedness or fainting.

Muscular Activity and Venous Valves

When a person who is recumbent stands but remains at rest, the pressure rises in the veins in the dependent regions of the body. The venous pressure in the legs increases gradually, and it does not reach an equilibrium value until almost 1 minute after standing. The slowness of this rise in P_v is attributable to the venous valves, which permit flow only toward the heart. When the person stands, the valves prevent blood in the veins from actually falling toward the feet. Hence the column of venous blood is supported at numerous levels by these valves; temporarily, the venous column consists of many discontinuous segments. However, blood continues to enter the column from many venules and small tributary veins, and the pressure continues to rise. As soon as the pressure in one segment exceeds that in the segment just above it, the intervening valve is forced to open. Ultimately, all the valves are open and the column is continuous. This state resembles that in the outflow limbs of the U tubes shown in Figures 10-23 and 10-24.

Precise measurement reveals that the final level of P_v in the feet during quiet standing is only slightly greater than that in a static column of blood extending from the right atrium to the feet. This finding indicates that the pressure drop caused by blood flow from the foot veins to the right atrium is very small. This very low resistance justifies regarding all the veins as a common venous compliance in the circulatory system model illustrated in Figure 10-8.

CLINICAL BOX

The superficial veins in the neck are ordinarily partially collapsed when a normal individual is upright. Blood returns to the heart from the head mainly through the deeper cervical veins. However, when central venous pressure is abnormally elevated, the superficial neck veins are distended and do not collapse even when the subject sits or stands. Such cervical venous distention is an important clinical sign of **congestive heart failure.**

When an individual who has been standing quietly begins to walk, the venous pressure in the legs decreases appreciably (Figure 10-25). Blood is forced from the veins toward the heart because of the intermittent venous compression exerted by the contracting leg muscles and because of the presence of the venous

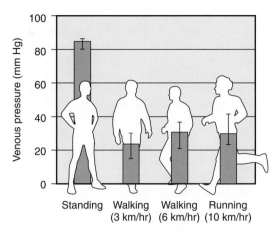

FIGURE 10-25 ■ Mean pressures (± 95% confidence intervals) in the foot veins of 18 people during quiet standing, walking, and running. *(From Stick C, Jaeger H, Witzleb E: Measurements of volume changes and venous pressure in the human lower leg during walking and running.* J Appl Physiol *72:2063, 1992.)*

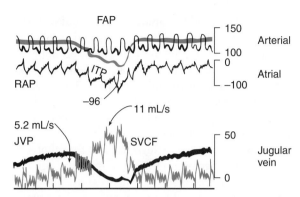

FIGURE 10-26 ■ During a normal inspiration, intrathoracic (ITP), right atrial (RAP), and jugular venous (JVP) pressures decrease, and flow in the superior vena cava (SVCF) increases (from 5.2 to 11 mL/second [s]). All pressures are in millimeters of water, except for femoral arterial pressure (FAP), which is in millimeters of mercury. *(Modified from Brecher GA:* Venous return, *New York, 1956, Grune & Stratton.)*

valves (see Figure 12-2). Hence, muscular contraction lowers the mean venous pressure in the legs, and it serves as an auxiliary pump. Furthermore, it prevents venous pooling and lowers capillary hydrostatic pressure, thereby reducing the tendency for edema fluid to collect in the feet during standing.

CLINICAL BOX

This auxiliary pumping mechanism is not very effective in people with **varicose veins** in their legs. The valves in such veins do not operate properly, and therefore when the leg muscles contract, the blood in the leg veins is forced in the retrograde as well as in the antegrade direction. Thus, when an individual with varicose veins stands or walks, the venous pressure in the ankles and feet is excessively high. The consequent high capillary pressure leads to the accumulation of edema fluid in the ankles and feet.

Respiratory Activity

The normal, periodic activity of the respiratory muscles causes rhythmic variations in vena caval blood flow. Thus, respiration constitutes an auxiliary pump to promote venous return. Coughing, straining at stool, and other activities that require respiratory muscle exertion may affect cardiac output substantially.

The changes in blood flow in the superior vena cava during the normal respiratory cycle are shown in Figure 10-26. During normal respiration, the reduction in intrathoracic pressure is transmitted to the lumina of the intrathoracic blood vessels. Central venous pressure is reduced during inspiration, increasing the pressure gradient between extrathoracic and intrathoracic veins. The consequent acceleration of venous return to the right atrium is displayed in Figure 10-26 as an increase in superior vena caval blood flow, from 5.2 mL/second (s) during expiration to 11 mL/s during inspiration.

An exaggerated reduction in intrathoracic pressure achieved by a strong inspiratory effort against a closed glottis (called **Müller maneuver**) does not increase venous return proportionately. The extrathoracic veins collapse near their entry into the chest when their internal pressures fall below the ambient level. As the veins collapse, flow into the chest momentarily stops. The cessation of flow raises pressure upstream, thereby forcing the collapsed segment to open again. The process is repetitive; the venous segments adjacent to the chest alternately open and close.

During normal expiration, flow into the central veins decelerates. However, the mean rate of venous return during normal respiration exceeds the flow during a brief period of **apnea** (**cessation of respiration**). Hence normal inspiration apparently facilitates venous return more than normal expiration impedes it. This effect must be partly attributable to the valves in the veins of the extremities and neck. These valves prevent any reversal of flow during expiration. Thus, the respiratory muscles and venous valves constitute an **auxiliary pump** for venous return.

Sustained expiratory efforts increase intrathoracic pressure and thereby impede venous return. Straining against a closed glottis (termed **Valsalva maneuver**) regularly occurs during coughing, defecation, and heavy lifting. Intrathoracic pressures in excess of 100 mm Hg have been recorded in trumpet players, and pressures over 400 mm Hg have been observed during paroxysms of coughing. Such pressure increases are transmitted directly to the lumina of the intrathoracic arteries. After coughing ceases, the arterial blood pressure may fall precipitously because of the preceding impediment to venous return.

tendency to impede venous return momentarily. During certain diagnostic procedures, such as coronary angiography and electrophysiological testing, patients are at increased risk for **ventricular fibrillation.** Such patients have been trained to cough rhythmically on command. If ventricular fibrillation does occur, substantial arterial blood pressure increments are generated by each cough, and enough cerebral blood flow may be promoted to sustain consciousness and to preserve the viability of the cerebral tissues. The cough raises the intravascular pressure equally in intrathoracic arteries and veins. Blood is propelled through the extrathoracic tissues, however, because the increased pressure is transmitted to the extrathoracic arteries but not to the extrathoracic veins. The venous valves prevent transmission of the intrathoracic pressure to the extrathoracic veins.

CLINICAL BOX

The intense, brief increases in intrathoracic pressure induced by coughing constitute an **auxiliary pumping mechanism** for the blood, despite the concurrent

Artificial Respiration

In most forms of artificial respiration (mouth-to-mouth resuscitation, mechanical respiration), lung inflation is achieved by applying endotracheal pressures above atmospheric pressure, and expiration occurs by passive recoil of the thoracic cage. Thus, lung inflation is accompanied by an appreciable rise in

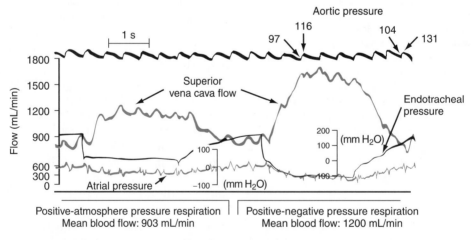

FIGURE 10-27 ■ During intermittent positive-pressure respiration, the flow in the superior vena cava is approximately 30% greater when the lungs are deflated actively by application of negative endotracheal pressure *(right side)* than when they are allowed to deflate passively against atmospheric pressure *(left side)*. *(Modified from Brecher GA:* Venous return, *New York, 1956, Grune & Stratton.)*

intrathoracic pressure. Vena caval flow decreases sharply during the phase of positive-pressure lung inflation (indicated by the progressive rise in endotracheal pressure in the central portion of Figure 10-27). When negative endotracheal pressure (indicated by

the abrupt decrease in endotracheal pressure in the right side of Figure 10-27) is used to facilitate deflation, vena caval flow accelerates more than when the lungs are allowed to deflate passively (near the left border of Figure 10-27).

SUMMARY

- Two important relationships between cardiac output (CO) and central venous pressure (P_v) prevail in the cardiovascular system. One applies to the heart and the other to the vascular system.
- With respect to the heart, CO varies directly with P_v (or preload) over a very wide range of P_v. This relationship is represented by the cardiac function curve and expresses the Frank-Starling mechanism.
- With respect to the vascular system, P_v varies inversely with CO. This relationship is represented by the vascular function curve, and it reflects the fact that as CO increases, for example, a greater fraction of the total blood volume resides in the arteries and a smaller volume resides in the veins.
- The principal mechanism that governs the cardiac function curve is the change in the affinity of the contractile proteins for calcium. This effect is evoked by changes in the cardiac filling pressure (preload).
- The principal factors that govern the vascular function curve are the arterial and venous compliances, the peripheral vascular resistance, and the total blood volume.
- The equilibrium values of CO and P_v that prevail under a given set of conditions are determined by the intersection of the cardiac and vascular function curves.
- At very low and very high heart rates, the heart is unable to pump an adequate CO. At very low rates, the increment in filling during diastole cannot compensate for the small number of cardiac contractions per minute. At very high rates, the large number of contractions per minute cannot compensate for the inadequate filling time.
- Gravity influences CO because the veins are so compliant, and substantial quantities of blood tend to pool in the veins of the dependent portions of the body.

- Respiration changes the pressure gradient between the intrathoracic and extrathoracic veins. Hence respiration serves as an auxiliary pump, which may alter the mean level of CO and may induce rhythmic changes in stroke volume during the various phases of the respiratory cycle.

ADDITIONAL READING

Arbab-Zadeh A, Dijk E, Prasad A, et al: Effect of aging and physical activity on left ventricular compliance, *Circulation* 110:1799, 2004.

Brengelmann GL: A critical analysis of the view that right atrial pressure determines venous return, *J Appl Physiol* 94:849, 2003.

Jacob G, Ertl AC, Shannon JR, et al: Effect of standing on neurohumoral responses and plasma volume in healthy subjects, *J Appl Physiol* 84:914, 1998.

McGee SR: Physical examination of venous pressure: A critical review, *Am Heart J* 136:10, 1998.

Pang CC: Autonomic control of the venous system in health and disease: Effects of drugs, *Pharmacol Ther* 90:179, 2001.

Rowell LB, O'Leary DS, Kellogg DL Jr: Integration of cardiovascular control systems in dynamic exercise. In Rowell LB, Shepherd JT, editors: *Handbook of Physiology, Section 12: Exercise: Regulation and Integration of Multiple Systems*, New York, 1996, Oxford University Press.

Tyberg JV, Belenkie I, Manyari DE, et al: Ventricular interaction and venous capacitance modulate left ventricular preload, *Can J Cardiol* 12:1058, 1996.

Uemura K, Sugimachi M, Kawada T, et al: A novel framework of circulatory equilibrium, *Am J Physiol* 286:H2376, 2004.

Uemura K, Kawada T, Kamiya A, et al: Prediction of circulatory equilibrium in response to changes in stressed blood volume, *Am J Physiol* 289:H301, 2005.

CASE 10-1

HISTORY

A 44-year-old woman with severe cardiac failure caused by coronary artery disease was treated by cardiac transplantation. She recovered very well, and

1 month after surgery her cardiovascular function was entirely normal, even though her new heart was entirely denervated. About 3 months after surgery, she developed a bleeding duodenal ulcer and was estimated to have lost about 600 mL of blood in 1 hour. After hospitalization for acute blood loss, her physician treated her with diet and antibiotics, and her ulcer was cured in about 2 weeks. The patient was healthy for 3 years, but then her strength and energy gradually diminished. Her physician determined that the cardiac transplant was slowly being rejected, and he began to treat her with a new drug that specifically increases myocardial contractility. Occasionally the patient experienced brief periods of tachycardia with a rate of 250 beats/min; the electrocardiogram indicated that the tachycardia originated in the AV junction.

QUESTIONS

1. The acute blood loss from her duodenal ulcer can be expected to:
   a. decrease central venous pressure and increase cardiac output.
   b. increase central venous pressure and decrease mean arterial pressure.
   c. decrease central venous pressure and decrease cardiac output.
   d. increase mean arterial pressure and decrease cardiac output.
   e. decrease central venous pressure and increase aortic pulse pressure.

2. Administration of a drug that acts specifically to improve myocardial contractility would:
   a. decrease central venous pressure and increase cardiac output.
   b. decrease central venous pressure and decrease mean arterial pressure.
   c. increase central venous pressure and increase aortic pulse pressure.
   d. decrease central venous pressure and decrease cardiac output.
   e. increase central venous pressure and increase arterial compliance.

3. Strapping the patient to a tilt-table and tilting her to the vertical, head-up position would:
   a. increase the pressure in a foot vein and increase the central venous pressure.
   b. decrease the pressure in a foot vein and decrease the cardiac output.
   c. decrease the central venous pressure and increase the mean arterial pressure.
   d. decrease the pressure in a foot vein and decrease the arterial pulse pressure.
   e. increase the pressure in a foot vein and decrease the cardiac output.

4. When the patient was experiencing the tachycardia at 250 beats per minute, the critical hemodynamic changes would be expected to be:
   a. an increase in mean arterial blood pressure and an increase in central venous pressure.
   b. a decrease in stroke volume and a decrease in cardiac output.
   c. an increase in stroke volume and an increase in aortic compliance.
   d. an increase in central venous pressure and an increase in cardiac output.
   e. a decrease in central venous pressure and an increase in arterial pulse pressure.

11

CORONARY CIRCULATION

OBJECTIVES

1. Delineate the physical, neural, and metabolic factors that affect coronary blood flow.

2. Explain the relative importance of these factors in the regulation of the coronary circulation.

3. Compare the oxygen requirements of the heart during pressure work versus volume work.

4. Discuss the metabolic changes caused by ischemia and the role of interstitial adenosine in ameliorating the effects of ischemia.

5. Describe the development of coronary collateral vessels.

FUNCTIONAL ANATOMY OF THE CORONARY VESSELS

The right and left coronary arteries, which arise at the root of the aorta behind the right and left cusps of the aortic valve, respectively, provide the entire blood supply to the myocardium. The right coronary artery supplies principally the right atrium and ventricle. The left coronary artery, which divides near its origin into the anterior descending and the circumflex branches, supplies principally the left ventricle and atrium, but there is some overlap. In humans, the right coronary artery is dominant in 50% of individuals, and the left coronary artery is dominant in another 20%. The flows delivered by the two main arteries are about equal in the remaining 30%. The epicardial distribution of the coronary arteries and veins is illustrated in Figure 11-1.

The microcirculatory unit of coronary vessels consists of terminal arterioles, precapillary sinuses, capillaries, and venules. Cardiac myocytes are surrounded by capillaries that, in general, are aligned with them. The average length of the microcirculatory unit is about 350 μm. During diastole, precapillary sinuses may serve as a blood reservoir. During systole, these sinuses disgorge the blood so as to sustain myocyte perfusion.

After the blood passes through the capillary beds, most of the venous blood returns to the right atrium through the coronary sinus. However, some of the blood reaches the right atrium by way of the anterior coronary veins. There are also vascular communications between the vessels of the myocardium and the cardiac chambers. These constitute the **arteriosinusoidal, arterioluminal, and thebesian vessels.** The arteriosinusoidal channels consist of small arteries or

223

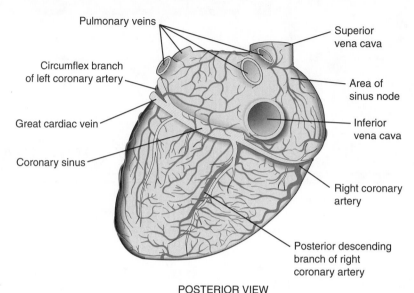

Pulmonary veins

Superior
vena cava

Circumflex branch
of left coronary artery

Area of
sinus node

Great cardiac vein

Inferior
vena cava

Coronary sinus

Right coronary
artery

Posterior descending
branch of right
coronary artery

POSTERIOR VIEW

FIGURE 11-1 ■ Anterior and posterior views of the heart, illustrating the location and distribution of the principal coronary vessels.

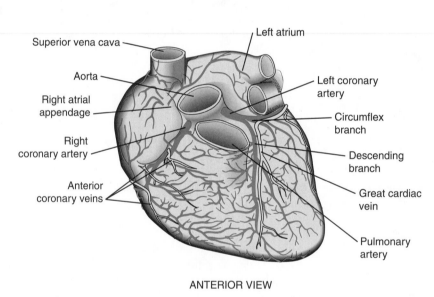

Superior vena cava

Left atrium

Aorta

Left coronary
artery

Right atrial
appendage

Circumflex
branch

Right
coronary artery

Descending
branch

Anterior
coronary veins

Great cardiac
vein

Pulmonary
artery

ANTERIOR VIEW

arterioles. These vessels lose their arterial structure as they penetrate the chamber walls and divide into irregular, endothelium-lined sinuses (50 to 250 μm). These sinuses anastomose with other sinuses and with capillaries, and they communicate with the cardiac chambers. The arteriosinusoidal vessels are small arteries or arterioles that open directly into the atria and ventricles. The thebesian vessels are small veins that connect capillary beds directly with the cardiac chambers, and they also communicate with cardiac veins and other thebesian veins. On the basis of anatomical studies, *intercommunication appears to exist among all the minute vessels of the myocardium in the form of an extensive plexus of subendocardial vessels.* However, the myocardium does not receive significant nutritional blood flow directly from the cardiac chambers.

CORONARY BLOOD FLOW IS REGULATED BY PHYSICAL, NEURAL, AND METABOLIC FACTORS

Physical Factors

The principal factor responsible for perfusion of the myocardium is the aortic pressure, which is generated by the heart itself. Changes in aortic pressure generally evoke parallel changes in coronary blood flow. If a cannulated coronary artery is perfused by blood from a pressure-controlled reservoir, perfusion pressure can be altered without changing aortic pressure and cardiac work. Under these conditions, abrupt variations in perfusion pressure produce equally abrupt changes in coronary blood flow in the same direction. However, maintenance of the perfusion pressure at the new level is associated with a return of blood flow toward the level observed before the induced change in perfusion pressure (Figure 11-2). This phenomenon is an example of **autoregulation of blood flow.** As discussed in Chapter 9, autoregulation in coronary arteries is mediated by a myogenic mechanism, by the metabolic activity of cardiac muscle, and by the endothelium. Thus, autoregulation depends on the interplay of activities of vascular smooth muscle and cardiac muscle. Under normal conditions, blood pressure is kept within relatively narrow limits by the baroreceptor reflex mechanisms.

However, alterations of cardiac work, produced by an increase or decrease in aortic pressure, have a considerable effect on coronary resistance. Increased metabolic activity of the heart decreases the coronary vascular resistance, and a reduction in cardiac metabolism increases the coronary resistance. The position of the autoregulatory region is affected by the metabolic state of cardiac muscle (Figure 11-3). Hence, *changes in coronary blood flow are caused mainly by caliber changes of the coronary resistance vessels in response to metabolic demands of the heart.* Coronary flow reserve is the difference between maximal flow as caused by a vasodilator drug and the flow in the physiological range.

In addition to providing the head of pressure to drive blood through the coronary vessels, the heart also influences its blood supply by the squeezing effect of the contracting myocardium on the blood vessels that course through it (**extravascular compression** or **extracoronary resistance**). This force is so great

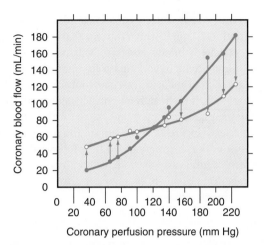

FIGURE 11-2 ▪ Pressure-flow relationships in the coronary vascular bed. At constant aortic pressure, cardiac output, and heart rate, coronary artery perfusion pressure was abruptly increased or decreased from the control level indicated by the point where the two *lines* cross. The *closed circles* represent the flows that were obtained immediately after the change in perfusion pressure; the *open circles* represent the steady-state flows at the new pressures. There is a tendency for flow to return toward the control level (autoregulation of blood flow), which is most prominent over the intermediate pressure range (about 60 to 180 mm Hg). *(From Berne RM, Rubio R: Coronary circulation. In Berne RM, Sperelakis N (Eds), Handbook of physiology, section 2: The cardiovascular system—the heart, vol 1, Bethesda, Md, 1979, American Physiological Society.)*

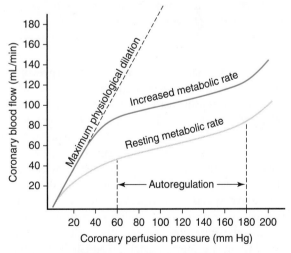

FIGURE 11-3 ▪ Illustration of autoregulation in coronary vasculature and the effect of metabolic activity on the position of the autoregulatory region. When cardiac metabolism increases, as during exercise, autoregulation persists as the pressure-flow relation shifts upward.

during early ventricular systole that blood flow, as measured in a large coronary artery that supplies the **left ventricle,** is briefly reversed. Maximal left coronary inflow occurs in early diastole, when the ventricles have relaxed and extravascular compression of the coronary vessels is virtually absent. This flow pattern is seen in the phasic coronary flow curve for the left coronary artery (Figure 11-4). After an initial reversal in early systole, left coronary blood flow follows the aortic pressure until early diastole, when it rises abruptly and then declines slowly as aortic pressure falls during the remainder of diastole.

CLINICAL BOX

The minimal extravascular resistance and absence of left ventricular work during diastole can be used to improve myocardial perfusion in patients with damaged myocardium and low blood pressure. The method, called **counterpulsation,** consists of the insertion of an inflatable balloon into the thoracic aorta through a femoral artery. The balloon is inflated during ventricular diastole and deflated during systole. This procedure enhances coronary blood flow during diastole by raising diastolic pressure at a time when coronary extravascular resistance is lowest. Furthermore, it reduces cardiac energy requirements by lowering aortic pressure (afterload) during ventricular ejection.

Left ventricular intramural pressure (**pressure within the wall of the left ventricle**) is greatest near the endocardium and least near the epicardium. However, under normal conditions this pressure gradient does not impair endocardial blood flow, because a greater blood flow to the endocardium during diastole compensates for the greater blood flow to the epicardium during systole. In fact, when 10-μm-diameter radioactive spheres are injected into the coronary arteries, their distribution indicates that the blood flows to the epicardial and endocardial halves of the left ventricle are approximately equal (slightly higher in the endocardium) under normal conditions. The equality of epicardial and endocardial blood flows indicates that the tone of the endocardial resistance vessels is less than the tone of the epicardial vessels

because extravascular compression is greatest at the endocardial surface of the ventricle.

CLINICAL BOX

Under abnormal conditions, when diastolic pressure in the coronary arteries is low (such as in **severe hypotension, partial coronary artery occlusion,** and **severe aortic stenosis**), the ratio of endocardial to epicardial blood flow falls below a value of 1. This change indicates that blood flow to the endocardial regions is more severely impaired than that to the epicardial regions of the left ventricle. Reduced blood flow to the endocardium is also reflected in an increase in the gradient of myocardial lactic acid and adenosine concentrations from epicardium to endocardium. Thus, the myocardial damage observed in the left ventricle after occlusion of a major coronary artery is greater in the inner wall than in the outer wall of the ventricle.

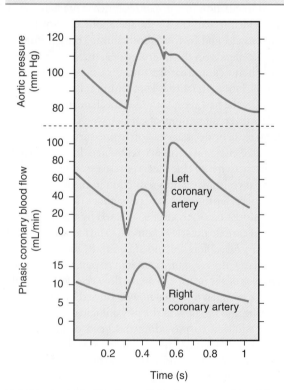

FIGURE 11-4 ■ Comparison of phasic coronary blood flow in the left and right coronary arteries.

Flow in the right coronary artery shows a similar pattern (see Figure 11-4). However, because of the lower pressure developed during systole by the thin right ventricle, reversal of blood flow does not occur in early systole, and systolic blood flow constitutes a much greater proportion of total coronary inflow than it does in the left coronary artery.

The extent to which extravascular compression restricts coronary inflow can readily be detected when the heart is suddenly arrested in diastole, or with the induction of ventricular fibrillation. Figure 11-5 illustrates the changes in mean left coronary flow when the vessel was perfused with blood at a constant pressure from a reservoir. At the arrow in Figure 11-5A, ventricular fibrillation was electrically induced, and blood flow increased immediately and substantially. Subsequent increase in coronary resistance over a period of 30 minutes reduced myocardial blood flow to below the level that existed before induction of ventricular fibrillation (Figure 11-5B, before stellate ganglion stimulation).

Tachycardia and bradycardia have dual effects on coronary blood flow. A change in heart rate is accomplished chiefly by shortening or lengthening of diastole. During tachycardia, the proportion of time spent in systole, and consequently the period of restricted inflow, increases. However, this mechanical reduction in mean coronary flow is overridden by the coronary vasodilation that is associated with the greater metabolic activity that prevails when the heart is beating rapidly. When bradycardia prevails, the opposite is true. Coronary inflow is less restricted (more time in diastole), but the metabolic (O_2) requirements of the myocardium are also diminished.

Neural and Neurohumoral Factors

Stimulation of the sympathetic nerves to the heart elicits a marked increase in coronary blood flow. However, the increase in flow is associated with cardiac acceleration and a forceful systole. A greater fraction of time is spent in systole because of the stronger myocardial contractions and the tachycardia. This situation tends to restrict coronary flow, whereas the increase in myocardial metabolic activity, as evidenced by the rate and contractility changes, tends to dilate the coronary resistance vessels. The increase in coronary blood flow observed with cardiac sympathetic nerve stimulation constitutes the algebraic sum of these factors. In perfused hearts, the mechanical effects of extravascular compression are eliminated by cardiac arrest or by ventricular fibrillation. An

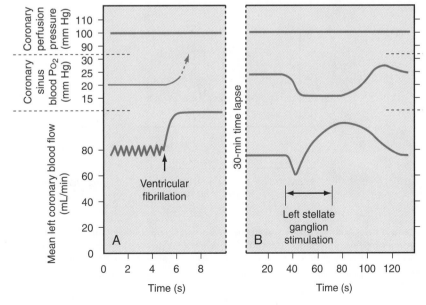

FIGURE 11-5 ■ **A,** Unmasking of the restricting effect of ventricular systole on mean coronary blood flow by induction of ventricular fibrillation during constant pressure perfusion of the left coronary artery. **B,** Effect of cardiac sympathetic nerve stimulation on coronary blood flow and coronary sinus blood O_2 tension in the fibrillating heart during constant pressure perfusion of the left coronary artery. *(From Berne RM: Unpublished observations.)*

initial coronary vasoconstriction is often observed with cardiac sympathetic nerve stimulation, before the vasodilation attributable to the metabolic effect comes into play (Figure 11-5B). Furthermore, after the β-adrenergic receptors are blocked to eliminate the positive chronotropic and inotropic effects, direct reflex activation of the sympathetic nerves to the heart increases coronary resistance. *These observations indicate that the main action of the sympathetic nerve fibers on the coronary resistance vessels is vasoconstriction.*

The **α-** and **β-adrenergic drugs** and their respective blocking agents reveal the presence of **α-adrenoceptors (constrictors)** and **β-adrenoceptors (dilators)** on the coronary vessels as in other blood vessels (see Chapter 9). Furthermore, the coronary resistance vessels participate in the baroreceptor and chemoreceptor reflexes, and the sympathetic constrictor tone of the coronary arterioles can be modulated reflexly. Nevertheless, coronary resistance is predominantly under local nonneural control. Vagus nerve stimulation or intracoronary acetylcholine causes slight dilation of coronary resistance vessels and, at constant perfusion pressure, increases coronary blood flow (Figure 11-6). The vasodilation is initiated at **muscarinic receptors** on endothelial cells that release nitric oxide (NO) (see Figure 8-4). When NO synthase is inhibited by nitro-L-arginine methyl ester (L-NAME), vagal stimulation and acetylcholine are less able to increase coronary flow (Figure 11-6). Activation of the carotid and aortic chemoreceptors can also elicit a small decrease in coronary resistance via the vagus nerves to the heart.

Reflexes that originate in the myocardium and that alter vascular resistance in the peripheral systemic vessels include the coronary vessels. However, the existence of extracardiac reflexes, with the coronary resistance vessels as the effector sites, has not been established.

Metabolic Factors

One of the most striking characteristics of the coronary circulation is the close parallelism between the level of myocardial metabolic activity and the magnitude of the coronary blood flow (Figure 11-7). This relationship is also found in the denervated heart and in the completely isolated heart, regardless of whether the heart is beating or fibrillating.

The nature of the links between cardiac metabolic rate and coronary blood flow remains unsettled. *However, it appears that a decrease in the ratio of O_2 supply to O_2 demand (whether produced by a reduction in O_2 supply or by an increment in O_2 demand)*

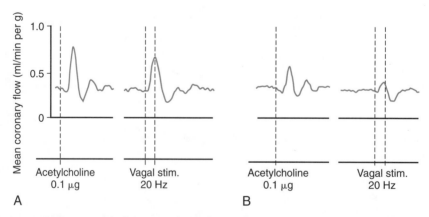

FIGURE 11-6 ■ **A,** Intracoronary acetylcholine or vagal stimulation (stim.) increases mean coronary blood flow at constant coronary perfusion pressure. **B,** Inhibition of nitric oxide (NO) synthase by nitro-L- arginine methyl ester greatly reduced the effects of acetylcholine and vagal stim. *(Redrawn from Broten TP, Miyashiro JK, Moncada S, Feigl EO: Role of endothelium-derived relaxing factor in parasympathetic coronary vasodilation. Am J Physiol 262:H1579, 1992.)*

releases vasodilator substances from the myocardium into the interstitial fluid, where they can relax the coronary resistance vessels. As diagrammed in Figure 11-8, a decrease in arterial blood O_2 content or in the coronary blood flow, or an increase in cardiac metabolic rate, decreases the O_2 supply/demand ratio. This releases vasodilator substances, such as adenosine and NO, which dilate the arterioles and thereby adjust O_2 supply to demand. A decrease in O_2 demand would reduce the release of vasodilators and permit greater expression of basal tone.

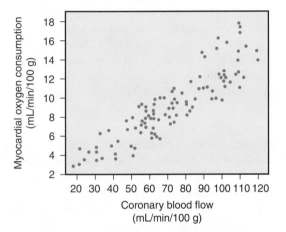

FIGURE 11-7 ■ Relationship between myocardial oxygen consumption and coronary blood flow during a variety of interventions that increased or decreased myocardial metabolic rate. *(Redrawn from Berne RM, Rubio R: Coronary circulation. In Berne RM, Sperelakis N (Eds), Handbook of physiology, section 2: The cardiovascular system—the heart, vol 1, Bethesda, Md, 1979, American Physiological Society.)*

Numerous agents, generally referred to as metabolites, have been suggested as mediators of the vasodilation observed with increased cardiac work. Among the factors implicated are CO_2, O_2 (reduced O_2 tension), hydrogen ions (lactic acid), K^+, adenosine, prostaglandins, NO, and opening of adenosine triphosphate (ATP)–sensitive K (K_{ATP}) channels.

Of these agents, the key factors appear to be **adenosine, NO,** and **opening of the K_{ATP} channels.** The contribution of each of these factors, and their interaction under basal conditions and during increased myocardial activity, is complex and has not been clearly delineated. A reduction of oxidative metabolism in vascular smooth muscle reduces ATP, which, in turn, opens K_{ATP} channels and causes hyperpolarization. This potential change reduces Ca^{++} entry and relaxes coronary vascular smooth muscle to increase flow. In endothelial cells, hypoxia activates K_{ATP} channels that signal an increased release of NO to relax vascular smooth muscle. A reduction of ATP also opens K_{ATP} channels in cardiac muscle and generates an outward current that reduces action potential duration and limits entry of Ca^{++} during phase 2 of the action potential. This action is thought to serve a protective role during periods of imbalance between O_2 supply and demand. Additionally, the release of vasodilators such as NO and adenosine dilates the arterioles and thereby adjusts the O_2 supply to the O_2 demand. For example, at low concentrations, adenosine appears to activate *endothelial* K_{ATP} channels and to enhance NO release. Conversely, at higher concentrations, adenosine acts directly on *vascular smooth muscle* to activate K_{ATP} channels. A decreased O_2 demand would sustain

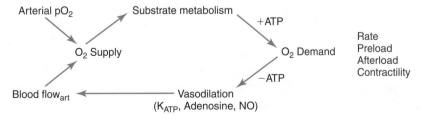

FIGURE 11-8 ■ Oxygen supply is determined by arterial blood flow (Blood flow$_{art}$) and its O_2 content. O_2 demand is a function of rate, preload, afterload, and contractility. Substrate metabolism provides adenosine triphosphate (ATP) to support cardiac work, whereas reduced ATP formation leads to vasodilation by various mechanisms. Imbalance in the O_2 supply/O_2 demand ratio alters coronary blood flow by the rate of release of vasodilator metabolites from the cardiomyocytes. A decrease in the ratio elicits an increase in vasodilator release, whereas an increase in the ratio has the opposite effect.

the ATP level and also reduce the amount of vasodilator substances released and permit greater expression of basal tone. If all three agents are inhibited, coronary blood flow is reduced, both at rest and during exercise. Furthermore, contractile dysfunction and signs of myocardial ischemia become evident.

DIMINISHED CORONARY BLOOD FLOW IMPAIRS CARDIAC FUNCTION

Most of the O_2 in the coronary arterial blood is extracted during one passage through the myocardial capillaries. Thus the O_2 supply to the myocardial cells is **flow limite**d. Myocardial ischemia occurs when the coronary blood flow is insufficient to support the required rate of myocardial O_2 consumption. Myocardial substrate metabolism during ischemia depends upon the severity of ischemia. Complete elimination of flow quickly results in depletion of high-energy phosphates and accumulation of lactate. Also, contractile akinesis occurs; over time, this akinesis evolves into myocardial infarction and tissue necrosis. On the other hand, a more modest reduction in flow (20%-60%) causes a decrease in myocardial O_2 consumption ($\approx$10%-50%), a transient increased dependence on anaerobic glycolysis (glycogen depletion and lactate production), oxidation of free fatty acids at a reduced rate, and modest to severe contractile dysfunction. Depending on the metabolic demand, these modest reductions in flow do not necessarily lead to irreversible tissue damage. The classic symptom of myocardial ischemia is chest pain, or angina pectoris.

(The relation between O_2 consumption and the work performed by the heart is discussed in Chapter 4.)

In myocardial ischemia, intracellular acidosis occurs, and Na^+ accumulates in the myocytes. The high H^+ concentration activates Na^+-H^+ exchange, and H^+ is extruded from the cells in exchange for Na^+. In addition, the ischemia inhibits Na^+,K^+-ATPase, thereby reducing Na^+ extrusion. The increased intracellular Na^+ content enhances Na^+-Ca^{++} exchange, so that as Na^+ leaves the cells, Ca^{++} enters (see Figure 4-8). The result is Ca^{++} overload, which impairs myocardial contraction, possibly leading to cell death. Inhibition of Na^+-H^+ exchange or of Na^+-Ca^{++} exchange hastens recovery from ischemia during reperfusion.

Reductions in coronary blood flow (**myocardial ischemia**) may critically impair the mechanical and electrical behavior of the heart. Diminished coronary blood flow as a consequence of coronary artery disease (usually **coronary atherosclerosis**) is one of the most common causes of serious cardiac disease. The ischemia may be global (i.e., affecting an entire ventricle) or regional (i.e., affecting some fraction of the ventricle). The impairment of the mechanical contraction of the affected myocardium is produced not only by the diminished delivery of O_2 and metabolic substrates but also by the accumulation of potentially deleterious substances (e.g., K^+, lactic acid, H^+) in the cardiac tissues. If the reduction of coronary flow to any region of the heart is sufficiently severe and prolonged, necrosis (death) of the affected cardiac cells results.

During myocardial ischemia, the rate of oxidative phosphorylation is reduced, and the concentration of ATP falls. The adenosine diphosphate (ADP) that is formed is further hydrolyzed to adenosine monophosphate (AMP) and converted to *adenosine* by the enzyme 5′-nucleotidase (Figure 11-9). Adenosine readily leaves the cardiomyocyte and exerts both autocrine and paracrine effects on cardiomyocytes and vascular smooth muscle in the local vicinity. Myocardial ischemia results in about a 100-fold increase in interstitial adenosine, and adenosine receptors are stimulated. These effects are mediated by two types of adenosine receptors, A_1 and A_{2a}.

The adenosine A_1 receptor, located on the plasma membrane of cardiomyocytes, inhibits adenylyl cyclase (AC) through the guanine nucleotide inhibitory protein (G_i) (see Figure 11-9). Stimulation of adenosine A_1 receptors results in an "antiadrenergic" effect on cardiomyocytes, decreasing guanine nucleotide stimulatory protein (G_s)-mediated adrenergic stimulation of AC activity and the production of cyclic AMP (cAMP). In the sinoatrial (SA) node pacemaker, adenosine A_1 receptor stimulation results in a decrease in heart rate via the same path as acetylcholine (see Figure 5-8). In ventricular cardiomyocytes, adenosine A_1 receptor stimulation also decreases AC and cAMP, especially

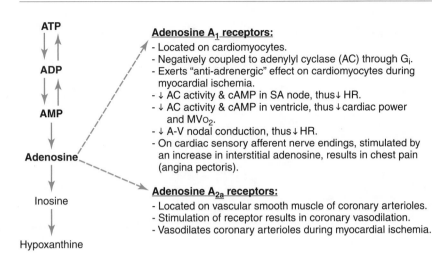

ATP
ADP
AMP
Adenosine
Inosine
Hypoxanthine

Adenosine A₁ receptors:
- Located on cardiomyocytes.
- Negatively coupled to adenylyl cyclase (AC) through G_i.
- Exerts "anti-adrenergic" effect on cardiomyocytes during myocardial ischemia.
- ↓ AC activity & cAMP in SA node, thus↓ HR.
- ↓ AC activity & cAMP in ventricle, thus ↓ cardiac power and MVO_2.
- ↓ A-V nodal conduction, thus↓ HR.
- On cardiac sensory afferent nerve endings, stimulated by an increase in interstitial adenosine, results in chest pain (angina pectoris).

Adenosine A₂ₐ receptors:
- Located on vascular smooth muscle of coronary arterioles.
- Stimulation of receptor results in coronary vasodilation.
- Vasodilates coronary arterioles during myocardial ischemia.

FIGURE 11-9 ▪ The metabolic path for adenosine production and degradation together with the cellular targets of adenosine. ADP, adenosine diphosphate; ATP, adenosine triphosphate; A-V atrio-ventricular, cAMP, cyclic adenosine monophosphate; G_i, guanine nucleotide inhibitory protein; HR, heart rate; MVO_2, maximal rate of O_2 consumption; SA, sinoatrial; ↓, decrease in.

under conditions of high adrenergic stimulation, thereby reducing the rate of O_2 consumption. This mechanism is particularly important during myocardial ischemia, when adenosine formation is greatly increased. Intravenous injections of adenosine are used to treat "superventricular tachycardia"; adenosine administration stimulates A_1 receptors on the atrioventricular (AV) node and rapidly reduces the ventricular rate like acetylcholine does (see Figure 3-10).

Adenosine A_1 receptors are also on cardiac sensory nerve endings; stimulation of these receptors can result in the sensation of pain in the chest, or angina pectoris. Thus during ischemia, the rise in adenosine links the reduction of O_2 delivery, oxidative phosphorylation, and ATP content to the clinical symptom of angina pectoris.

The adenosine A_{2a} receptor, located on vascular smooth muscle cells of coronary arterioles (see Figure 11-9), causes coronary vasodilation when activated. Adenosine is a most effective endogenous coronary vasodilator. In healthy humans, an intracoronary infusion of adenosine can increase coronary blood flow fivefold. During myocardial ischemia, adenosine formation is dramatically increased in cardiomyocytes, resulting in an increase in interstitial adenosine. This increase stimulates A_{2a} receptors located on coronary arterioles, resulting in coronary vasodilation. Overall, adenosine reduces the severity of ischemia by increasing coronary blood flow and decreases the myocardial requirement for O_2 consumption by

decreasing the heart rate and contractility. In the normal healthy heart, the interstitial levels of adenosine are very low and adenosine receptors are not stimulated.

ENERGY SUBSTRATE METABOLISM DURING ISCHEMIA

A reduction in coronary blood flow results in a rapid and proportional reduction in mechanical work, a decrease in ATP and creatine phosphate concentrations, and a transient net output of lactate by the myocardium. Myocardial ischemia leads to an increase in the ability of cardiomyocytes to take up glucose. The uptake of extracellular glucose is regulated by the transmembrane glucose gradient and the concentration and activity of glucose transporters in the plasma membrane. Ischemia results in a translocation of GLUT 1 and GLUT 4 glucose transporters from an intracellular site into the plasma membrane, increasing membrane capacitance for glucose transport (see Figure 4-23). Glycogen depletion occurs and lactate accumulates; these effects increase as a function of the severity of ischemia (Figure 11-10). If the ischemia is of sufficient duration, myocardial infarction and necrosis follow. With complete elimination of blood flow there is no washout of lactate, intracellular pH decreases, and eventually a reduction in the rate of glycolysis occurs owing to H^+ inhibition of phosphofructokinase and

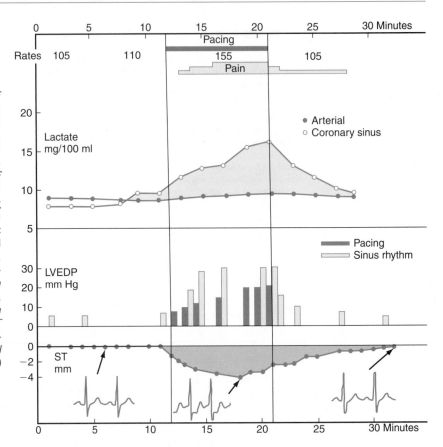

FIGURE 11-10 ■ Effects of increasing the heart rate by atrial pacing in a patient with typical stable angina. Pacing stress caused a rapid switch from lactate uptake to lactate production, a drop in the ST segment of the electrocardiogram, and chest pain. Cessation of pacing resulted in a rapid reversal from lactate production back to net uptake, elimination of pain, and a return to a normal ST segment. LVEDP, left ventricular end-diastolic pressure; *(Modified from Parker JO, Chiong MA, West RO, Case RB: Sequential alterations in myocardial lactate metabolism, S-T segments, and left ventricular function during angina induced by atrial pacing. Circulation 40:113, 1969.)*

a decreased flux through glycerol phosphate dehydrogenase due to a low cytosolic ratio of nicotinamide adenine dinucleotide (NAD^+) to the reduced form of NAD^+ (NADH) (see Figure 4-25). Complete elimination of flow differs from partial reductions in flow, in that there is no residual resynthesis of ATP by oxidative phosphorylation, complete dependence on endogenous substrate, and no washout of noxious metabolites (e.g., H^+). The sole source of glycolytic substrate under these conditions becomes glycogen, because there is no blood flow to deliver glucose to the tissue.

Substantial but temporary mechanical dysfunction of the heart may occur if the reduction of coronary flow is neither too prolonged nor too severe to cause myocardial necrosis. A relatively brief period of severe ischemia, followed by reperfusion, may be associated with pronounced mechanical dysfunction

(called **myocardial stunning**) of the heart, which can eventually fully recover after a period of hours to days.

Myocardial stunning can be prevented by preconditioning. This procedure consists of one or more brief occlusions of a coronary artery. A prolonged occlusion in the absence of the brief occlusions would impair contractile force. Preconditioning appears to involve adenosine release from the myocardium in short (minutes) responses, and it involves protein synthesis in the myocardium in late (2 to 3 days) responses. Protection from the ischemia-induced impairment of cardiac function can be achieved by long-term administration of **dipyridamole,** a drug that blocks the cellular uptake of adenosine, which raises the blood levels of adenosine. Administration of an adenosine A_1 receptor antagonist abolishes the protective action of dipyridamole.

CLINICAL BOX

Myocardial stunning may be evident in patients who have had an **acute coronary artery occlusion** (a so-called heart attack). If the patient is treated sufficiently early by **coronary bypass surgery** or **balloon angioplasty** and if adequate blood flow is restored to the ischemic region, the myocardial cells in this region may eventually recover fully. However, the contractility of the myocardium in the affected region may be grossly subnormal for many days or even weeks.

CORONARY COLLATERAL VESSELS DEVELOP IN RESPONSE TO IMPAIRMENT OF CORONARY BLOOD FLOW

In the normal human heart there are virtually no functional intercoronary channels, whereas in the dog heart there are a few small vessels that link branches of the major coronary arteries. Abrupt occlusion of a coronary artery, or of one of its branches, in a human or dog leads to ischemic necrosis and eventually to fibrosis of the areas of myocardium that are supplied by the occluded vessel. However, if narrowing of a coronary artery occurs slowly and progressively over a period of days, weeks, or longer, collateral vessels develop. These vessels may furnish sufficient blood to the ischemic myocardium to prevent or reduce the extent of necrosis. The development of collateral coronary vessels has been extensively studied in dogs, and the clinical picture of coronary atherosclerosis as it occurs in humans can be simulated by gradual narrowing of a normal dog's coronary arteries. Collateral vessels develop between branches of occluded and nonoccluded arteries. They originate from preexisting arterioles that undergo proliferative changes of the endothelium and smooth muscle by a process of arteriogenesis.

Myocardial hibernation also occurs, mainly in patients with coronary artery disease. Their coronary blood flow is diminished persistently and significantly, and the mechanical function of the heart is impaired concomitantly. However, the metabolic activity of the heart does not reflect the extent of the ischemia; the process is called "hibernation" because the downregulation of metabolism tends to preserve the viability of the cardiac tissues. If coronary blood flow is restored to normal by bypass surgery or angioplasty, mechanical function returns to normal.

The stimulus to **arteriogenesis** is the shear stress caused by the enhanced blood flow velocity that occurs in the arterioles proximal to the site of occlusion. With occlusion of a coronary artery, the pressure gradient along the proximal arterioles increases because of a greater perfusion pressure upstream from the occlusion. The stress-activated endothelium upregulates expression of monocyte chemoattractant protein-1 (MCP-1), which attracts monocytes that then invade the arterioles. Other adhesion molecules and growth factors participate with MCP-1 in inflammatory reactions and cell death in the potential collateral vessels. This stage is followed by remodeling and development of new and enlarged collateral vessels that are indistinguishable from normal arteries after several months.

CLINICAL BOX

Numerous surgical attempts have been made to enhance the development of coronary collateral vessels. However, the techniques used do not increase the collateral circulation over and above that produced by coronary artery narrowing alone. When discrete occlusions or severe narrowing occurs in coronary arteries, as in coronary atherosclerosis, the lesions can be bypassed with an artery (internal mammary) or a vein graft. In many cases the narrow segment can be dilated by insertion of a balloon-tipped catheter into the diseased vessel via a peripheral artery and inflation of the balloon. Distention of the vessel by balloon inflation (**angioplasty**) can produce lasting dilation of a narrowed coronary artery, especially when a drug-eluting stent is inserted to maintain patency of the diseased vessel (Figure 11-11).

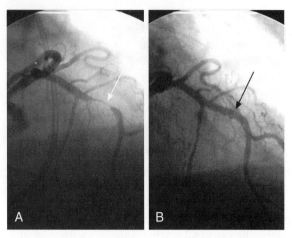

FIGURE 11-11 ■ **A,** Angiogram (intracoronary radiopaque dye) of a person with marked narrowing of the left anterior descending branch of the left coronary artery *(arrow).* **B,** The same segment of the coronary artery after angioplasty *(arrow). (Courtesy of Dr. Michael Azrin.)*

CLINICAL BOX

Many drugs are available for use in patients with coronary artery disease to relieve **angina pectoris,** the chest pain associated with myocardial ischemia. Many of these compounds are organic nitrates and nitrites. They do not dilate the coronary vessels selectively. The vasodilation arises from the production of NO, which has effects on the arterial and venous circulations. Moreover, organic nitrates and nitrites have little effect on autoregulation in the coronary circulation.

The arterioles in the ischemic heart that would dilate in response to the drugs are undoubtedly already maximally dilated by the ischemia responsible for the symptoms. In a patient with marked narrowing of a coronary artery, administration of certain vasodilators can fully dilate

normal vessel branches parallel to the narrowed segment and reduce the head of pressure to the partially occluded vessel. This effect further compromises blood flow to the ischemic myocardium and elicits pain and electrocardiographic changes indicative of tissue injury. This phenomenon is known as **coronary steal,** and it can be observed with vasodilator drugs such as dipyridamole, which acts by blocking cellular uptake and metabolism of endogenous adenosine. Also, dipyridamole reduces or eliminates coronary autoregulation because it dilates small resistance vessels. Nitrites and nitrates alleviate angina pectoris, at least partly, by reducing cardiac work and myocardial O_2 requirements by relaxing the great veins (decreased preload) and decreasing blood pressure (decreased afterload). In short, the reduction in pressure work and O_2 requirements must be greater than the reduction in coronary blood flow and O_2 supply consequent to the lowered coronary perfusion pressure. It has also been demonstrated that nitrites and endogenous NO dilate large coronary arteries and coronary collateral vessels, thus increasing blood flow to ischemic myocardium and alleviating precordial pain.

Capillary proliferation is stimulated by vascular endothelial growth factor (VEGF), whose expression is upregulated by hypoxia. The enhanced production of VEGF is mediated in part by adenosine release caused by the hypoxia. Drug-induced chronic bradycardia can also enhance capillary density by greater expression of VEGF protein. The role of VEGF in development of collateral arterial vessels continues to be an exciting research area.

SUMMARY

- The physical factors that influence coronary blood flow are the viscosity of the blood, the frictional resistance of the vessel walls, the aortic pressure, and the extravascular compression of the vessels within the walls of the left ventricle. Left coronary blood flow is restricted during ventricular systole as a result of extravascular compression, and flow is greatest during diastole when the intramyocardial vessels are not compressed.

- Neural regulation of coronary blood flow is much less important than metabolic regulation. Activation of the cardiac sympathetic nerves directly constricts the coronary resistance vessels. However, the enhanced myocardial metabolism caused by the associated increase in heart rate and contractile force produces vasodilation, which overrides the direct constrictor effect of sympathetic nerve stimulation. Stimulation of the cardiac branches of the vagus nerves slightly dilates the coronary arterioles.

- A striking parallelism exists between metabolic activity of the heart and coronary blood flow. A decrease in O_2 supply or an increase in O_2 demand apparently releases vasodilators that decrease coronary resistance. Of the several factors that mediate this response, the key ones are adenosine, nitric oxide, and activation of the ATP-sensitive K^+ channels.

- Moderate, sustained reductions in coronary blood flow may evoke myocardial hibernation, which is a reversible impairment of mechanical performance associated with a downregulation of cardiac metabolism. Transient periods of severe ischemia followed by reperfusion may induce myocardial stunning, which is a temporary stage of impaired mechanical performance by the heart.

- Prolonged, severe reduction in coronary blood flow leads to changes in substrate metabolism such that glucose uptake increases as does glycolysis; lactate accumulates in the tissue. Acidosis and the ischemia lead to myocardial infarction and cell necrosis. Arrhythmias can occur that, as with the necrosis, impair cardiac contraction.

- In response to gradual occlusion of a coronary artery, collateral vessels from adjacent unoccluded arteries develop and supply blood to the compromised myocardium distal to the point of occlusion.

- The stimulus for the development of coronary collateral arteries is the shear stress caused by the enhanced blood flow in arterioles proximal to the occlusion.

ADDITIONAL READING

Buschmann I, Schaper W: Arteriogenesis versus angiogenesis: Two mechanisms of vessel growth, *News Physiol Sci* 14:121, 1999.

Duncker DJ, Bache RJ: Regulation of coronary blood flow during exercise, *Physiol Rev* 88:1009, 2008.

Gödecke A, Decking UKM, Ding Z, et al: Coronary hemodynamics in endothelial NO synthase knockout mice, *Circ Res* 82:186, 1998.

Hein TW, Kuo L: cAMP-independent dilation of coronary arterioles to adenosine: Role of nitric oxide, G proteins, and K_{ATP} channels, *Circ Res* 85:634, 1999.

Heusch G, Schulz R: The biology of myocardial hibernation, *Trends Cardiovasc Med* 10:108, 2000.

Imahashi K, Kusuoka H, Hashimoto K, et al: Intracellular sodium accumulation during ischemia as the substrate for reperfusion injury, *Circ Res* 84:1401, 1999.

Kaneko N, Matsuda R, Toda M, Shimamoto K: Three-dimensional reconstruction of the human capillary network and the intramyocardial micronecrosis, *Am J Physiol* 300:H754, 2011.

Kiriazis H, Gibbs CL: Effects of aging on the work output and efficiency of rat papillary muscle, *Cardiovasc Res* 48:111, 2000.

Knaapen P, Camici PG, Marques KM, et al: Coronary microvascular resistance: methods for its quantification in humans, *Basic Res Cardiol* 104:485, 2009.

Rizri A, Tang X-L, Qiu Y, et al: Increased protein synthesis is necessary for the development of late preconditioning against myocardial stunning, *Am J Physiol* 277:H874, 1999.

Westerhof N, Boer C, Lamberts RR, Sipkema P: Cross-talk between cardiac muscle and coronary vasculature, *Physiol Rev* 86:1263, 2006.

Zheng W, Brown MD, Brock TA, et al: Bradycardia-induced coronary angiogenesis is dependent on vascular endothelial growth factor, *Circ Res* 85:192, 1999.

CASE 11-1

HISTORY

A 70-year-old man with a long history of angina pectoris had been treated successfully with nitroglycerin. He entered the hospital because of short episodes of lightheadedness and occasional loss of consciousness. Physical examination was not remarkable, except for a pulse rate of 35. Blood pressure was 130/50. Electrocardiogram showed an atrial rate of 72 and a ventricular rate of 35, with complete dissociation of the P and R waves. Chest x-ray showed a moderately enlarged heart. The diagnosis was coronary artery disease with complete (third-degree) heart block. A pacemaker was inserted, and the patient was discharged from the hospital.

QUESTIONS

1. The severe bradycardia produced:
   a. myogenic constriction of the coronary vessels.
   b. metabolic dilation of the coronary vessels.
   c. reflex dilation of the coronary vessels.
   d. a decrease and an increase in coronary resistance.
   e. reversal of the endocardial to epicardial blood flow ratio.

Within 2 to 3 months after leaving the hospital, the patient experienced more frequent and more severe bouts of angina pectoris, and he was admitted again to the hospital for study. An angiogram showed advanced coronary disease with almost complete occlusion of the three main coronary arteries. He was then scheduled for coronary bypass surgery.

2. During the operation, the surgeon electrically stimulated the right and left stellate ganglia. This stimulation resulted in:
   a. no change in coronary blood flow.
   b. an increase in ventricular rate and a decrease in atrial rate.
   c. a decrease in ventricular rate and an increase in atrial rate.
   d. a sustained coronary dilation in one of the partially occluded vessels.
   e. a sustained coronary constriction in one of the partially occluded vessels.

3. Shortly after bypass surgery, the reactivity of the patient's coronary vessels was tested by intracoronary administration (via a catheter) of several vasoactive agents. Which of the following substances elicited an increase in coronary resistance?
   a. Nitroglycerin
   b. Endothelin
   c. Prostacyclin
   d. Adenosine
   e. Acetylcholine

4. Despite the coronary bypass surgery, the patient's cardiac function progressively deteriorated. He became severely short of breath (dyspneic), and intractable cardiac failure developed. A suitable donor was found, and he received a heart transplant. Following cardiac transplantation, the:
   a. coronary blood flow increased with vagus nerve stimulation.
   b. coronary blood flow decreased with sympathetic nerve stimulation.
   c. heart rate increased with inspiration.
   d. heart rate decreased with inspiration.
   e. stroke volume increased with exercise.

12

SPECIAL CIRCULATIONS

OBJECTIVES

1. Describe the regulation of cutaneous blood flow and its role in maintaining a constant body temperature.

2. Indicate the relative importance of the local and neural factors in adjustments of skeletal muscle blood flow at rest and during exercise.

3. Describe the regulation of cerebral blood flow.

4. Explain the regulation of the pulmonary circulation.

5. Describe the characteristics of the renal circulation.

6. Relate the intestinal and hepatic components of the splanchnic circulation.

7. Explain the changes in the fetal circulation that occur at birth.

Previous chapters describe how the heart and vessels function to provide the tissues of the body with O_2 and nutrients and how CO_2 and waste products are removed. This chapter on special circulations is included because the circulations of the various body organs differ to some degree with respect to their function and regulation.

CUTANEOUS CIRCULATION

The O_2 and nutrient requirements of the skin are relatively small. Unlike most other body tissues, the supply of these essential materials is not the chief governing factor in the regulation of cutaneous blood flow. The primary function of the cutaneous circulation is to maintain a constant body temperature. Consequently, the skin shows wide fluctuations in blood flow, depending on the need for loss or conservation of body heat. Mechanisms responsible for alterations in

skin blood flow are primarily activated by changes in ambient and internal body temperatures.

Skin Blood Flow Is Regulated Mainly by the Sympathetic Nervous System

There are essentially two types of resistance vessels in skin: arterioles and arteriovenous (AV) anastomoses. The arterioles are similar to those found elsewhere in the body. AV anastomoses shunt blood from the arterioles to the venules and venous plexuses; hence they bypass the capillary bed. The anastomoses are found primarily in the fingertips, palms of the hands, toes, soles of the feet, ears, nose, and lips. The anastomoses differ morphologically from the arterioles, in that they are either short, straight vessels, or long, coiled vessels about 20 to 40 μm in lumen diameter. The thick muscular walls are richly supplied with nerve fibers (Figure 12-1). These vessels are almost exclusively under

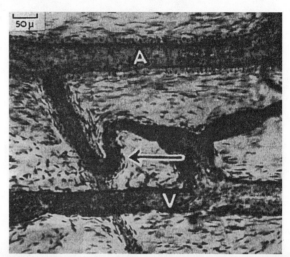

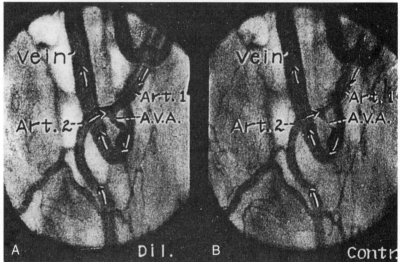

FIGURE 12-1 ■ *Top,* Arteriovenous (AV) anastomosis in the human ear injected with Berlin blue. The walls of the AV anastomosis in the finger-tips are thicker and more cellular. *Arrow* points to AV anastomosis. A, Artery; V, Vein. *Bottom,* Two frames from a motion picture record of the same relatively large AV anastomosis (A.V.A.) in a stable rabbit ear chamber installed 3.5 months previously. On this day the lumen of the A.V.A. measured 51 μm dilated and 5 μm contracted at its narrowest point. **A,** A.V.A. dilated; **B,** A.V.A. contracted. Art., artery. *(Top illustration from Prichard MML, Daniel PM: Arteriovenous anastomoses in the human external ear.* J Anat *90:309, 1956; bottom illustration from Clark ER, Clark EL:* Am J Anat *54:229, 1934.)*

sympathetic neural control, and they become maximally dilated when their nerve supply is interrupted.

Conversely, reflex stimulation of the sympathetic fibers to these vessels may cause them to constrict to the point of obliteration of the vascular lumen. Although AV anastomoses do not exhibit basal tone (tonic activity of the vascular smooth muscle that is independent of innervation), they are highly sensitive to vasoconstrictor agents such as epinephrine and norepinephrine. Furthermore, AV anastomoses do not appear to be under metabolic control, and they fail to show reactive hyperemia or autoregulation of blood flow. *Thus the regulation of blood flow through anastomotic channels is governed principally by the nervous system, in response to reflex activation by temperature receptors or by higher centers of the central nervous system.*

In contrast to AV anastomoses, the resistance vessels in the skin exhibit some basal tone. These resistance vessels are under dual control of the sympathetic nervous system and local regulatory factors, in much the same manner as are resistance vessels in other vascular beds. However, in the case of skin, neural control plays a more important role than local factors. Stimulation of sympathetic nerve fibers to skin blood vessels (**arteries, veins, and arterioles**) induces vasoconstriction, and severance of the sympathetic nerves induces vasodilation. With chronic denervation of the cutaneous blood vessels, the degree of tone that existed before denervation is gradually regained over a period of several weeks. This is accomplished by an enhancement of basal tone that compensates for the degree of tone previously contributed by sympathetic nerve fiber activity. Epinephrine and norepinephrine elicit only vasoconstriction in cutaneous vessels. Denervation of the skin vessels enhances sensitivity to circulating catecholamines (**denervation hypersensitivity**).

Parasympathetic vasodilator nerve fibers do not innervate the cutaneous blood vessels. However, stimulation of the sweat glands, which are innervated by cholinergic fibers of the sympathetic nervous system, dilates the resistance vessels in the skin. Sweat contains an enzyme that acts on a protein moiety in the tissue fluid to produce **bradykinin,** a polypeptide with potent vasodilator properties. Bradykinin, formed in the tissue, acts locally to dilate the arterioles and increase blood flow to the skin.

The skin vessels in certain regions, particularly the head, neck, shoulders, and upper chest, are influenced by higher centers of the central nervous system. **Blushing,** in response to embarrassment or anger, and **blanching,** as with fear or anxiety, are examples of cerebral inhibition and stimulation, respectively, of the sympathetic nerve fibers to the affected regions.

In contrast to AV anastomoses in the skin, the cutaneous resistance vessels show autoregulation of blood flow and reactive hyperemia. If the arterial inflow to a limb is stopped with an inflated blood pressure cuff for a brief period, the skin becomes very red below the point of vascular occlusion when the cuff is deflated. This increased cutaneous blood flow (**reactive hyperemia**) is also manifested by distention of the superficial veins in the erythematous extremity. Autoregulation of blood flow in the skin is best explained by a myogenic mechanism (see p. 179).

Ambient Temperature and Body Temperature Play Important Roles in the Regulation of Skin Blood Flow

The primary function of the skin is to preserve the internal milieu and to protect it from adverse changes in the environment. The vasculature of the skin is chiefly influenced by environmental temperature because ambient temperature is a very important external variable with which the body must contend. Exposure to cold elicits a generalized cutaneous vasoconstriction that is most pronounced in the hands and feet. This response is principally mediated by the nervous system. Arrest of the circulation to a hand with a pressure cuff, and immersion of that hand in cold water, results in vasoconstriction in the skin of the other extremities that are exposed to room temperature. With the circulation to the chilled hand intact, the reflex vasoconstriction is caused in part by the cooled blood that returns to the general circulation. This cooling stimulates the temperature-regulating center in the anterior hypothalamus. Direct cooling of this region of the brain produces cutaneous vasoconstriction.

The skin vessels of the cooled hand also show a direct response to cold. Moderate cooling or exposure for brief periods to severe cold (0° C to 15° C) causes constriction of the resistance and capacitance vessels, including AV anastomoses. However, prolonged exposure of the hand to severe cold has a secondary vasodilator effect. Prompt vasoconstriction and severe pain are elicited by immersion of the hand in water near 0° C, but the responses are soon followed by dilation of the skin vessels, reddening of the immersed part, and alleviation of the pain. With continued immersion of the hand, alternating periods of constriction and dilation occur, but the skin temperature rarely drops as low as it did in response to the initial vasoconstriction.

Prolonged severe cold causes tissue damage. The rosy faces of people working or playing in a cold environment are examples of cold vasodilation. However, the blood flow through the skin of the face may be greatly reduced, despite the flushed appearance. The red color of the slowly flowing blood is in large measure the result of reduced O_2 uptake by the cold skin and by the cold-induced shift to the left of the oxyhemoglobin dissociation curve (see Figure 1-5).

Direct application of heat to the skin produces not only local vasodilation of resistance and capacitance vessels and AV anastomoses but also reflex dilation in other parts of the body. The local effect is independent of the vascular nerve supply, whereas the reflex vasodilation is a combination of anterior hypothalamic stimulation by the returning warmed blood and of stimulation of the receptors in the heated part. However, evidence of a reflex from peripheral temperature receptors is not as definitive for warm stimulation as it is for cold stimulation.

The close proximity of the major arteries and veins to each other permits considerable heat exchange (counter-current) between artery and vein. Cold blood that flows toward the heart in veins from a cooled hand takes up heat from adjacent arteries. This results in warming of the venous blood and cooling of the arterial blood. Heat exchange is in the opposite direction with exposure of the extremity to heat. Thus, heat conservation is enhanced and heat gain is minimized during exposure of extremities to cold and warm environments, respectively.

> The fingers (and sometimes the toes) of some individuals are very sensitive to cold. When exposed to cold, the arteries and arterioles to the hands constrict, producing ischemia of the fingers characterized by blanching of the skin, which is associated with tingling, numbness, and pain. The blanching is followed by cyanosis and later by redness as the arterial spasm subsides. This condition, called **Raynaud disease,** is of unknown cause and occurs most frequently in young women.

Skin Color Depends on the Volume and Flow of Blood in the Skin and on the Amount of O_2 Bound to Hemoglobin

The color of the skin is determined in large part by pigment, in all but very dark skin. The degree of pallor or ruddiness is mainly a function of the amount of blood in the skin. With little blood in the venous plexus, the skin appears pale. However, with moderate to large quantities of blood in the venous plexus, the skin displays color. Whether this color is bright red, blue, or some shade between is determined by the degree of oxygenation of the blood in the subcutaneous vessels. As examples, a combination of vasoconstriction and reduced hemoglobin can produce an ashen gray color of the skin, and a combination of venous engorgement and reduced hemoglobin can produce a dark purple hue. *Skin color provides little information about the rate of cutaneous blood flow.* Rapid blood flow and pale skin may coexist when the AV anastomoses are open, and slow blood flow and red skin when the extremity is exposed to cold.

SKELETAL MUSCLE CIRCULATION

The rate of blood flow in skeletal muscle varies directly with the contractile activity of the tissue and the type of muscle. Blood flow and capillary density in red, slow-twitch, highly oxidative muscles are greater than in white, fast-twitch, slowly oxidative muscle. In resting muscle, the precapillary arterioles exhibit asynchronous, intermittent contractions and relaxations. Hence, at any given moment, a large fraction of the capillary bed is not perfused. Consequently, total blood flow through quiescent skeletal muscle is low (1.4 to 4.5 mL/min/100 g). During exercise, the resistance vessels relax and muscle blood flow may increase manyfold (up to about 20 times the resting level); the magnitude of the increase depends largely on the severity of the exercise.

Regulation of Skeletal Muscle Circulation

As with all tissues, physical factors such as arterial pressure, tissue pressure, and blood viscosity influence muscle blood flow. However, another physical factor operates during exercise; that is, the squeezing effect of the active muscle on the vessels. When the contractions are intermittent, inflow is restricted, and venous outflow is enhanced during each brief contraction (Figure 12-2). The presence of the venous valves prevents backflow of blood in the veins between contractions, thus aiding the forward propulsion of the blood (see also p. 218). With strong, sustained contractions, the vascular bed can be compressed to the point at which blood flow actually ceases temporarily.

Neural Factors
Although the resistance vessels of muscle possess a high degree of basal tone, they also display tone attributable to continuous low-frequency activity in the sympathetic vasoconstrictor nerve fibers. The basal frequency of firing in the sympathetic vasoconstrictor fibers is quite low (about 1 to 2 per second), and maximal vasoconstriction is observed at frequencies as low as 8 to 10 per second. Stimulation of the sympathetic nerve fibers to skeletal muscle elicits vasoconstriction that is caused by

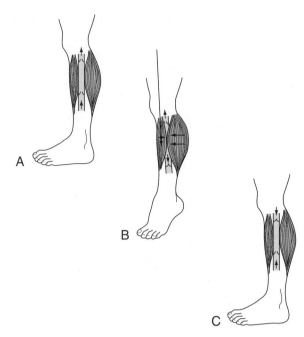

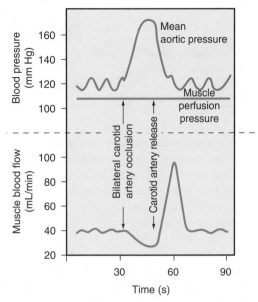

FIGURE 12-3 ■ Evidence for participation of the muscle vascular bed in vasoconstriction and vasodilation mediated by the carotid sinus baroreceptors after common carotid artery occlusion and release. In this preparation the sciatic and femoral nerves constituted the only direct connection between the hind leg muscle mass and the rest of the dog. The muscle was perfused by blood at a constant pressure that was completely independent of the animal's arterial pressure. *(Redrawn from Jones RD, Berne RM: Vasodilation in skeletal muscle. Am J Physiol 204:461, 1963.)*

FIGURE 12-2 ■ Action of the muscle pump in venous return from the legs. **A,** Standing at rest, the venous valves are open and blood flows upward toward the heart by virtue of the pressure generated by the heart and transmitted through the capillaries to the veins from the arterial side of the vascular system (*vis a tergo*). **B,** Contraction of the muscle compresses the vein so that the increased pressure in the vein drives blood toward the thorax through the upper valve and closes the lower valve in the uncompressed segment of the vein just below the point of muscular compression. **C,** Immediately after muscle relaxation, the pressure in the previously compressed venous segment falls, and the reversed pressure gradient causes the upper valve to close. The valve below the previously compressed segment opens because pressure below it exceeds that above it, and the segment fills with blood from the foot. As blood flow continues from the foot, the pressure in the previously compressed segment rises. When it exceeds the pressure above the upper valve, this valve opens, and continuous flow occurs as in **A.**

norepinephrine release at the fiber endings. Skeletal muscle vessels have α_1-adrenergic receptors (vasoconstriction) and β_2-adrenergic receptors (vasodilation). Intraarterial injection of norepinephrine elicits only vasoconstriction (α_1-adrenergic receptor activation), whereas low doses of epinephrine produce vasodilation (β_2-adrenergic receptor activation) in muscle, and large doses cause vasoconstriction (α_1-adrenergic receptor

activation). Thus, the type and amount of catecholamine determine the resultant vascular effect (see Chapter 9 and Figure 9-4).

Baroreceptors reflexes greatly influence the tonic activity of the sympathetic nerves. An increase in carotid sinus pressure results in dilation of the muscle vascular bed, and a decrease in carotid sinus pressure elicits vasoconstriction (Figure 12-3). When the existing sympathetic constrictor tone is high, as in the experiment illustrated in Figure 12-3, the decrease in blood flow associated with common carotid artery occlusion is small, but the increase after the release of occlusion is large. The vasodilation produced by baroreceptor stimulation is caused by inhibition of sympathetic vasoconstrictor activity. Because muscle is the major body component on the basis of mass and thereby represents the largest vascular bed, the participation of its resistance vessels in vascular reflexes plays an important role in maintaining a constant arterial blood pressure.

When the valves of the superficial leg veins are incompetent, as may occur with pregnancy, thrombophlebitis, or obesity, the veins become dilated and tortuous. Such **varicose veins** can be treated by surgical removal, by injection of sclerosing solutions, or merely by the use of elastic stockings.

A comparison of the vasoconstrictor and vasodilator effects of the sympathetic nerves to blood vessels of muscle and skin is summarized in Figure 12-4. Note the lower basal tone of the skin vessels, their greater constrictor response, and the absence of active cutaneous vasodilation.

Local Factors

Whether neural or local factors predominate in the regulation of skeletal muscle blood flow depends on the activity of the muscle. Neural factors predominate in resting muscle, and neurogenic vasoconstrictor tone is superimposed on the nonneural basal tone (see Figure 12-4). This is evidenced by the facts that cutting the sympathetic nerves or administration of α-adrenergic receptor antagonists to muscle abolishes the neural component of vascular tone and unmasks the intrinsic basal tone of the blood vessels. During exercise however, some (but not necessarily all) muscles must contract and perform work. The blood flow to the working skeletal muscles must increase greatly in order to meet their greater metabolic needs. As a consequence of their increased metabolism, the working muscles produce more metabolites, and these metabolic factors, which are vasodilatory, override the intrinsic sympathetic vasoconstriction and allow greatly increased local blood flow. Thus, working, but not nonworking skeletal muscles (which are not producing increased metabolites) receive an increased blood flow. Local factors underlying this vasodilation (see Chapter 9) in skeletal muscle involve the action of metabolites (e.g., H^+, K^+, prostaglandins, adenosine triphosphate [ATP], CO_2, and nitric oxide [NO]). The rhythmic contraction of exercising muscle provides a physical component to the local factors regulating blood flow. *In summary, neural and local blood flow–regulating mechanisms oppose each other, and during muscle contraction the local vasodilator mechanism overrides the neural vasoconstrictor mechanism.* Nevertheless, tonic sympathetic nerve activity persists during exercise, in part via reflexes initiated at carotid chemoreceptors. This sympathetic nerve activity, which produces vasoconstriction only in the nonworking muscles, limits the extent of metabolite-induced vasodilation and, together with the action of the muscle pump, is essential to sustain mean arterial pressure.

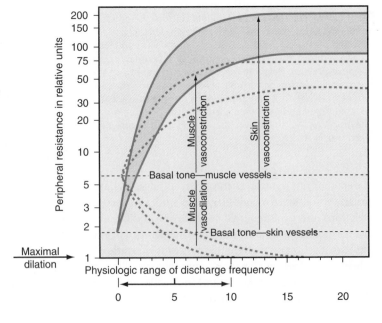

FIGURE 12-4 ■ Basal tone and the range of response of the resistance vessels in muscle (*dashed lines*) and skin (*shaded area*) to stimulation and section of the sympathetic nerves. Peripheral resistance is plotted on a logarithmic scale. (*Redrawn from Celander O, Folkow B: A comparison of the sympathetic vasomotor fibre control of the vessels within the skin and the muscles.* Acta Physiol Scand 29:241, 1953.)

CLINICAL BOX

Disease of the arterial walls can lead to obstruction of the arteries and symptoms, called **intermittent claudication** when it occurs in the legs. The symptoms consist of leg pain that occurs during walking or climbing stairs and is relieved by rest. The disease, called thromboangiitis obliterans, is seen most frequently in men who are smokers. With minimal walking, the resistance vessels become maximally dilated by local metabolite release; when the O_2 demand of the muscles increase with further walking, blood flow cannot increase sufficiently to meet the muscle needs for O_2, and pain caused by muscle ischemia results.

CEREBRAL CIRCULATION

Blood reaches the brain through the internal carotid and vertebral arteries. The latter vessels join to form the basilar artery, which, in conjunction with branches of the internal carotid arteries, forms the circle of Willis. A unique feature of the cerebral circulation is that it all lies within a rigid structure, the cranium. Because intracranial contents are incompressible, any increase in arterial inflow, as with arteriolar dilation, must be associated with a comparable increase in venous outflow. The volume of blood and extravascular fluid varies considerably in most tissues. In the brain, the volume of blood and of extravascular fluid is relatively constant; changes in either of these fluid volumes must be accompanied by a reciprocal change in the other. Unlike the rate of blood flow in most other organs, the rate of total cerebral blood flow is held within a relatively narrow range; in humans it averages 55 mL/min per 100 g of brain.

Local Factors Predominate in the Regulation of Cerebral Blood Flow

At rest, the brain consumes 20% of total body O_2 and 25% of total body glucose. Of the various body tissues, the brain is the least tolerant of ischemia. Interruption of cerebral blood flow for as little as 5 seconds results in loss of consciousness. Ischemia that lasts just a few minutes may cause irreversible tissue damage. Fortunately, regulation of the cerebral circulation is primarily under the direction of the brain itself. Local regulatory mechanisms and reflexes that originate in the brain tend to maintain a relatively constant cerebral circulation in the presence of such adverse effects as sympathetic vasomotor nerve activity, circulating humoral vasoactive agents, and changes in arterial blood pressure. Under certain conditions, the brain also regulates its blood flow by initiating changes in systemic blood pressure.

Neural Factors

The extrinsic innervation of cerebral (pial) vessels consists of components of the autonomic nervous system. Cervical sympathetic nerve fibers that accompany the internal carotid and vertebral arteries into the cranial cavity innervate the cerebral vessels. Relative to other vascular beds, sympathetic control of the cerebral vessels is weak and the contractile state of the cerebrovascular smooth muscle depends primarily on local metabolic factors. The density of α_1-adrenergic receptors is less than in other vascular beds. The cerebral vessels are not innervated appreciably by sympathetic vasodilator nerves, but the vessels do receive parasympathetic fibers from the facial nerve. These parasympathetic fibers produce a slight vasodilation on stimulation.

Local Factors

Generally, total cerebral blood flow is constant. Cerebral blood flow autoregulation involves interplay among myogenic, metabolic and neural mechanisms much as described for peripheral vessels (see Chapter 9). However, regional cortical blood flow is associated with regional neural activity, an example of intrinsic innervation. For example, movement of one hand results in increased blood flow only in the hand area of the contralateral sensorimotor and premotor cortex. Also, talking, reading, and other stimuli to the cerebral cortex are associated with increased blood flow in the appropriate regions of the contralateral cortex (Figure 12-5). Stimulation of the retina with flashes of light increases blood flow only in the visual cortex. Glucose uptake also corresponds with regional cortical neuronal activity. For example, when the retina is stimulated by light, uptake of ^{14}C-2-deoxyglucose is enhanced in the visual cortex.

Production of vasoactive compounds is thought to link increased neuronal activity to greater uptake of O_2 and glucose. Astrocytes participate in this through a phenomenon termed "neurovascular coupling." At one

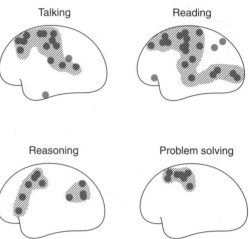

FIGURE 12-5 ▨ Effects of different stimuli on regional blood flow in the contralateral human cerebral cortex. Sens 1, low-intensity electrical stimulation of the hand; Sens 2, high-intensity electrical stimulation of the hand (pain). *(Redrawn from Ingvar DH: Functional landscapes of the dominant hemisphere.* Brain Res *107:181, 1976.)*

pole, astrocytes surround presynaptic and postsynaptic neurons at synapses. At the other pole, astrocytes converge upon vascular smooth muscle and endothelial cells of cerebral vessels. When this neurovascular unit is activated by the neurotransmitter glutamate, astrocytes produce inositol triphosphate (IP_3), which releases Ca^{++} that, in turn, activates K^+ channels. The released K^+ (0.5-10 mM) causes hyperpolarization of smooth muscle by activating the Na-K pump and increasing the conductance of inwardly rectifying K^+ channels. The hyperpolarization reduces Ca^{++} entry in vascular smooth muscle. With respect to K^+, stimuli such as hypoxia, electrical stimulation of the brain, and seizures elicit rapid increases in cerebral blood flow, and they are associated with increases in perivascular K^+. The increments in K^+ are similar to those that produce pial arteriolar dilation when K^+ is applied topically to these vessels. When extracellular K^+ exceeds 15 mM, smooth muscle cells depolarize, and Ca^{++} entry is increased to cause contraction and vasoconstriction. Thus, K^+ has a dual effect on smooth muscle function that derives from its actions on K^+ conductance and the K^+ concentration gradient.

The cerebral vessels (pial and parenchymal) are very sensitive to CO_2 tension. Increases in arterial blood CO_2 tension ($Paco_2$) elicit marked cerebral vasodilation; inhalation of 7% CO_2 results in a twofold increment in cerebral blood flow. Similarly, decreases in $Paco_2$, such as those elicited by hyperventilation, produce a decrease in cerebral blood flow. Carbon dioxide evokes changes in arteriolar resistance by altering perivascular pH (and probably also by altering intracellular vascular smooth muscle pH). By changing $Paco_2$ and bicarbonate concentration independently, some researchers have demonstrated that pial vessel diameter and pH (and presumably blood flow) are inversely related, regardless of the level of the $Paco_2$. Acidosis initiates a marked vasodilation of brain arterioles. The vasodilation is mediated by a very localized release of Ca^{++} from the endoplasmic reticulum (Ca "sparks"). This local Ca^{++} signal activates large-conductance K^+ channels (BK_{Ca}); the ensuing hyperpolarization stabilizes the vascular smooth muscle cell and opposes vasoconstriction.

Carbon dioxide can diffuse to the vascular smooth muscle from the brain tissue or from the lumen of the vessels, whereas H^+ in the blood is prevented from reaching the arteriolar smooth muscle by the **blood-brain barrier.** Hence the cerebral vessels dilate when the H^+ concentration of the cerebrospinal fluid is increased. However, the vessels show only minimal dilation in response to an increase in the H^+ concentration in the arterial blood. Chemical regulation of cerebral blood flow by $Paco_2$ is impaired in human subjects with endothelial dysfunction (diabetes, hypertension); the relative roles of H^+ and NO in response to changes in $Paco_2$ are not clear. However, in humans with normal endothelial cell function, inhibition of NO production has no effect on pressure-dependent autoregulation.

Adenosine levels of the brain rise with ischemia, hypoxemia, hypotension, hypocapnia, electrical stimulation of the brain, and induced seizures. Topically applied **adenosine** is a potent dilator of the pial arterioles. In short, any intervention that either reduces the O_2 supply to the brain or increases the O_2 requirements of the brain results in rapid (within 5 seconds) formation of adenosine in the cerebral tissue. Unlike pH or K^+ concentration, the adenosine concentration of the brain increases with initiation of the stimulus, and it remains elevated throughout the period of O_2 imbalance. The adenosine released into the cerebrospinal fluid during conditions associated with inadequate brain O_2 supply is available to the brain tissue for reincorporation into cerebral tissue adenine nucleotides.

Three factors—pH, K^+, and adenosine—may act in concert to adjust the cerebral blood flow to the metabolic activity of the brain. The cerebral circulation shows reactive hyperemia and excellent autoregulation when the pressures are between about 60 and 160 mm Hg. Mean arterial pressures below 60 mm Hg result in reduced cerebral blood flow and syncope, whereas mean pressures above 160 may lead to increased permeability of the blood-brain barrier and cerebral edema. Autoregulation of cerebral blood flow is abolished by hypercapnia and any other potent vasodilator. None of the candidates for metabolic regulation of cerebral blood flow has been shown to be responsible for this phenomenon. Hence autoregulation of cerebral blood flow is probably attributable to a myogenic mechanism, although experimental proof is still lacking.

Elevation of intracranial pressure results in an increase in systemic blood pressure. This response, called **Cushing' phenomenon,** is apparently caused by ischemic stimulation of vasomotor regions in the medulla. It helps maintain cerebral blood flow in such conditions as expanding intracranial tumors.

THE PULMONARY AND SYSTEMIC CIRCULATIONS ARE IN SERIES WITH EACH OTHER

Under steady-state conditions, the total pulmonary and systemic blood flows are virtually identical (see Chapter 10). Despite this similarity in the rate of blood flow, the anatomic, hemodynamic, and physiological characteristics of these two sections of the cardiovascular system differ substantially.

Functional Anatomy

Pulmonary Vasculature

The pulmonary vascular system is a low-resistance network of highly distensible vessels. The main pulmonary artery is much shorter than the aorta. The walls of the pulmonary artery and its branches are much thinner than the walls of the aorta, and they contain less smooth muscle and elastin. Unlike systemic arterioles, which have very thick walls composed mainly of circularly arranged smooth muscle, pulmonary arterioles are thin and contain little smooth muscle. The pulmonary arterioles do not have the same capacity for vasoconstriction as do their counterparts in the systemic circulation. The pulmonary venules and veins are also very thin and possess little smooth muscle.

The pulmonary capillaries differ markedly from the systemic capillaries. Whereas the systemic capillaries constitute an interconnecting network of tubular vessels, the pulmonary capillaries are aligned so that the blood flows in thin sheets between adjacent alveoli (Figure 12-6). Hence the capillary blood is exposed optimally to the alveolar gases. The total surface area for exchange between alveoli and blood is about 50 to 70 m^2. Only thin layers of vascular and alveolar endothelium separate the blood and alveolar gas. The thickness of the sheets of blood between

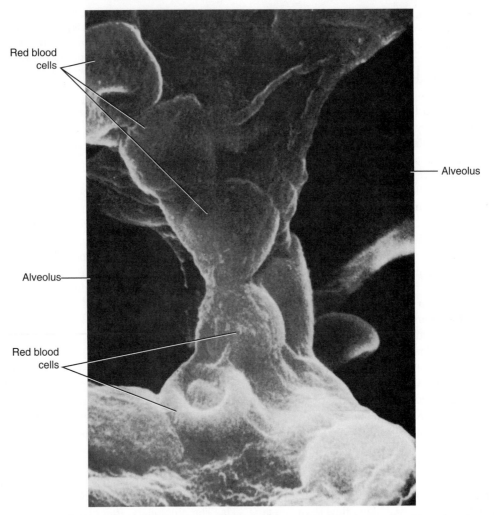

Red blood cells

Alveolus

Alveolus

Red blood cells

FIGURE 12-6 ■ Scanning electron micrograph of mouse lung to show an interalveolar septum. Note that the membranes that separate an alveolus from a capillary are so thin that the shapes of the erythrocytes in the capillary can easily be discerned. *(From Greenwood MF, Holland P: The mammalian respiratory tract surface. A scanning electron microscopic study.* Lab Invest *27:296, 1972.)*

adjacent alveoli depends on the intravascular and intraalveolar pressures. Ordinarily, the width of an interalveolar sheet of blood is about equal to the diameter of a red blood cell (see Figure 12-6). During pulmonary vascular congestion, as when the left atrial pressure is elevated, the width of the sheet may increase severalfold. Conversely, when local alveolar pressure exceeds the adjacent capillary pressure, the capillaries may collapse and blood will not flow to those alveoli. Hydrostatic factors participate in this phenomenon, particularly with respect to the regional

distribution of blood flow to the lungs, as described in the next section.

Bronchial Vasculature

The bronchial arteries are branches of the thoracic aorta. These arteries and their branches, down to the arterioles, have the structural characteristics of most systemic arteries. Hence they have much thicker walls and more smooth muscles than do the pulmonary arterial vessels of equivalent caliber. The bronchial vessels supply blood to the tracheobronchial tree down to the terminal bronchioles.

Pulmonary Hemodynamics

The bronchial veins drain partly into the pulmonary venous system, and partly into the azygos veins, which are a part of the systemic venous system. The bronchial circulation normally constitutes about 1% of the cardiac output. Therefore the fraction of the bronchial blood flow that returns to the left atrium (**via the pulmonary veins**) rather than to the right atrium (**via the azygos veins**) constitutes at most 1% of the venous return to the heart. This small quantity of bronchial venous blood, plus a small amount of coronary venous blood that drains directly into the left atrium or left ventricle, "contaminates" the pulmonary venous blood, which is ordinarily fully saturated with O_2. Hence, the aortic blood is very slightly desaturated. This small quantity of venous drainage directly into the left side of the heart also accounts for the fact that, under true steady-state conditions, the output of the left ventricle slightly exceeds that of the right ventricle.

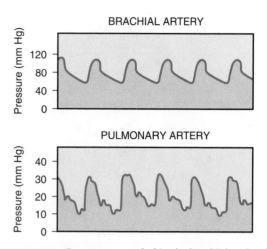

FIGURE 12-7 ▪ Pressures recorded in the brachial and pulmonary arteries of a normal human subject. *(Modified from Harris P, Heath D:* Human pulmonary circulation, *Edinburgh, 1962, E & S Livingstone.)*

Pressures in the Pulmonary Circulation

In normal individuals, the average systolic and diastolic pressures in the pulmonary artery are about 25 and 10 mm Hg, respectively, and the mean pressure is about 15 mm Hg (Figure 12-7). These pressures are much lower than those in systemic arteries because the pulmonary vascular resistance is only about one tenth the resistance of the systemic vascular bed. The mean pressure in the left atrium is normally about 5 mm Hg, and so the total pulmonary arteriovenous pressure gradient is only about 10 mm Hg. The mean hydrostatic pressure in the pulmonary capillaries lies between the pulmonary arterial and pulmonary venous values but somewhat closer to the latter.

Pulmonary Blood Flow

Under steady-state conditions the pulmonary and systemic blood flows are equal, except for the small disparity contributed by the bronchial circulation. Gravity affects the regional distribution of blood flow in the lungs because of the low pressures in the pulmonary blood vessels and their great distensibility.

Three distinct flow patterns may be found at different hydrostatic levels in the lung, as illustrated in Figure 12-8. Consider that the pulmonary artery delivers blood at a steady pressure of 15 mm Hg, and that pulmonary venous pressure remains constant at 5 mm Hg. In those pulmonary arterial and venous branches that are 13 cm

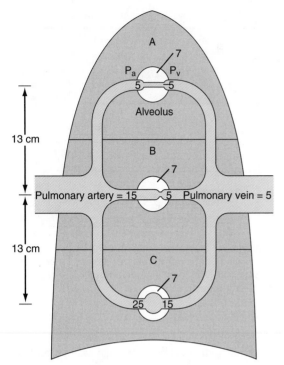

FIGURE 12-8 ■ Schematic representation of the three types of flow regimens that might exist in the pulmonary circulation. In zone A, alveolar pressure exceeds intravascular pressures. Pulmonary capillaries in this zone will not be perfused. In zone B, alveolar pressure is intermediate between pulmonary arterial and venous pressures. Pulmonary capillaries will flutter between the open and closed states. In zone C, intravascular pressures exceed alveolar pressure. The pulmonary capillaries are always open, but the flow resistances in individual vessels vary with the hydrostatic pressure in the vessel. P_a, pulmonary artery pressure; P_v, pulmonary vein pressure; alveolar pressure is 7 mm Hg in all zones. All pressures are in mm Hg.

below (zone C) the hydrostatic level of the main pulmonary vessels, the respective pressures will be 10 mm Hg, which is equivalent to 13 cm of blood greater than those in the main vessels, by virtue of the gravitational effects. Conversely, in pulmonary arterial and venous branches that are 13 cm above (zone A) the main vessels, the respective pressures will be 10 mm Hg less than those in the main vessels. At the same hydrostatic level (zone B) as the main vessels, the respective pressures in the branches will be approximately equal to those in the main vessels.

Consider that the alveolar pressure equals 7 mm Hg in all alveoli. Such an alveolar pressure might exist in

an individual who is receiving positive-pressure ventilation. In zone A in Figure 12-8, the alveolar pressure would exceed the local arterial and venous pressures. The pulmonary capillary pressures lie between the pressures of the arteries and veins, and therefore alveolar pressure would also exceed capillary pressure. Capillaries lying between adjacent alveoli would collapse. Those alveoli would not be perfused, and gas would not be exchanged.

Ordinarily, the mean pressure in the alveoli is atmospheric. Therefore the conditions depicted in zone A in Figure 12-8 do not ordinarily prevail in any region of the lungs. In **hypovolemic shock,** however, the mean pulmonary artery pressure is often very low. Therefore, vascular pressures in the lung apices might be subatmospheric. The atmospheric pressure in the alveoli would then compress the apical capillaries, so that virtually no blood would flow to that zone from the pulmonary circulation. However, the bronchial circulation, which operates at much higher pressures, would be unaffected.

In zone B in Figure 12-8, the alveolar pressure lies between the local arterial and venous pressures. Again, if alveolar pressure equals 7 mm Hg, a capillary in that region will flutter between the open and closed states. When the capillary is open, blood will flow through it, and the capillary pressure will decrease progressively from the arterial to the venous end. The pressure at the venous end will be less than the alveolar pressure, and therefore the capillary will collapse at that end. When flow ceases, the arterial and capillary pressures will equalize at a given hydrostatic level. Thus the capillary pressure will quickly rise to that in the small local arteries, which exceeds the prevailing alveolar pressure. The capillary will then be forced open. With the restitution of flow, however, the pressure will drop along the length of the capillary. As the pressure at the venous end drops below the ambient alveolar pressure, the capillary will again close. Hence the capillary will flutter between the open and closed states.

The critical pressure gradient for flow in zone B is the arterioalveolar pressure difference, not the arteriovenous pressure difference, as it is for most vessels in the body. As long as venous pressure is less than alveolar pressure, venous pressure does not influence the flow. Such a flow condition is called a **waterfall effect** because the height of a waterfall has no influence on the flow.

In zone C in Figure 12-8, the arterial and venous pressures both exceed the alveolar pressure. Hence the pressure everywhere along the capillary exceeds the alveolar pressure, and the capillary remains permanently open. In this zone, the flow is determined by the arteriovenous pressure gradient, and the resistance may be calculated by the hydraulic analog of Ohm's law.

The large and small pulmonary vessels, including the capillaries, are very distensible, as previously noted. The pressure difference that determines the caliber of a distensible tube is the **transmural pressure;** that is, the difference between the internal and external pressures. In an erect individual, the intravascular pressures in the lungs increase from apex to base. The transmural pressures increase accordingly, and the diameter of the pulmonary vessels increases from apex to base. Because resistance to flow varies inversely with vessel caliber, in zone C resistance decreases and flow increases in the apex-to-base direction. Such predicted changes in flow have been verified in humans.

Regulation of the Pulmonary Circulation

The total volume of blood pumped by the heart passes through the pulmonary circulation. Therefore the various cardiac and vascular factors that determine cardiac output in general also determine total pulmonary blood flow. These factors have been discussed in Chapter 10.

The autonomic nervous system innervates the pulmonary blood vessels. Although the small pulmonary vessels contain little smooth muscle, small changes in smooth muscle tone may alter vascular resistance substantially because the pressures in the pulmonary circulation are so low. Baroreceptor stimulation can dilate the pulmonary resistance vessels reflexly. Conversely, peripheral chemoreceptor stimulation constricts the pulmonary vessels; however, the importance of such neural regulation remains to be established.

Hypoxia has the most important influence on pulmonary vasomotor tone. Acute or chronic hypoxia increases pulmonary vascular resistance (Figure 12-9). Regional reductions in alveolar O_2 tension constrict the nearby arterioles. This response helps maintain an optimal **ventilation-perfusion ratio.** The O_2 tension in poorly ventilated alveoli approaches the Po_2 in the

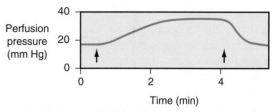

FIGURE 12-9 ▦ Effect of hypoxia on vascular resistance of an isolated rat lung. The lung was perfused with blood at a constant flow. When the O_2 tension of the inspired air was reduced *(between the arrows),* the pulmonary resistance vessels constricted, as indicated by the substantial rise in perfusion pressure. *(Modified from Grover RF, Wagner WW Jr, Mcmurtry IF, et al: Pulmonary circulation. In Shepherd JT Abboud FM, editors: Handbook of physiology, section 2: the cardiovascular system-peripheral circulation and organ blood flow, vol III, Bethesda, Md, 1983, American Physiological Society.)*

pulmonary arterial blood. Blood flowing by such alveoli is not well oxygenated, and therefore the O_2 tension of the blood returning to the left atrium decreases. Arteriolar vasoconstriction reduces the blood flow to poorly ventilated alveoli and thereby reduces the contamination of the pulmonary venous blood with poorly oxygenated blood. Thus this mechanism shunts pulmonary blood flow from the poorly ventilated regions to the better ventilated regions of the lungs and thereby improves the O_2 saturation of the systemic arterial blood.

The mechanism by which hypoxia raises pulmonary vascular resistance has received much attention. Isolated pulmonary artery smooth muscle cells have a "sensor" for O_2 because they contract in hypoxic conditions. The O_2 sensor is not known but is suspected to be mitochondria. The intact pulmonary artery is more sensitive to hypoxia than is the isolated cell. This greater sensitivity depends on the endothelium; the endothelial cells are thought to amplify rather than initiate the vasoconstrictor effect of hypoxia. Electrophysiological studies of pulmonary vascular smooth muscle cells indicate that hypoxia inhibits an outward K^+ current. The resulting depolarization of the cell membrane augments the influx of Ca^{++} into the smooth muscle cells and thereby induces contraction. The mechanism for the contraction involves the calcium-calmodulin system that causes phosphorylation of myosin light chains (see Figure 9-2). These results suggest that in an intact pulmonary blood vessel, hypoxia would lead to vasoconstriction. Chronic hypoxia results in proliferation of vascular smooth muscle, which thickens the blood vessel wall and culminates in pulmonary hypertension. Again, increased Ca^{++} entry is thought to be involved, because sustained elevation of cytosolic Ca^{++} activates a signal transduction process to activate genes involved in regulation of cell division.

THE RENAL CIRCULATION AFFECTS THE CARDIAC OUTPUT

Anatomy

The primary branches of the **renal artery** divide into a number of interlobar arteries. These **interlobar branches** (Figure 12-10) proceed radially from the hilus to the **corticomedullary junction,** which lies between the adjacent medullary pyramids. As an interlobar artery approaches the corticomedullary junction, it branches into a number of **arcuate arteries.** These travel in various directions over the bases of the adjacent medullary pyramids, in the zone between the cortex and the medulla. The arcuate branches that arise from adjacent interlobar arteries do not interconnect. Hence occlusion of an interlobar artery destroys a pyramid-shaped region of the kidney.

From the arcuate arteries, a number of **interlobular branches** travel toward the capsular surface of the kidney (see Figure 12-10). The **afferent arterioles** to the

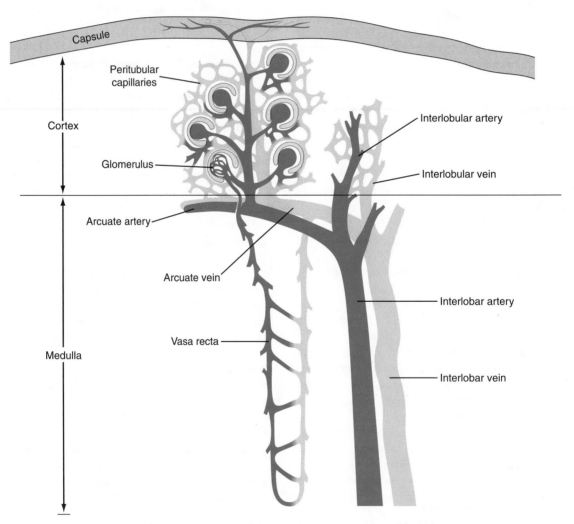

FIGURE 12-10 ■ Anatomy of the vasculature to one lobe of the kidney.

glomeruli are branches of these interlobular arteries. Each human kidney has approximately 1 million glomeruli. The afferent arteriole to each glomerulus divides into several vessels that form discrete capillary loops (Figure 12-11). The proximal and distal limbs of each loop are interconnected by many smaller capillaries. The distal limbs of each capillary loop within a glomerulus rejoin to form the efferent arteriole. The diameter of these arterioles is usually less than that of the afferent arteriole. The entire glomerular capillary tuft is enveloped by **Bowman capsule,** which collects the glomerular filtrate.

The efferent arterioles divide into another capillary network, the **peritubular capillaries** (Figure 12-12). The architecture of the peritubular capillary network varies, depending on whether the efferent arteriole arises from glomeruli close to the medullary border (**juxtamedullary glomeruli**) or from glomeruli in the more peripheral regions of the renal cortex (see Figure 12-10).

Capillaries that originate from the regular cortical glomeruli surround relatively short renal tubules, which are located almost entirely in the renal cortex. The capillary networks of neighboring cortical nephrons communicate freely with one another. Most of the capillaries arising from the efferent arterioles of juxtamedullary glomeruli form long hairpin loops (**vasa recta**) that accompany the loops of Henle deep into the renal medulla. Sometimes these loops extend to the tips of the renal papillae (see Figure 12-10). The vasa recta participate in the countercurrent exchange system, which is responsible for concentrating the urine. In general, the renal venous system parallels the arterial distribution to the renal tissues.

FIGURE 12-11 ■ Scanning electron micrograph of the mammalian glomerulus. An interlobular artery branches with two afferent arterioles (af) proceeding into the glomerular tuft and emerging in efferent arterioles (ef). The afferent arterioles are 15 to 20 μm in diameter. *(From Kimura K, Hirata Y, Nanba S et al: Effects of atrial natriuretic peptide on renal arterioles: morphometric analysis using microvascular casts.* Am J Physiol 259:F936, 1990.)

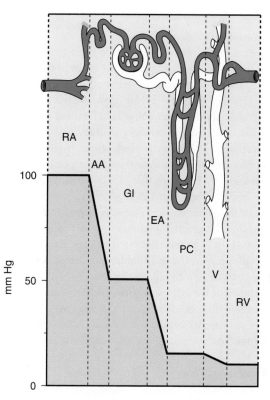

FIGURE 12-12 ■ Intravascular pressures in the renal artery (RA), afferent arterioles (AA), glomerular capillaries (GI), efferent arterioles (EA), peritubular capillaries (PC), venules (V), and renal vein (RV). *(From Frohnert PP: Renal blood flow. In Knox FG, editor:* Textbook of Renal Pathophysiology, *Hagerstown, MD, 1978, Harper & Row. Based on data from Brenner BM: The dynamics of glomerular ultrafiltration in the rat.* J Clin Invest 50:1776, 1971.)

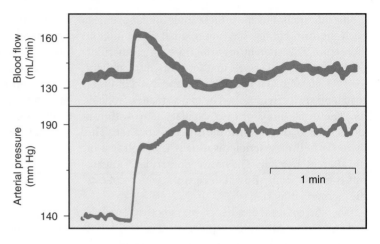

FIGURE 12-13 ■ Changes in renal blood flow evoked by a sudden increase in arterial perfusion pressure from 140 to 190 mm Hg in an isolated dog kidney. The kidney was perfused from a peripheral artery of another dog. *(Modified from Semple SJG, deWardener HE: Effect of increased renal venous pressure on circulatory autoregulation of isolated dog kidneys.* Circ Res 7:643, 1959.)

Renal Hemodynamics

Segmental Resistance

The pressure drops only slightly in the interlobar, arcuate, and interlobular arteries: the main preglomerular resistance resides in the afferent arterioles (see Figure 12-12). The pressure in the glomerular capillaries is normally about 50 to 60 mm Hg. Thus the net balance of forces across the capillary wall favors the outward filtration of plasma water along the entire length of the capillary loop. The filtration coefficient of the glomerular capillaries exceeds that of most other capillaries in the body. *Hence about 20% of the plasma water that enters the glomerular capillaries is filtered into Bowman capsule.* The greatest hydraulic resistance in the renal circulation is in the efferent arterioles. Consequently, the pressure in the peritubular capillaries is normally about 10 to 20 mm Hg. Such pressures favor net reabsorption of the large quantities of fluid that pass from the renal tubules to the interstitial spaces of the kidney. *The peritubular capillaries are also considerably more permeable than most of the other capillaries in the body.*

Renal Blood Flow

The weight of the kidneys constitutes only about 0.5% of total body weight, yet the kidneys receive about 20% of cardiac output. Most of this rich blood supply perfuses the renal cortex; and blood flow per unit weight to the inner medulla and papillae is only about one tenth that to the cortex. *Nevertheless, these medullary tissues receive as much blood per unit weight as does the brain.*

The kidney has one of the highest metabolic rates in the body. However, the large renal blood flow is not essential to subserve the high metabolic rate. The kidney extracts less than 10% of the O_2 present in the renal arterial blood. Therefore the renal blood flow is at least ten times greater than that needed to deliver the required O_2 and nutrients. The very high renal blood flow is important because it delivers large volumes of blood to the glomeruli for the process of ultrafiltration.

The Renal Circulation Is Regulated by Intrinsic Mechanisms

Autoregulation

Renal blood flow tends to remain constant despite fluctuations in arterial perfusion pressure. In the experiment illustrated in Figure 12-13, for example, arterial pressure was suddenly raised from 140 to 190 mm Hg. This stepwise change in pressure rapidly increased the renal blood flow from 135 to 165 mL/min. The rise in renal blood flow was transitory, however, and flow returned close to the control level in less than 1 minute. Over a pressure range of about 75 to 170 mm Hg, the steady-state level of renal blood flow is relatively insensitive to changes in arterial pressure (Figure 12-14). Beyond this range, however, renal blood flow varies directly with perfusion pressure.

This ability of the renal blood flow to remain constant despite fluctuations in perfusion pressure is a process intrinsic to the kidney itself. The steady flow has been demonstrated even in isolated kidney preparations

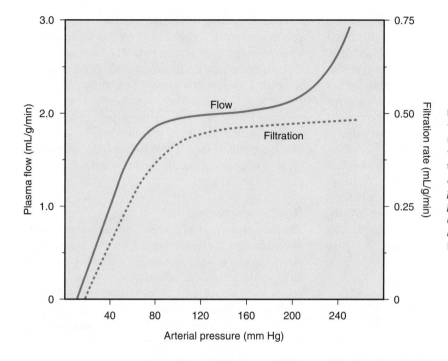

FIGURE 12-14 ■ Renal plasma flow and glomerular filtration rate as functions of arterial perfusion pressure in an anesthetized dog. *(Adapted from Shipley RE, Study RS: Changes in renal blood flow, extraction of inulin, glomerular filtration rate, tissue pressure and urine flow with acute alterations of renal artery blood pressure.* Am J Physiol *167:676, 1951.)*

(see Figure 12-13). Concomitant measurement of **glomerular filtration rate** (**GFR**) reveals that the tendency for GFR to be autoregulated is equally pronounced (see Figure 12-14). Therefore the resistance change induced by an alteration in perfusion pressure must occur mainly in the afferent arteriole. As the perfusion pressure is raised, for example, afferent arteriolar constriction not only limits the increase in renal blood flow but also restricts the rise in glomerular capillary pressure and the concomitant increment in GFR.

Renal autoregulation has been studied extensively, but its mechanism remains controversial. The two principal mediators appear to be the **myogenic mechanism** and **tubuloglomerular feedback.** The myogenic mechanism is the intrinsic property of vascular smooth muscle to contract in response to a stretching force, such as an increase in transmural pressure (see Chapter 9). Tubuloglomerular feedback involves a feedback loop, in which a change in the flow of renal tubular fluid is detected by the **macula densa** of the juxtaglomerular apparatus, and the juxtaglomerular apparatus then sends a signal to the afferent arterioles to restore basal levels of renal blood flow and GFR.

The precise nature of the signal that regulates the caliber of the afferent arterioles is controversial. Many vasoactive substances, such as prostaglandins, catecholamines, adenosine, NO, and the components of the **renin-angiotensin system,** may participate in the process of tubuloglomerular feedback. The juxtaglomerular apparatus is the source of one of the principal humoral mechanisms, the renin-angiotensin system, which is involved in the regulation of blood volume and blood pressure. In response to various types of signals, such as a reduction in GFR, the juxtaglomerular apparatus releases the enzyme **renin.** This enzyme acts on a substrate, **angiotensinogen,** which circulates in the blood, to release the decapeptide **angiotensin I.** This peptide is then split by a **converting enzyme found on endothelial cell surfaces** mainly in the lungs and kidney, to form an octapeptide, **angiotensin II.** This peptide not only is a potent arteriolar vasoconstrictor but also affects many other vital functions, such as the regulation of certain renal tubular transport processes and the release of aldosterone, an adrenocortical hormone that affects renal excretion of Na^+ and water.

Neural Regulation

Stimulation of the renal sympathetic nerves decreases renal blood flow substantially but reduces GFR only slightly. The neural activity constricts the afferent and efferent arterioles and the proximal segments of the vasa recta. Presumably the reduction of renal blood flow exceeds the reduction of GFR, because the postglomerular constriction exceeds the preglomerular constriction.

In resting subjects, the basal level of renal sympathetic tone is low; abolition of that tone scarcely affects renal blood flow. The arterial baroreceptor reflexes influence the renal vasculature only slightly. Activation of low-pressure vascular receptors elicits much larger reflex effects on the renal circulation. A reduction in left atrial pressure, for example, increases renal nerve activity and renal vascular resistance greatly. Emotional reactions such as anxiety, fear, and rage also curtail renal blood flow dramatically.

THE SPLANCHNIC CIRCULATION PROVIDES BLOOD FLOW TO THE GASTROINTESTINAL TRACT, LIVER, SPLEEN, AND PANCREAS

Several features distinguish the splanchnic circulation, the most noteworthy being that two large capillary beds are partially in series with each other. The small splanchnic arterial branches supply the capillary beds in the gastrointestinal tract, spleen, and pancreas. From these capillary beds, the venous blood ultimately flows into the portal vein, which normally provides most of the blood supply to the liver. However, the hepatic artery also supplies blood to the liver.

Intestinal Circulation

Anatomy

The gastrointestinal tract is supplied by the **celiac, superior mesenteric, and inferior mesenteric arteries.** The superior mesenteric artery is the largest of all the aortic branches and carries more than 10% of the cardiac output. Small mesenteric arteries form an extensive vascular network in the submucosa (Figure 12-15). Their branches penetrate the longitudinal and circular muscle layers, and they give rise to third- and fourth-order arterioles. Some third-order arterioles in the submucosa become the main arterioles to the tips of the villi.

The direction of the blood flow in the capillaries and venules in a villus is opposite to that in the main arteriole (Figure 12-16). This arrangement constitutes a **countercurrent exchange system.** An effective countercurrent multiplier in the villus facilitates the absorption of Na^+ and water. The countercurrent exchange also permits diffusion of O_2 from arterioles to venules. At low flow rates, a substantial fraction of the O_2 may be shunted from arterioles to venules near the base of the villus. Thus the supply of O_2 to the mucosal cells at the tip of the villus may be curtailed. When intestinal blood flow is reduced, the shunting of O_2 is exaggerated, possibly causing extensive necrosis of the intestinal villi.

Neural Regulation

The neural control of the mesenteric circulation is almost exclusively sympathetic. Increased sympathetic activity constricts the mesenteric arterioles, precapillary sphincters, and capacitance vessels. These responses are mediated by **α_1-adrenergic receptors,** which are dominant in the mesenteric circulation; **β_2-adrenergic receptors** are also present. Infusion of a β-adrenergic receptor agonist, such as isoproterenol, causes vasodilation.

In response to **fighting,** or to **artificial stimulation of the hypothalamic "defense" area,** vasoconstriction becomes pronounced in the mesenteric vascular bed. This shifts blood flow from the temporarily less important intestinal circulation to the more crucial skeletal muscles, heart, and brain.

Autoregulation

Autoregulation in the intestinal circulation is not as well developed as it is in certain other vascular beds, such as those in the brain and kidney. The principal mechanism responsible for autoregulation is metabolic, although a myogenic mechanism probably also participates (see Chapter 9). The adenosine concentration in the mesenteric venous blood rises fourfold after brief arterial occlusion. Adenosine is a potent vasodilator in the mesenteric vascular bed, and it may be the principal metabolic mediator of autoregulation. However, K^+ and altered osmolality may also contribute to the overall response.

The O_2 consumption of the small intestine is more rigorously controlled than is the blood flow. In one series of experiments, the O_2 uptake of the small intestine remained constant when arterial perfusion pressure was varied between 30 and 125 mm Hg.

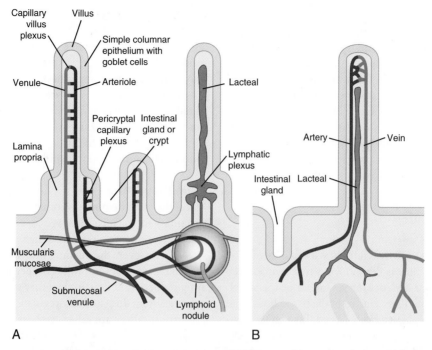

FIGURE 12-15 ■ Diagrammatic view of the microcirculation of the small intestine. **A,** Arterioles in the villus and in the crypt give rise to capillaries; blood flows to venules that eventually enter the portal circulation. **B,** Lymphatic vessels (lacteals) are found in the villus and form a plexus at the base of the villus where lymphoid nodules are located. *(Redrawn from Kierszenbaum A:* Histology and cell biology: an introduction to pathology, *Philadelphia, Mosby, 2002.)*

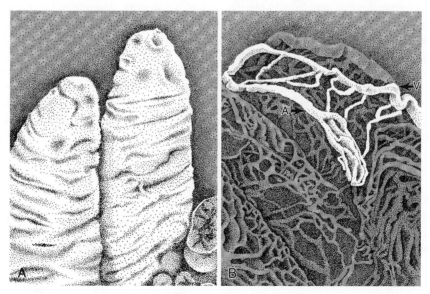

FIGURE 12-16 ■ Scanning electron micrographs of rabbit intestinal villi *(A)* and corrosion cast of the microcirculation in the villus *(B)*. A, arteriole; V, venule. *(From Gannon BJ, Gore RW, Rogers PAW: Is there an anatomical basis for a vascular counter-current mechanism in rabbit and human intestinal villi?* Biomed Res *2(Suppl):235, 1981.)*

Functional Hyperemia

Food ingestion increases **intestinal blood flow.** The secretion of certain gastrointestinal hormones contributes to this hyperemia. **Gastrin** and **cholecystokinin** augment intestinal blood flow, and these **hormones** are secreted when food is ingested. The absorption of food affects intestinal blood flow. Undigested food has no vasoactive influence, whereas several products of digestion are potent vasodilators. Among the various constituents of chyme, the principal mediators of mesenteric hyperemia are **glucose** and **fatty acids.**

Hepatic Circulation

Anatomy

The blood flow to the liver is normally about 25% of cardiac output. The flow is derived from two sources: the **portal vein** and the **hepatic artery.** Ordinarily, the portal vein provides about three fourths of the blood flow. The portal venous blood has already passed through the gastrointestinal capillary bed, and therefore much of the O_2 has already been extracted. The hepatic artery delivers the remaining one fourth of the blood, which is fully saturated with O_2. Hence about three fourths of the O_2 used by the liver is derived from the hepatic arterial blood.

The small branches of the portal vein and hepatic artery give rise to terminal portal venules and hepatic arterioles (Figure 12-17). These terminal vessels enter the **hepatic acinus** (the functional unit of the liver) at its center. Blood flows from these terminal vessels into the sinusoids, which constitute the capillary network of the liver. The sinusoids radiate toward the periphery of the acinus, where they connect with the terminal hepatic venules. Blood from these terminal venules drains into progressively larger branches of the hepatic veins, which are tributaries of the inferior vena cava.

Hemodynamics

The mean blood pressure in the portal vein is about 10 mm Hg, and that in the hepatic artery is about 90 mm Hg. The resistance of the vessels upstream to the hepatic sinusoids is considerably greater than is that of the downstream vessels. Consequently, the pressure in the sinusoids is only 2 or 3 mm Hg greater than that in the hepatic veins and inferior vena cava.

The ratio of **presinusoidal** resistance to **postsinusoidal** resistance in the liver is much greater than the ratio of **precapillary** resistance to **postcapillary** resistance in almost any other vascular bed. Hence, drugs and other interventions that alter the presinusoidal resistance usually affect the pressure in the sinusoids only slightly. Such changes in presinusoidal resistance have little effect on the fluid exchange across the sinusoidal wall. Conversely, changes in hepatic venous (and in central venous) pressure are transmitted almost quantitatively to the hepatic sinusoids and profoundly affect the transsinusoidal exchange of fluids.

Regulation of Blood Flow

Blood flows in the **portal venous** and **hepatic arterial systems** vary reciprocally. When blood flow is curtailed in one system, the flow increases in the other system. However, the ensuing increase in flow in one system usually does not fully compensate for the initiating reduction in flow in the other system. The portal venous system does not autoregulate. As portal venous pressure and flow are raised, resistance either remains constant or decreases. However, the hepatic arterial system displays autoregulation.

The liver tends to maintain a constant O_2 consumption because the extraction of O_2 from the hepatic blood is very efficient. As the rate of O_2 delivery to the liver is varied, the liver compensates with an appropriate change in the fraction of O_2 that is extracted from the blood. This extraction is facilitated by the distinct separation of the presinusoidal vessels at the acinar center from the postsinusoidal vessels at the periphery of the acinus (see Figure 12-17). The substantial distance between these types of vessels prevents a countercurrent exchange of O_2, contrary to the condition that exists in an intestinal villus (see Figure 12-16).

CLINICAL BOX

When central venous pressure is elevated, as in **congestive heart failure,** large quantities of plasma water transude from the liver into the peritoneal cavity; such a fluid accumulation in the abdomen is known as ascites. Extensive fibrosis of the liver, as in the various types of **hepatic cirrhosis,** leads to a pronounced increase in hepatic vascular resistance, which raises the pressure substantially in the portal venous system. The consequent increase in capillary hydrostatic pressure throughout the splanchnic circulation also leads to extensive fluid transudation into the abdominal

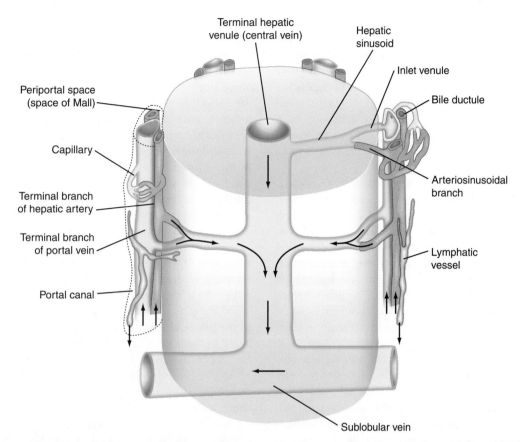

FIGURE 12-17 ■ Microcirculation in a hepatic acinus. The *arrows* indicate the direction of blood flow from the hepatic artery and portal vein to the hepatic sinusoids. The admixture of blood flows through the terminal hepatic venule and then into the sublobular vein. *(Redrawn from Ross MH, Pawling W:* Histology: A text and atlas: with correlated cell and molecular biology, *Philadelphia, Lippincott William & Wilkins, 2006.)*

cavity (i.e., ascites). Furthermore, the pressure may rise substantially in other veins that anastomose with the portal vein. A noteworthy example is that of the esophageal veins. These veins may enlarge considerably to form **esophageal varices,** which may rupture and thereby lead to severe, and frequently fatal, internal bleeding. To obviate these grave problems associated with elevated portal venous pressure, an anastomosis (**portacaval shunt**) is often created surgically between the portal vein and the inferior vena cava to decrease portal venous pressure.

The sympathetic nerves constrict the presinusoidal resistance vessels in the portal venous and hepatic arterial systems. Neural effects on the capacitance vessels are more important, however. The liver contains about 15% of the total blood volume of the body. Under appropriate conditions, such as in response to hemorrhage, about half of the hepatic blood volume can be rapidly expelled by virtue of a constriction of the capacitance vessels. Hence the liver constitutes an important blood reservoir in humans. In certain other species, such as the dog, the spleen is a more important blood reservoir.

FETAL CIRCULATION

The circulation in the fetus displays various differences from that in the postnatal infant. The fetal lungs are functionally inactive, and the fetus depends completely on the placenta for O_2 and nutrient supply. Oxygenated fetal blood from the placenta passes through the umbilical vein to the liver. Approximately half passes through the liver, and the remainder bypasses the liver and reaches the inferior vena cava through the **ductus venosus** (Figure 12-18). In the inferior vena cava, blood from the ductus venosus joins blood returning from the lower trunk and extremities, and this combined stream is in turn joined by blood from the liver through the hepatic veins.

The streams of blood tend to maintain their identity in the inferior vena cava, and they are divided into two streams of unequal size by the edge of the interatrial septum (**crista dividens**). The larger stream, which is mainly blood from the umbilical vein, is shunted to the left atrium through the **foramen ovale,** which lies between the inferior vena cava and the left atrium (see inset, Figure 12-18). The other stream passes into the right atrium, where it is joined by superior vena caval blood that returns from the upper parts of the body and by blood from the myocardium.

Unlike in the adult, in whom the right and left ventricles pump in series, the ventricles in the fetus operate essentially in parallel. Only one tenth of right ventricular output goes through the lungs, because of the large pulmonary resistance. Fetal oxygenation is derived from gas exchange in the placenta; O_2 tension in the alveoli is low. The low O_2 tension causes tonic pulmonary artery vasoconstriction. The hypoxia also results in dilation of the **ductus arteriosus.** This dilation shunts the remaining blood from the pulmonary artery to the aorta, at a point that is distal to the origins of the arteries to the head and upper extremities (see Figure 12-18). Blood flows from pulmonary artery to the aorta because the pulmonary resistance is great and the diameter of the ductus arteriosus is as large as that of the descending aorta.

The large volume of blood coming through the foramen ovale into the left atrium is joined by blood returning from the lungs. The blood from these sources is pumped out by the left ventricle into the aorta. Most of the blood in the ascending aorta goes to the head, upper thorax, and arms; the remainder joins blood from the ductus arteriosus and supplies the rest of the body and the placenta. The amount of blood pumped by the **left ventricle** is about half that pumped by the **right ventricle.** The major fraction of the blood that passes down the descending aorta comes from the ductus arteriosus and right ventricle, and it flows by way of the two umbilical arteries to the placenta.

Figure 12-18 illustrates the O_2 saturations of the blood at various points of the fetal circulation. Fetal blood leaving the placenta is 80% saturated. However, the O_2 saturation of the blood passing through the foramen ovale is reduced to 67% by mixing with the desaturated blood returning from the lower part of the body and the liver. Addition of the desaturated blood from the lungs reduces the O_2 saturation of left ventricular blood to 62%, which is the level of saturation of the blood that reaches the head and upper extremities.

The blood in the right ventricle, a mixture of desaturated superior vena caval blood, coronary venous blood, and inferior vena caval blood, is only 52% saturated with O_2. When the major portion of this blood traverses the ductus arteriosus and joins that pumped out by the left ventricle, the resulting O_2 saturation of blood traveling to the lower part of the body and back to the placenta is 58%. Thus, the tissues that receive blood of the highest O_2 saturation are the liver, heart, and upper parts of the body, including the head.

At the placenta, the chorionic villi dip into the maternal sinuses, and the O_2, CO_2, nutrients, and metabolic waste products are exchanged across the membranes. The barrier to exchange is quite large, and the equilibrium of Po_2 between the two circulations is not reached at normal rates of blood flow. Therefore the O_2 tension of the fetal blood leaving the placenta is very low. Were it not true that fetal hemoglobin has a greater affinity for O_2 than does adult hemoglobin, the fetus would not receive an adequate O_2 supply. The **fetal oxyhemoglobin dissociation curve** is shifted to the left, so that at equal pressures of O_2, fetal blood carries significantly more O_2 than does maternal blood. In early fetal life, the high **cardiac glycogen levels** that prevail may protect the heart from acute periods of hypoxia. The glycogen levels decrease in late fetal life and reach adult levels by term.

If the mother is subjected to hypoxia, the reduced blood O_2 tension is reflected in the fetus by tachycardia and an increase in blood flow through the umbilical vessels. If the hypoxia persists or if flow through the umbilical vessels is impaired, fetal distress occurs and is first manifested as bradycardia.

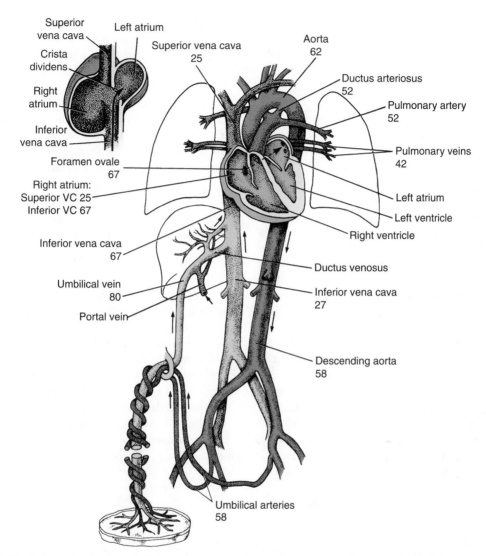

FIGURE 12-18 ▪ Schematic diagram of the fetal circulation. The *numbers* represent the percentages of O_2 saturation of the blood flowing in the indicated blood vessels. The *inset* at upper left illustrates the direction of flow of a major portion of the inferior vena cava (VC) blood through the foramen ovale to the left atrium. *(Values for O_2 saturations are from Dawes GS, Mott JC, Widdicombe JG: The foetal circulation in the lamb.* J Physiol *126:563, 1954.)*

Changes in the Circulatory System at Birth

The umbilical vessels have thick muscular walls that are very reactive to trauma, tension, sympathomimetic amines, bradykinin, angiotensin, and changes in Po_2. In animals in which the umbilical cord is not tied, hemorrhage of the newborn is prevented by constriction of these large vessels in response to various stimuli. Closure of the umbilical vessels increases the total peripheral resistance and the blood pressure. When blood flow ceases through the umbilical vein, the ductus venosus closes. This structure is a thick-walled vessel with a muscular sphincter. The event that closes the ductus venosus is still unknown.

The asphyxia that starts with constriction or clamping of the umbilical vessels, together with the cooling of the body, activates the respiratory center of the newborn infant. As the lungs fill with air, pulmonary vascular resistance decreases to about one tenth of the value that exists before lung expansion. This resistance change is not caused by the presence of O_2 in the lungs, because the change is just as great if the lungs are filled with nitrogen. However, filling the lungs with liquid does not reduce pulmonary vascular resistance.

The left atrial pressure is raised above the pressure in the inferior vena cava and right atrium by (1) the decrease in pulmonary resistance, with the resulting large flow of blood through the lungs to the left atrium; (2) the reduction of flow to the right atrium caused by occlusion of the umbilical vein; and (3) the increased resistance to left ventricular output produced by occlusion of the umbilical arteries. This reversal of the pressure gradient across the atria abruptly closes the valve over the foramen ovale, and the septal leaflets fuse over several days.

With the decrease in pulmonary vascular resistance, the pressure in the pulmonary artery falls to about one half its previous level (to about 35 mm Hg). This change in pressure, coupled with a slight increase in aortic pressure, reverses the flow of blood through the ductus arteriosus. However, within several minutes the large ductus arteriosus begins to constrict. This response produces turbulent flow, which is manifested as a murmur in the newborn. Constriction of the ductus arteriosus is progressive, and it is usually complete within 1 to 2 days after birth. Closure of the ductus arteriosus appears to be initiated by (1) the high O_2 tension of the arterial blood that passes through it and (2) the pulmonary ventilation with O_2 that closes the ductus. Furthermore, ventilation with air low in O_2 opens this shunt vessel. Whether O_2 acts directly on the ductus or through the release of a vasoconstrictor substance is not known.

> The ductus arteriosus occasionally fails to close after birth. This failure constitutes a congenital cardiovascular abnormality that is amenable to surgical correction.

At birth the walls of the two ventricles are approximately of the same thickness, with a possibly slight preponderance of the right ventricle. Also, in the newborn the muscle layer of the pulmonary arterioles is thick, a feature that is partly responsible for the high pulmonary vascular resistance of the fetus. After birth the thickness of the walls of the right ventricle diminishes, as does the muscle layer of the pulmonary arterioles; the left ventricular walls become thicker. These changes are progressive over a period of weeks after birth.

SUMMARY

SKIN CIRCULATION

- Most of the resistance vessels in the skin are under dual control of the sympathetic nervous system and local vasodilator metabolites, but the arteriovenous anastomoses found in the hands, feet, and face are solely under neural control.
- The main function of skin blood vessels is to aid in the regulation of body temperature by constricting to conserve heat and dilating to lose heat.
- Skin blood vessels dilate directly and reflexly in response to heat and constrict directly and reflexly in response to cold.

SKELETAL MUSCLE CIRCULATION

- Skeletal muscle blood flow is regulated centrally by the sympathetic nerves and regulated locally by the release of vasodilator metabolites.
- At rest, neural regulation of blood flow is paramount, but it yields to metabolic regulation during muscle contractions.

CEREBRAL CIRCULATION

- Cerebral blood flow is predominantly regulated by metabolic factors, especially H^+, CO_2, K^+, and adenosine.

- Increased regional cerebral activity produced by stimuli such as touch, pain, hand motion, talking, reading, reasoning, and problem solving is associated with enhanced blood flow in the activated areas of the contralateral cerebral cortex.

PULMONARY CIRCULATION

- The pulmonary circulation consists of the pulmonary vasculature, whose function is to promote the exchange of O_2 and CO_2 across the pulmonary capillaries, and the bronchial vasculature, whose function is to deliver O_2 and nutrients to the airways.
- The resistance of the pulmonary vasculature is low. The distribution of blood flow to different regions of the lungs is affected by the body's position in space because of the low pulmonary vascular pressures.
- The smooth muscles in the pulmonary arterioles constrict in response to hypoxia. This response tends to shift blood flow to the well-ventilated alveoli and away from the poorly ventilated alveoli.

RENAL CIRCULATION

- Renal blood flow is very high (about 20% of cardiac output), and the chief resistance to blood flow in the kidneys resides in the afferent and efferent arterioles.
- Glomerular capillary pressure is high (about 50 to 60 mm Hg), and the glomerular capillaries are very permeable to water; these two factors favor the filtration of large quantities of water from the blood to Bowman' capsule.

INTESTINAL CIRCULATION

- The microcirculation in the intestinal villi constitutes a countercurrent exchange system for O_2. This arrangement puts the villi in jeopardy in states of low blood flow.
- The splanchnic resistance and capacitance vessels are very responsive to changes in sympathetic neural activity.

HEPATIC CIRCULATION

- The liver receives about 25% of cardiac output; about three fourths of this comes via the portal vein and about one fourth via the hepatic artery. When flow is diminished in either the portal or hepatic system, flow in the other system usually increases, but not proportionately.

- The liver tends to maintain a constant O_2 consumption, in part because its mechanism for extracting O_2 from the blood is so efficient.
- The liver normally contains about 15% of total blood volume. It serves as an important blood reservoir for the body.

FETAL CIRCULATION

- In the fetus a large percentage of right atrial blood passes through the foramen ovale to the left atrium, and a large percentage of pulmonary artery blood passes through the ductus arteriosus to the aorta.
- At birth the umbilical vessels, ductus venosus, and ductus arteriosus close by contraction of their muscle layers. The reduction in pulmonary vascular resistance caused by lung inflation is the main factor that reverses the pressure gradient between the atria, thereby closing the foramen ovale.

ADDITIONAL READING

Ainslie PN, Duffin J: Integration of cerebrovascular CO_2 reactivity and chemoreflex control of breathing: mechanisms of regulation, measurement, and interpretation, *Am J Physiol Regul Integr Comp Physiol* 296:R1473, 2009.

Baschat AA, Gembruch U, Harman CR: Coronary blood flow in fetuses with intrauterine growth restriction, *J Perinat Med* 26:143, 1998.

Dabertrand F, Nelson MT, Brayden JE: Acidosis dilates brain parenchymal arterioles by conversion of calcium waves to sparks to activate BK channels, *Circ Res* 110:285, 2012.

Delp MD, O'Leary DS: Integrative control of the skeletal muscle microcirculation in the maintenance of arterial pressure during exercise, *J Appl Physiol* 97:1112, 2004.

Faraci FM, Heistad DD: Regulation of the cerebral circulation: Role of endothelium and potassium channels, *Physiol Rev* 78:53–97, 1998.

Granger DN, Kvietys PR, Korthuis RJ, et al: Microcirculation of the intestinal mucosa. In Schultz SG, editor: *Handbook of Physiology, Section 6: The Gastrointestinal System-Motility and Circulation*, vol I, Bethesda, Md, 1989, American Physiological Society.

Greenway CV, Lautt WW: Hepatic circulation. In Schultz SG, editor: *Handbook of Physiology, Section 6: The Gastrointestinal System-Motility and Circulation*, vol I, Bethesda, Md, 1989, American Physiological Society.

Kiserud T, Acharya G: The fetal circulation, *Prenat Diagn* 24:1049, 2004.

Mauban JR, Remillard CV, Yuan JX: Hypoxic pulmonary vasoconstriction: Role of ion channels, *J Appl Physiol* 98:415, 2005.

Mortensen SP, González-Alonso J, Bune LT, et al: ATP-induced vasodilation and purinergic receptors in the human leg: roles of nitric oxide, prostaglandins, and adenosine, *Am J Physiol Regul Integr Comp Physiol* 296:R1140, 2009.

Rychik J: Fetal cardiovascular physiology, *Pediatr Cardiol* 25:201, 2004.

Stamler JS, Meissner G: Physiology of nitric oxide in skeletal muscle, *Physiol Rev* 81:209, 2001.

Stickland MK, Miller JD, Smith CA, Dempsey JA: Carotid chemoreceptor modulation of regional blood flow distribution during exercise in health and chronic heart failure, *Circ Res* 100:1371, 2007.

Straub SV, Nelson MT: Astrocytic calcium signaling: The information currency coupling neuronal activity to the cerebral microcirculation, *Tr Cardiovasc Med* 17:183, 2007.

Thomas GD, Segal SS: Neural control of muscle blood flow during exercise, *J Appl Physiol* 97:731, 2004.

Toda N, Ayajiki K, Okamura T: Cerebral blood flow regulation by nitric oxide: recent advances, *Pharmacol Rev* 61:62, 2009.

Waypa GB, Schumacker PT: Hypoxic pulmonary vasoconstriction: Redox events in oxygen sensing, *J Appl Physiol* 98:404, 2005.

CASE 12-1

HISTORY

A 53-year-old man has consumed substantial amounts of alcohol over the past 3 decades. For the past 2 or 3 years, he has noticed that his belt size has progressively increased and that his abdomen is distended. His physician was able to evoke a fluid wave across the patient's abdomen by tapping it. The physician made the diagnosis of hepatic cirrhosis, which is associated with extensive fibrosis of the liver.

Question

1. The reason for the large accumulation of fluid in the patient's abdomen is that:
   a. the hydrostatic pressure in the splanchnic capillaries was abnormally high.
   b. the hydrostatic pressure in the hepatic artery was abnormally high.
   c. the hydrostatic pressure in the hepatic veins exceeded that in the portal vein.
   d. the hydrostatic pressure in the hepatic veins exceeded that in the splenic vein.
   e. the hepatic resistance was subnormal.

CASE 12-2

HISTORY

A 6-year-old boy was referred by his family physician to a pediatric cardiologist because of chronic fatigue, effort intolerance, and a heart murmur. On physical examination, the boy appeared slightly small for his age, and had normal skin color, no clubbing of the fingers, and a harsh murmur throughout systole that was heard best in the fourth intercostal space to the left of the sternum but extending over the entire precordium. An x-ray revealed an enlarged heart, especially the right ventricle. An ear oximeter showed normal oxygenation of arterial blood. Hematocrit was normal. Cardiac catheterization data were as follows:

Mean right atrial pressure: 5 mm Hg
Right ventricular systolic pressure: 30 mm Hg
Right ventricular diastolic pressure: 3 mm Hg
Right atrial blood P_{O_2}: 40 mm Hg
Right ventricular blood P_{O_2}: 60 mm Hg

Question

1. The patient was admitted to the cardiac surgery unit for repair of:
   a. coarctation of the aorta.
   b. interventricular septal defect.
   c. pulmonic stenosis.
   d. tetralogy of Fallot.
   e. patent ductus arteriosus.

CASE 12-3

HISTORY

A 55-year-old man visits his family physician and presents with a chief complaint of pain in his left leg when he walks about 2 blocks from his home to the grocery store. The pain subsides when he rests for a few minutes but it returns when he walks home. He has hypertension for which he takes amlodipine and a diuretic. He had a mild heart attack 4 years ago. Since that time, he has had occasional angina, which is treated with oral nitrates. Although counseled to stop smoking, he continues his one pack per day habit. He has a resting blood pressure of 140/95 mm Hg and an ankle-brachial index (ABI) of 0.5 in the left leg and of 1.1 in the right leg (see Chapter 7). He is diagnosed with intermittent claudication due to peripheral vascular disease in the left leg.

Question

1. What is the systolic pressure in dorsal pedal artery of the afflicted left leg?
   a. 140 mm Hg
   b. 110 mm Hg
   c. 95 mm Hg
   d. 70 mm Hg
   e. 55 mm Hg

13

INTERPLAY OF CENTRAL AND PERIPHERAL FACTORS THAT CONTROL THE CIRCULATION

OBJECTIVES

1. Describe the sequence of cardiovascular events during exercise.
2. Describe how most cardiovascular functions are integrated in exercise.
3. Describe the effects of blood loss on the cardiovascular system.
4. Explain the various compensatory mechanisms that protect against hemorrhagic shock.
5. Explain the various decompensatory mechanisms that intensify the effects of blood loss.

The primary function of the circulatory system is to deliver the supplies needed for tissue metabolism and growth and to remove the products of metabolism. To explain how the heart and blood vessels serve this function, the circulatory system has been analyzed morphologically and functionally. Furthermore, the mechanisms of the component parts that maintain adequate tissue perfusion under different physiological conditions have been discussed.

Once the functions of the various individual components are understood, it is essential to consider the interrelationships in the overall operation of the circulatory system. Tissue perfusion depends on the arterial pressure and the local vascular resistance. Furthermore, the arterial pressure in turn depends on cardiac output and total peripheral resistance (TPR). Arterial pressure is maintained within a relatively narrow range in normal individuals, a feat accomplished by reciprocal changes in cardiac output and TPR (see Chapter 7). However, cardiac output and peripheral resistance are each influenced by a number of factors, and the interplay among these factors determines the level of these two variables. Acutely, the autonomic nervous system and the baroreceptors play the key role in regulating blood pressure (see Chapter 9). However, from a long-range point of view, the control of fluid balance by the kidneys, adrenal cortex, and central nervous system, along with the maintenance of a constant blood volume, is crucial.

In a well-regulated system, one way to study the extent and sensitivity of the regulatory mechanisms is to disturb the system and then to observe its response in restoring the preexisting steady state. Disturbances in the form of physical exercise and hemorrhage are used to illustrate the effects of the various factors involved in the regulation of the circulatory system.

EXERCISE

The cardiovascular adjustments in exercise consist of a combination and an integration of neural and local chemical factors. The neural factors consist of (1) central command, (2) reflexes originating in the contracting muscle, and (3) the baroreceptor reflex. **Central command** is the cerebrocortical activation of the sympathetic nervous system that produces cardiac acceleration, increased myocardial contractile force, and peripheral vasoconstriction (see Chapter 5).

Reflexes can be activated intramuscularly by stimulation of mechanoreceptors (**by stretch, tension**) and of chemoreceptors (**by-products of metabolism**) in response to muscle contraction. Impulses from these receptors travel centrally via small myelinated (group III) and unmyelinated (group IV) afferent nerve fibers. The group IV unmyelinated fibers may represent the muscle chemoreceptors; no morphological chemoreceptor has been identified. The central connections of this reflex are unknown, but the efferent limb is composed of the sympathetic nerve fibers to the heart and peripheral blood vessels.

The baroreceptor reflex and the local factors that influence skeletal muscle blood flow (**metabolic vasodilators**) are described in Chapters 9 and 12. Vascular chemoreceptors play a significant role in regulation of the cardiovascular system in exercise. This assertion is supported by the observation that the pH, Pco_2, and Po_2 of arterial blood are normal during exercise, and the vascular chemoreceptors are located on the arterial side of the circulatory system.

Mild to Moderate Exercise

In humans and in trained animals, anticipation of physical activity inhibits vagus nerve impulses to the heart; this withdrawal of vagal nerve activity underlies the initial increase in heart rate. Eventually, sympathetic nerve discharge also increases. The concerted inhibition of parasympathetic areas and activation of sympathetic areas of the medulla increase the heart rate and myocardial contractility. The tachycardia and the enhanced contractility increase the cardiac output, in turn raising the arterial pressure.

Exercise can be understood with the help of cardiac function and vascular function curves described in

Chapter 10. An example is shown in Figure 13-1. From the interactions described in Chapter 10, Figure 13-1 can be seen as a composite that illustrates the effects of two changes. First, along with tachycardia, there is increased contractility caused by norepinephrine released from cardiac sympathetic nerves (see also Figures 5-23 and 10-15). Second, there is a change in the vascular function curve that results from vasodilation (Figure 13-1; see also Figure 10-13). In this closed circulatory system, TPR is reduced as a result of vasodilation in the skeletal muscle vascular bed. The vascular function curve is shifted upward, as is the contractility curve, because cardiac output and venous return are two measures of the same parameter.

Peripheral Resistance Declines during Exercise

At the same time that the heart is stimulated, the sympathetic nervous system elicits vascular resistance changes in the periphery. In skin, kidneys, splanchnic regions, and inactive muscle, sympathetically mediated vasoconstriction increases vascular resistance,

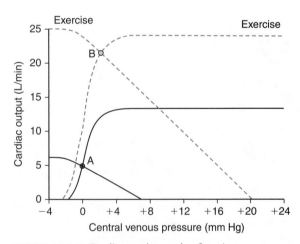

FIGURE 13-1 ■ Cardiac and vascular function curves are greatly altered during strenuous exercise, allowing an increase in cardiac output of fourfold to fivefold. The operating point of the cardiovascular system moves from A to B. The cardiac function curve during strenuous exercise is the result of increased heart rate, stroke volume, and contractility. The vascular function curve reflects greatly decreased total peripheral resistance and increased mean circulatory pressure (see Chapter 10). At the new operating point (B), cardiac output is increased more than fourfold, but filling pressure is increased only slightly.

diverting blood away from these areas (Figure 13-2). This greater resistance in vascular beds of inactive tissues persists throughout the period of exercise.

The increase in blood flow in the active muscles at the onset of exercise cannot be attributed to a neural mechanism, because a chemical block of the autonomic nervous system does not alter this blood flow response. This increase in muscle blood flow may be caused by the modest elevation of blood pressure or by some unknown mechanism.

As cardiac output and blood flow to active muscles increase with progressive increments in the intensity of exercise, visceral blood flow (**splanchnic and renal vasculatures**) decreases. Blood flow to the myocardium increases, whereas that to the brain is unchanged (see Figure 13-2). Skin blood flow initially decreases during exercise. It then increases, as body temperature

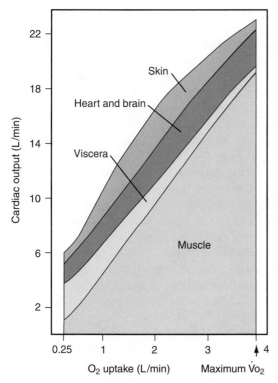

rises with increments in duration and intensity of the exercise. Skin blood flow finally decreases when the skin vessels constrict, as the total body O_2 consumption ($\dot{V}O_{2\,max}$) nears maximum.

The major circulatory adjustment to prolonged exercise involves the vasculature of the active muscles. Local formation of vasoactive metabolites induces marked dilation of the resistance vessels, which progresses as the intensity level of exercise increases. **Potassium** is one of the substances released by contracting muscle, and it may be in part responsible for the initial decrease in vascular resistance in the active muscles. Elevated interstitial K^+ can cause vasodilation by stimulation of the Na-K pump and by activation of the conductance of inwardly rectifying K^+ channels. Either action causes hyperpolarization of vascular smooth muscle membrane, thereby reducing Ca^{++} entry. Other contributing factors are the release of **adenosine** and **nitric oxide** (**NO**), the activation of adenosine triphosphate–sensitive potassium channels (**K_{ATP} channels),** and a decrease in pH during sustained exercise. All of these factors can act locally to dilate arterioles in contracting muscle. Adenosine release and K_{ATP} channel activation are thought to act at more distal arterioles to increase blood flow. The mechanism for the transmission of the dilating effect to distal arterioles is not understood.

The local accumulation of metabolites relaxes the terminal arterioles. Blood flow through the muscle may rise 15 to 20 times above the resting level (see Figure 13-2). This metabolic vasodilation of the precapillary vessels in active muscles occurs very soon after the onset of exercise. Furthermore, the decrease in TPR enables the heart to pump more blood at a lesser load and more efficiently (**less pressure work;** see Chapter 4) than if TPR were unchanged. Only a small percentage of the capillaries is perfused at rest, whereas in actively contracting muscle, nearly all of the capillaries contain flowing blood (**capillary recruitment**).

The surface available for exchange of gases, water, and solutes is increased many-fold. Furthermore, the hydrostatic pressure in the capillaries increases because of the relaxation of the resistance vessels. Hence there is a net movement of water and solutes into the muscle tissue. Interstitial pressure rises, and it remains elevated during exercise, as fluid continues to move out of the capillaries and is carried away by the lymphatics.

FIGURE 13-2 ■ Approximate distribution of cardiac output at rest and at different levels of exercise up to the maximal O_2 consumption ($\dot{V}O_2$) in a normal young man. *(Redrawn from Ruch HP, Patton TC: Physiology and biophysics, 12th ed, Philadelphia, Saunders, 1974.)*

Lymph flow is increased as a result of both the rise in capillary hydrostatic pressure and the massaging effect of the contracting muscles on the valve-containing lymphatic vessels (see Chapter 8).

The contracting muscle avidly extracts O_2 from the perfusing blood (**increased Ao_2–Vo_2 difference**) (Figure 13-3), and the release of O_2 from the blood is facilitated by the nature of oxyhemoglobin dissociation. The reduction in pH caused by the high concentration of CO_2 and the formation of lactic acid and the increase in temperature in the contracting muscle all contribute to shifting the **oxyhemoglobin dissociation curve** to the right, an example of the Bohr effect (see Figure 1-5). At any given partial pressure of O_2, less O_2 is bound by the hemoglobin in the red blood cells; consequently, O_2 removal from the blood is facilitated. *Oxygen consumption may increase as much as*

60-fold, with only a 15-fold increase in muscle blood flow. Muscle myoglobin serves as a limited O_2 store in exercise; it can release attached O_2 at very low partial pressures. Hence, it facilitates O_2 transport from capillaries to mitochondria by serving as an O_2 carrier.

Cardiac Output Can Increase Substantially in Exercise

The enhanced sympathetic drive and the reduced parasympathetic inhibition of the sinoatrial node continue during exercise, and consequently tachycardia persists. If the workload is moderate and constant, the heart rate will reach a certain level and remain there throughout the period of exercise. However, if the workload increases, a concomitant rise in heart rate occurs until a plateau is reached during severe exercise at about 180 beats per minute (beats/min) (see Figure 13-3). With moderate exercise, there is a substantial increase in stroke volume of about 10% to 35% (see Figure 13-3), the larger values occurring in trained individuals. (In very well-trained distance runners, whose cardiac outputs can reach six to seven times the resting level, stroke volume reaches about twice the resting value.) The increase in stroke volume has been ascribed to the Frank-Starling mechanism because left ventricular end-diastolic pressure and end-diastolic volume increase (see Chapter 4). This is seen in the rightward shift of the equilibrium point B in Figure 13-1. (The importance of greater ventricular filling in the response of cardiac output during exercise is underscored by the observation that increasing the heart rate alone through pacing is associated with reduced stroke volume and a constant cardiac output.) Contractility also increases during moderate exercise, an indication of sympathetic activation (see Figure 13-1; see also Chapter 5). When exercise is strenuous, cardiac output increases largely as a result of tachycardia. Stroke volume remains at a plateau or may even diminish slightly (see Figure 13-3) while contractility remains elevated.

Thus, it is apparent that the increase in cardiac output observed with exercise is correlated with an increase in heart rate. If the baroreceptors are denervated, the cardiac output and heart rate responses to exercise are sluggish in comparison with the changes in animals with normally innervated baroreceptors. However, exercise still elicits an increment in cardiac output in the absence of autonomic innervation of the heart, as occurs

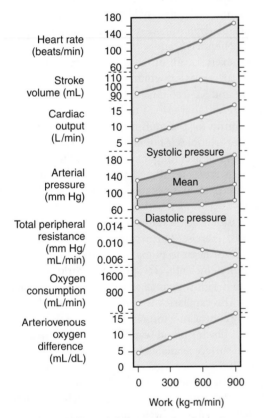

FIGURE 13-3 ■ Effect of different levels of exercise on several cardiovascular variables. *(From Carlsten A, Grimby G: The circulatory response to muscular exercise in man, Springfield, Ill, Charles C Thomas, 1966.)*

when a donor heart is prepared for transplantation. Resting heart rate is elevated to about 100 beats/min because parasympathetic innervation is lacking. The increment in cardiac output is less than that observed in normal subjects, and it is achieved principally by means of a gradual increase in heart rate. The stroke volume also increases but is below the level seen in the normal heart. If a **β-adrenergic receptor–blocking agent** is given, exercise performance is impaired in subjects with transplanted hearts. The β-adrenergic receptor antagonist opposes the cardiac acceleration and enhanced contractility caused by increased amounts of circulating catecholamines. Hence the increase in cardiac output necessary for maximal exercise performance is limited.

Venous Return Is Enhanced in Exercise

In addition to the contribution made by sympathetically mediated constriction of the capacitance vessels in both exercising and non-exercising parts of the body, venous return is aided by the working skeletal muscles and the muscles of respiration (see Figure 13-1). The intermittently contracting muscles compress the vessels that course through them (see Figure 12-2). In the case of veins with their valves oriented toward the heart, blood is pumped back toward the right atrium. The flow of venous blood to the heart is also aided by the increase in the pressure gradient developed by the more negative intrathoracic pressure produced by deeper and more frequent respirations. In humans, there is little evidence that blood reservoirs such as skin, lungs, and liver contribute much to circulating blood volume. In fact, blood volume is usually reduced slightly during exercise, as evidenced by a rise in the hematocrit ratio, because of both water lost externally by sweating and enhanced ventilation, and movement of fluid into the contracting muscle.

The fluid loss from the vascular compartment into contracting muscle reaches a plateau as interstitial fluid pressure rises and opposes the increased hydrostatic pressure in the capillaries of the active muscle. The fluid loss is partially offset by movement of fluid from the splanchnic regions and inactive muscle into the bloodstream. This influx of fluid occurs as a result of a decrease in hydrostatic pressure in the capillaries of these tissues and an increase in plasma osmolarity due to movement of osmotically active particles into the blood from the contracting muscle. In addition,

reduced urine formation by the kidneys helps to conserve body water.

Arterial Pressure Increases Slightly during Exercise

If the exercise involves a large proportion of the body musculature, as in running or swimming, the reduction in total vascular resistance can be considerable (see Figure 13-3). Nevertheless, arterial pressure starts to rise with the onset of exercise, and the increase in blood pressure roughly parallels the intensity of the exercise performed (see Figure 13-3). Therefore the increase in cardiac output is proportionally greater than the decrease in TPR. The vasoconstriction produced in the inactive tissues by the sympathetic nervous system (and to some extent by the release of catecholamines from the adrenal medulla) is important for maintaining normal or increased blood pressure because sympathectomy or drug-induced block of the sympathetic adrenergic nerve fibers results in a decrease in arterial pressure (**hypotension**) during exercise.

Some sympathetically mediated vasoconstriction occurs in active muscle and increases during strenuous exercise, when more than half of the total body musculature is contracting. In experiments in which one leg is working at maximal levels and then the other leg starts to work, blood flow decreases in the first working leg. Furthermore, blood levels of norepinephrine rise significantly in exercise, and most is derived from the sympathetic nerve endings in the active muscles.

As body temperature rises during exercise, the skin vessels dilate in response to thermal stimulation of the heat-regulating center in the hypothalamus, and TPR decreases further (see Figure 13-3). This would result in a decline in blood pressure were it not for the increasing cardiac output and constriction of arterioles in the renal, splanchnic, and other tissues.

In general, mean arterial pressure rises during exercise, as a result of the increase in cardiac output (see Figure 13-3). However, the effect of enhanced cardiac output is offset by the overall decrease in TPR. Hence, the mean blood pressure rise is relatively small. Vasoconstriction in the inactive vascular beds contributes to the maintenance of a normal arterial blood pressure for adequate perfusion of the active tissues. The actual pressure attained represents a balance between cardiac output and TPR (see p. 140). Systolic pressure usually increases more than diastolic pressure, resulting in an increase in pulse pressure (see Figure 13-3). The larger pulse pressure is primarily attributable to a greater stroke volume and, to a lesser degree, to a more rapid ejection of blood by the left ventricle. Peripheral runoff is less during the brief ventricular ejection period.

Severe Exercise

When severe exercise is taken to the point of exhaustion, the compensatory mechanisms begin to fail. Heart rate attains a maximal level of about 180 beats/min, and stroke volume reaches a plateau. The stroke volume often decreases, resulting in a fall in blood pressure. Dehydration occurs, and sympathetic vasoconstrictor activity supersedes the vasodilator influence on the cutaneous vessels. The neural activity has the hemodynamic effect of a slight increase in effective blood volume. However, cutaneous vasoconstriction also reduces the

rate of heat loss. Body temperature is normally elevated in exercise, and reduction in heat loss through cutaneous vasoconstriction can, under these conditions, lead to very high body temperatures, with associated feelings of acute distress. The tissue and blood pH values decrease as a result of greater lactic acid and CO_2 production. The reduced pH is probably the key factor that determines the maximal amount of exercise a given individual can tolerate because of muscle pain, subjective feelings of exhaustion, and inability or loss of the will to continue. A summary of the neural and local effects of exercise on the cardiovascular system is schematized in Figure 13-4.

Postexercise Recovery

When exercise stops, sympathetic activity to the heart declines, and the heart rate and cardiac output decrease. Peripheral sympathetic activity also decreases, and coupled with resistance vessel dilation (**caused by the**

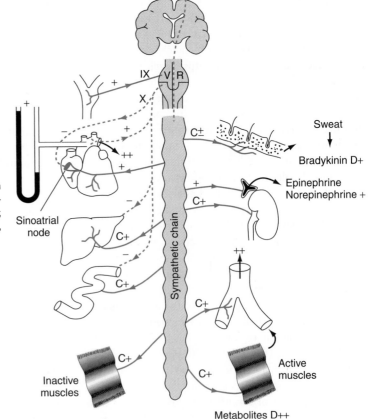

FIGURE 13-4 ■ Cardiovascular adjustments in exercise. C, vasoconstrictor activity; D, vasodilator activity; IX, glossopharyngeal nerve; VR, vasomotor region; X, vagus nerve; +, increased activity; −, decreased activity.

accumulated vasodilator metabolites), arterial pressure falls, often below the pre-exercise level. This hypotension is brief, and the baroreceptor reflexes restore the blood pressure to normal levels.

Limits of Exercise Performance

The two main forces that can limit skeletal muscle performance in humans are the rate of O_2 utilization by the muscles and the O_2 supply to the muscles. Muscle O_2 usage is probably not critical, because maximum O_2 consumption ($\dot{V}_{O_2max}$) during exercise by a large percentage of the body muscle mass either is unchanged or increases slightly when additional muscles are activated. In fact, during exercise of a large muscle mass, as in vigorous bicycling, commencement of bilateral arm exercise without change in the cycling efforts produces only a small increment in cardiac output and $\dot{V}_{O_2max}$. However, it causes a decrease in blood flow to the legs. This centrally mediated (**baroreceptor reflex**) vasoconstriction during maximal cardiac output prevents a fall in blood pressure. This drop in blood pressure would otherwise be caused by metabolically induced vasodilation in the active muscles. If muscle O_2 utilization were limiting, recruitment of more contracting muscle would use much more O_2 to meet the enhanced O_2 requirements (an amount about equal to the sum of O_2 consumption of the arms and legs exercised alone).

Limitation of O_2 supply may be caused by inadequate oxygenation of blood in the lungs or by limitation of the supply of O_2-laden blood to the muscles. Failure to fully oxygenate blood by the lungs can be excluded, because even with the most strenuous exercise at sea level, arterial blood is fully saturated with O_2. *Therefore O_2 delivery (or blood flow because arterial blood O_2 content is normal) to the active muscles appears to be the limiting factor in muscle performance.* This limitation could be caused by the inability to increase cardiac output beyond a certain level, as the result of a limitation of stroke volume, which might occur because heart rate reaches maximal levels before $\dot{V}_{O_2\ max}$ is reached. Hence the major factor is the pumping capacity of the heart.

Physical Training and Conditioning

The response of the cardiovascular system to regular exercise is to increase its capacity to deliver O_2 to the active muscles, and to improve the ability of the muscle to utilize O_2. The $\dot{V}_{O_2max}$ is quite reproducible in a given individual, and it varies with the level of physical conditioning. Training progressively increases the $\dot{V}_{O_2max}$, which reaches a plateau at the highest level of conditioning. Highly trained athletes have a lower resting heart rate, greater stroke volume, and lower peripheral resistance than they had before training or will have after deconditioning (i.e., **becoming sedentary**). The low resting heart rate is caused by a higher vagal tone and a lower sympathetic tone. With exercise, the maximal heart rate in the trained individual is the same as that in the untrained person, but it is attained at a higher level of exercise.

The trained athlete also exhibits a low vascular resistance that is inherent in the muscle. For example, if an individual exercises one leg regularly over an extended period and does not exercise the other leg, the vascular resistance is lower, and the $\dot{V}_{O_2max}$ higher, in the "trained" leg than in the "untrained" leg. Physical conditioning is associated with a greater extraction of O_2 from the blood (**greater Ao_2–Vo_2 difference**) by the muscles. With long-term training, capillary density and the numbers of mitochondria increase, as does the activity of the oxidative enzymes in the mitochondria. Also, it appears that **ATPase activity, myoglobin,** and **enzymes** involved in lipid metabolism increase with physical conditioning.

Endurance training, such as running or swimming, produces proportionate increases of left ventricular wall thickness (t) and of left ventricular chamber radius (r) such that the ratio, t/r, remains constant. In contrast, strength exercises, such as weight lifting, appear to produce some increase in left ventricular wall thickness (hypertrophy) with little effect on ventricular chamber radius. However, this increase in wall thickness is small relative to that observed in hypertension, in which there is a persistent elevation of afterload because of the high peripheral resistance.

HEMORRHAGE

In an individual who has lost a large quantity of blood, the principal system affected is the cardiovascular system.

The arterial systolic, diastolic, and pulse pressures diminish, and the arterial pulse is rapid and feeble. The cutaneous veins collapse and fill slowly when compressed centrally. The skin is pale, moist, and slightly cyanotic. Respiration is rapid, but the depth of respiration may be shallow or deep.

Hemorrhage Evokes Compensatory and Decompensatory Effects on the Arterial Blood Pressure

Cardiac output decreases as a result of blood loss (see Chapter 10). The amount (10%) of blood removed in a donation of blood is well tolerated; there is little change in mean arterial blood pressure. This is not the case when greater amounts are lost from the circulation. The changes in mean arterial pressure evoked by an acute hemorrhage in experimental animals are illustrated in Figure 13-5. If sufficient blood is withdrawn rapidly from a subject to bring mean arterial pressure to about 50 mm Hg, the pressure tends to rise spontaneously toward control over the subsequent 20 or 30 minutes. In some animals (curve A, Figure 13-5), this trend continues, and normal pressures are regained within a few hours. In other animals

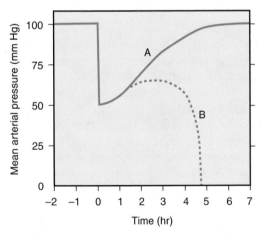

FIGURE 13-5 ■ Changes in mean arterial pressure after a rapid hemorrhage. At time 0, the animal is bled rapidly to a mean arterial pressure of 50 mm Hg. After a period in which the pressure returns toward the control level, some animals continue to improve until the control pressure is attained (curve A). However, in other animals the pressure will begin to decline until death ensues (curve B).

(curve B), after an initial pressure rise, the pressure begins to decline, and it continues to fall at an accelerating rate until death ensues. This progressive deterioration of cardiovascular function is termed **hemorrhagic shock.** At some point the deterioration becomes irreversible; a lethal outcome can be retarded only temporarily by any known therapy, including massive transfusions of donor blood.

The Compensatory Mechanisms are Neural and Humoral

The changes in arterial pressure immediately after an acute blood loss (see Figure 13-5) indicate that certain compensatory mechanisms must be operating. Any mechanism that senses the level of blood pressure and that raises the pressure toward normal in response to the reduction in pressure may be designated a **negative feedback mechanism.** It is termed "negative" because the direction of the secondary change in pressure is opposite to that of the initiating change. The following negative feedback responses are evoked: (1) baroreceptor reflexes, (2) chemoreceptor reflexes, (3) cerebral ischemic responses, (4) reabsorption of tissue fluids, (5) release of endogenous vasoconstrictor substances, and (6) renal conservation of salt and water.

Baroreceptor Reflexes

The reductions in mean arterial pressure and in pulse pressure during hemorrhage decrease the stimulation of the baroreceptors in the carotid sinuses and aortic arch (see Chapter 9). Several cardiovascular responses are thus evoked, all of which tend to restore the normal level of arterial pressure. Reduction of vagal tone and enhancement of sympathetic tone raise the heart rate and enhance myocardial contractility.

The increased sympathetic discharge also produces generalized **venoconstriction,** which has the same hemodynamic consequences as a transfusion of blood (see Chapter 10). Sympathetic activation constricts the vasculature in certain blood reservoirs. This vasoconstriction provides an autotransfusion of blood into the circulation. In humans, the cutaneous, pulmonary, and hepatic vasculatures probably constitute the principal blood reservoirs.

Generalized **arteriolar vasoconstriction** is a prominent response to the diminished baroreceptor stimulation during hemorrhage. The reflex increase in peripheral resistance minimizes the fall in arterial pressure that results from the reduction of cardiac output. Figure 13-6 shows the effect of an 8% blood loss on mean aortic pressure in a group of dogs. If both vagi are cut to eliminate the influence of the aortic arch baroreceptors, and only the carotid sinus baroreceptors are operative (*left panel*), this hemorrhage reduces mean aortic pressure by 14%. This pressure change does not differ significantly from the pressure decline (12%) evoked by the same hemorrhage before vagotomy (not shown). When the carotid sinuses are denervated and the aortic baroreceptor reflexes are intact, the 8% blood loss decreases mean aortic pressure by 38% (*middle panel* in Figure 13-6). Hence the carotid sinus baroreceptors are more effective than the aortic baroreceptors in attenuating the fall in pressure. The aortic baroreceptors must also be operative, however, because when both sets of afferent baroreceptor pathways are interrupted, an 8% blood loss reduces arterial pressure by 48% (*right panel* in Figure 13-6).

Although arteriolar vasoconstriction is widespread during hemorrhage, it is by no means uniform. Vasoconstriction is most severe in the cutaneous, skeletal muscle, and splanchnic vascular beds, and it is slight or absent in the cerebral and coronary circulations. In many instances the cerebral and coronary vascular resistances are diminished. *Thus the reduced cardiac output is redistributed to favor flow through the brain and the heart.*

In the early stages of mild to moderate hemorrhage, the changes in renal resistance are usually slight. The tendency for increased sympathetic activity to constrict the renal vessels is counteracted by autoregulatory mechanisms (see Chapter 12). With more prolonged and severe hemorrhage, however, renal vasoconstriction becomes intense. The reductions in renal circulation are most severe in the outer layers of the renal cortex. The inner zones of the cortex and outer zones of the medulla are spared.

The severe renal and splanchnic vasoconstriction during hemorrhage favors the heart and brain. However, if such constriction persists too long, it may be detrimental. Frequently, patients survive the acute hypotensive period only to die several days later from kidney failure because the prolonged renal ischemia causes acute tubular necrosis. Intestinal ischemia may also have dire effects. In the dog, for example, intestinal bleeding and extensive sloughing of the mucosa occur after only a few hours of hemorrhagic hypotension. Furthermore, the diminished splanchnic flow swells the centrilobular cells in the liver. The resulting obstruction of the hepatic sinusoids raises the portal venous pressure, intensifying the intestinal blood loss.

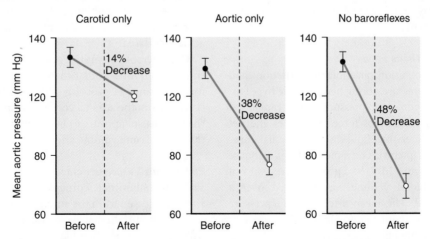

FIGURE 13-6 ■ Changes in mean aortic pressure (mean +/- SE) in response to an 8% blood loss in a group of eight dogs. *Left panel,* The carotid sinus baroreceptor reflexes were intact and the aortic reflexes were interrupted. *Middle panel,* The aortic reflexes were intact and the carotid sinus reflexes were interrupted. *Right panel,* All sinoaortic reflexes were abrogated. *(From Shepherd JT: Lewis A. Conner Memorial Lecture: The cardiac catheter and the American Heart Association.* Circulation 50:418, 1974; *derived from the data of Edis AJ: Aortic baroreflex function in the dog.* Am J Physiol 221:1352, 1971.)

Fortunately, the pathological changes in the liver and in the intestine are usually much less severe in humans than in dogs.

Chemoreceptor Reflexes

Reductions in arterial pressure below about 60 mm Hg do not evoke any additional responses through the baroreceptor reflexes, because this pressure level constitutes the threshold for stimulation (see Chapter 9). However, low arterial pressure may stimulate peripheral chemoreceptors, because inadequate local blood flow produces hypoxia in the chemoreceptor tissue. Chemoreceptor excitation enhances the already existing peripheral vasoconstriction evoked by the baroreceptor reflexes. Also, respiratory stimulation assists venous return by the auxiliary pumping mechanism described in Chapter 10.

Cerebral Ischemia

When the arterial pressure is below about 40 mm Hg, the resulting cerebral ischemia activates the sympathoadrenal system. The sympathetic nervous discharge is several times greater than the maximal neural activity that occurs when the baroreceptors cease to be stimulated. Therefore the vasoconstriction and facilitation of myocardial contractility may be pronounced. With more severe degrees of cerebral ischemia, however, the vagal centers also become activated. The resulting **bradycardia** may aggravate the hypotension that initiated the cerebral ischemia.

Reabsorption of Tissue Fluids

The arterial hypotension, arteriolar constriction, and reduced venous pressure during hemorrhagic hypotension lower the hydrostatic pressure in the capillaries. The balance of transmural forces promotes the net reabsorption of interstitial fluid into the vascular compartment (see Chapter 8). The rapidity of this response is displayed in Figure 13-7. In a group of cats, 45% of the estimated blood volume was removed over a 30-minute period. The mean arterial blood pressure declined rapidly to about 45 mm Hg. The pressure then returned quickly, but only temporarily, to near the control level. The plasma colloid osmotic pressure declined markedly during the bleeding and continued to decrease more gradually for several hours. The reduction in colloid osmotic pressure reflects the dilution of the blood

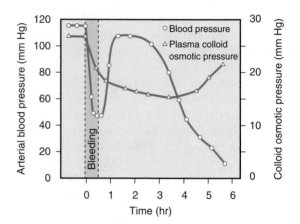

FIGURE 13-7 ■ Changes in arterial blood pressure and plasma colloid osmotic pressure in response to withdrawal of 45% of the estimated blood volume over a 30-minute period, beginning at time 0. The data are the average values for 23 cats. *(Redrawn from Zweifach BW: Mechanisms of blood flow and fluid exchange in microvessels: hemorrhagic hypotension model.* Anesthesiology *41:157, 1974.)*

by reabsorption of tissue fluids that contain little protein. The hematocrit is accordingly reduced, as is the O_2-carrying capacity of the blood.

Considerable quantities of fluid may thus be drawn into the circulation during hemorrhage. About 0.25 mL of fluid per minute per kilogram of body weight may be reabsorbed. Approximately 1 L of fluid per hour might be autoinfused into the circulatory system of an average individual from the interstitial spaces after an acute blood loss.

Considerable quantities of fluid may also be slowly shifted from intracellular to extracellular spaces. Thus fluid exchange is probably mediated by secretion of cortisol from the adrenal cortex in response to hemorrhage. Cortisol appears to be essential for a full restoration of plasma volume after hemorrhage.

Endogenous Vasoconstrictors

The **catecholamines, epinephrine, and norepinephrine** are released from the adrenal medulla in response to the same stimuli that evoke widespread sympathetic nervous discharge. Blood levels of catecholamines are high during and after hemorrhage. When animals are bled to an arterial pressure level of about 40 mm Hg, the concentration of catecholamines increases as much as 50 times.

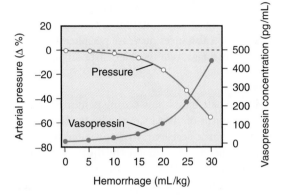

FIGURE 13-8 ■ Mean percentage changes in arterial blood pressure and in plasma vasopressin concentration in response to blood loss (0.5 mL/kg/min) in a group of 12 dogs; the maximal volume of blood withdrawn was 30 mL/kg. *(Redrawn from Shen Y-T, Cowley AW Jr, Vatner SF: Relative roles of cardiac and arterial baroreceptors in vasopressin regulation during hemorrhage in conscious dogs. Circ Res 68:1422, 1991.)*

Epinephrine comes almost exclusively from the adrenal medulla, whereas norepinephrine is derived from both the adrenal medulla and the peripheral sympathetic nerve endings. These humoral substances reinforce the effects of sympathetic nervous activity listed previously.

Vasopressin, a potent vasoconstrictor, is actively secreted by the posterior pituitary gland in response to hemorrhage. The plasma concentration of vasopressin rises progressively as the arterial blood pressure diminishes (Figure 13-8). The receptors responsible for the augmented release are the **sinoaortic baroreceptors** and **stretch receptors in the left atrium.**

The diminished renal perfusion during hemorrhagic hypotension leads to the secretion of **renin** from the juxtaglomerular apparatus (see Chapters 9 and 12). This enzyme acts on a plasma protein, **angiotensinogen,** to form **angiotensin I,** from which **angiotensin II,** a very powerful vasoconstrictor, is produced.

Renal Conservation of Salt and Water
During hemorrhage, the kidneys conserve fluid and electrolytes in response to various stimuli, including the increased secretion of vasopressin (**antidiuretic hormone**) noted previously (see Figure 13-8). The lower arterial pressure decreases the glomerular filtration rate and thus curtails the excretion of water and

electrolytes. Also, the diminished renal blood flow raises the blood levels of angiotensin II, as previously described. This polypeptide accelerates the release of **aldosterone** from the adrenal cortex. Aldosterone, in turn, stimulates sodium reabsorption by the renal tubules, and water accompanies the sodium that is actively reabsorbed.

The Decompensatory Mechanisms are Mainly Humoral, Cardiac, and Hematologic

In contrast to the negative feedback mechanisms just described, latent **positive feedback mechanisms** are also evoked by hemorrhage. Such mechanisms exaggerate any primary change initiated by the blood loss. Specifically, positive feedback mechanisms aggravate the hypotension induced by blood loss, and they tend to initiate vicious circles, which may lead to death. The result of the operation of positive feedback mechanisms is illustrated in curve B of Figure 13-5.

Whether a positive feedback mechanism will lead to a vicious circle depends on the gain of that mechanism. **Gain** is defined as the ratio of the secondary change evoked by a given mechanism to the initiating change itself. A gain greater than 1 induces a vicious circle; a gain less than 1 does not. For example, consider a positive feedback mechanism with a gain of 2. If, for any reason, mean arterial pressure were to decrease by 10 mm Hg, the positive feedback mechanism with a gain of 2 would then evoke a secondary pressure reduction of 20 mm Hg, which in turn would cause a further decrement of 40 mm Hg; that is, each change would induce a subsequent change that was twice as great. Hence mean arterial pressure would decline at an ever-increasing rate until death supervened, much as is depicted by curve B in Figure 13-5.

Conversely, a positive feedback mechanism with a gain of 0.5 would indeed exaggerate any change in mean arterial pressure, but it would not necessarily lead to death. For example, if arterial pressure suddenly decreased by 10 mm Hg, the positive feedback mechanism would initiate a secondary, additional fall of 5 mm Hg. This in turn would provoke a further decrease of 2.5 mm Hg. The process would continue in ever-diminishing steps, with the arterial pressure approaching an equilibrium value asymptotically.

Some of the more important positive feedback mechanisms are (1) cardiac failure, (2) acidosis, (3) central nervous system depression, (4) aberrations of blood clotting, and (5) depression of the reticuloendothelial system.

Cardiac Failure

The role of cardiac failure in the progression of shock during hemorrhage is controversial. All investigators agree that the heart fails terminally, but opinions differ concerning the importance of cardiac failure during earlier stages of hemorrhagic hypotension. Shifts to the right in ventricular function curves (Figure 13-9) constitute experimental evidence of a progressive depression of myocardial contractility during hemorrhage.

The hypotension induced by hemorrhage reduces the coronary blood flow and therefore depresses ventricular function. The consequent reduction in cardiac output leads to a further decline in arterial pressure, a classic example of a positive feedback mechanism.

Furthermore, the reduced blood flow to the peripheral tissues leads to an accumulation of vasodilator metabolites. These substances decrease peripheral resistance and therefore aggravate the fall in arterial pressure.

Acidosis

The inadequate blood flow during hemorrhage affects the metabolism of all cells in the body. The resulting stagnant anoxia accelerates the production of lactic acid and other acid metabolites by the tissues. Furthermore, impaired kidney function prevents adequate excretion of the excess H^+, and generalized metabolic acidosis ensues (Figure 13-10). The resulting depressant effect of acidosis on the heart (see Chapter 5) further reduces tissue perfusion, thus aggravating the metabolic acidosis. Acidosis also diminishes the reactivity of the heart and resistance vessels to neurally released and circulating catecholamines and thereby intensifies the hypotension.

Central Nervous System Depression

The hypotension in shock reduces cerebral blood flow. Moderate degrees of cerebral ischemia induce a pronounced sympathetic nervous stimulation of the heart, arterioles, and veins, as stated previously. With severe

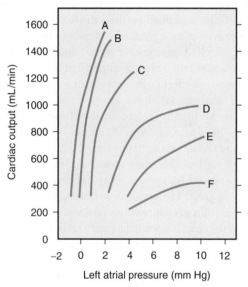

FIGURE 13-9 ■ Ventricular function curves for the left ventricles during the course of hemorrhagic shock. Curve A represents the control function curve. Curve B represents 117 min, curve C 247 min, curve D 280 min, curve E 295 min, and curve F 310 min after the initial hemorrhage. *(Redrawn from Crowell JW, Guyton AC: Further evidence favoring a cardiac mechanism in irreversible hemorrhagic shock. Am J Physiol 203:248, 1962.)*

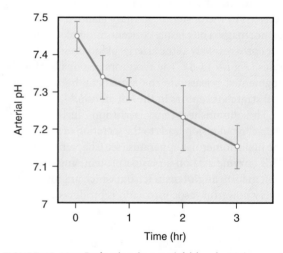

FIGURE 13-10 ■ Reduction in arterial blood pH (mean ± SD) in a group of 11 dogs whose blood pressure had been held at a level of 35 mm Hg by bleeding into a reservoir, beginning at time 0. *(Modified from Markov AK, Oglethorpe N, Young DB, et al: Irreversible hemorrhagic shock: treatment and cardiac pathophysiology. Circ Shock 8:9, 1981.)*

degrees of hypotension, however, the cardiovascular centers in the brainstem eventually become depressed because of inadequate blood flow to the brain. The resulting loss of sympathetic tone then reduces cardiac output and peripheral resistance. The consequent reduction in mean arterial pressure intensifies the inadequate cerebral perfusion.

Various endogenous **opioids,** such as **enkephalins** and **β-endorphin,** may be released into the brain substance and into the circulation in response to hemorrhage. Opioids exist, along with catecholamines, in secretory granules in the adrenal medulla and sympathetic nerve terminals. Also, they are released together in response to stress. Similar stimuli release β-endorphin and **adrenocorticotropic hormone** (**ACTH**) from the anterior pituitary gland. The opioids depress the medullary vasomotor center in the brainstem. Such centers mediate some of the compensatory autonomic adaptations to blood loss, endotoxemia, and other shock-provoking stresses. Conversely, the opioid antagonist **naloxone** improves cardiovascular function and survival in various forms of shock.

Aberrations of Blood Clotting

The alterations of blood clotting after hemorrhage are typically biphasic—an initial phase of hypercoagulability followed by a secondary phase of hypocoagulability and fibrinolysis. In the initial phase, platelets and leukocytes adhere to the vascular endothelium, and intravascular clots, or **thrombi,** develop within a few minutes of the onset of severe hemorrhage. Coagulation may be extensive throughout the minute blood vessels.

Thromboxane A_2 (TxA_2) may be released from various ischemic tissues. It aggregates platelets, and more TxA_2 is released from the trapped platelets, serving to trap additional platelets. This form of positive feedback intensifies and prolongs the clotting tendency. The mortality from certain standard shock-provoking procedures has been reduced considerably by anticoagulants such as **heparin.**

In the later stages of hemorrhagic hypotension, the clotting time is prolonged and fibrinolysis is prominent. As stated previously, hemorrhage into the intestinal lumen is common after several hours of hemorrhagic hypotension in dogs. Blood loss into the intestinal lumen would aggravate the hemodynamic effects of the original hemorrhage.

Depression of the Reticuloendothelial System

During the course of hemorrhagic hypotension, reticuloendothelial system (RES) function becomes depressed. The phagocytic activity of the RES is modulated by an **opsonic protein.** The opsonic activity in plasma diminishes during shock; this process may account in part for the depression of RES function. As a consequence, antibacterial and antitoxic defense mechanisms are impaired. Endotoxins from the normal bacterial flora of the intestine constantly enter the circulation. Ordinarily they are inactivated by the RES, principally in the liver. When the RES is depressed, these endotoxins invade the general circulation. *Endotoxins produce profound, generalized vasodilation, mainly by inducing the abundant synthesis of an isoform of NO synthase in the smooth muscle of blood vessels throughout the body.* The profound vasodilation aggravates the hemodynamic changes caused by blood loss.

In addition to their role in inactivating endotoxin, macrophages release many of the mediators that are associated with shock. These mediators include **acid hydrolases, neutral proteases, oxygen free radicals, certain coagulation factors,** and **arachidonic acid derivatives:** namely **prostaglandins, thromboxanes,** and **leukotrienes.** Macrophages also release certain **monokines** that modulate temperature regulation, intermediary metabolism, hormone secretion, and the immune system.

The Positive and Negative Feedback Mechanisms Interact

Hemorrhage provokes a multitude of circulatory and metabolic derangements. Some of these changes are compensatory, and others are decompensatory. Certain feedback mechanisms possess a high gain, and others a low gain. Furthermore, the gain of any specific mechanism varies with the severity of the hemorrhage. For example, with only a slight loss of blood, mean arterial pressure is within the range of normal, and the gain of the baroreceptor reflexes is high. With greater losses of blood, during which mean arterial pressure is below about 60 mm Hg (i.e., **below the threshold for the baroreceptors**), further reductions of pressure have no additional influence through the baroreceptor reflexes. Hence, below this critical pressure, the baroreceptor reflex gain is zero or near zero.

As a general rule, with minor degrees of blood loss, the gains of the negative feedback mechanisms are high, whereas those of the positive feedback mechanisms are low. The converse is true with more severe hemorrhages. The gains of the various mechanisms are additive algebraically. Therefore whether a vicious circle develops depends on whether the sum of the various gains exceeds 1. Total gains in excess of 1 are more likely when blood losses are severe. To avert a vicious circle, serious hemorrhages must be treated quickly and intensively, preferably by whole blood transfusions, before the process becomes irreversible.

SUMMARY

EXERCISE

- In anticipation of exercise, the vagus nerve impulses to the heart are inhibited and the sympathetic nervous system is activated by central command. The result is an increase in heart rate, myocardial contractile force, cardiac output, and arterial pressure.

- With exercise, vascular resistance increases in skin, kidneys, splanchnic regions, and inactive muscles and decreases in active muscles.

- The increase in cardiac output is accomplished mainly by the rise in heart rate. Stroke volume increases only slightly. In well-trained endurance athletes, stroke volume increases substantially during exercise.

- During exercise total peripheral resistance decreases, O_2 consumption and blood O_2 extraction increase, and systolic and mean blood pressures rise slightly.

- As body temperature rises during exercise, the skin blood vessels dilate. However, when the heart rate becomes maximal during severe exercise, the skin vessels constrict. This enlarges the effective blood volume but causes greater increases in body temperature and a feeling of exhaustion.

- The limiting factor in exercise performance is the delivery of blood to the active muscles.

HEMORRHAGE

- Acute blood loss induces tachycardia, hypotension, generalized arteriolar vasoconstriction, and generalized venoconstriction.

- Acute blood loss invokes a number of negative feedback (compensatory) mechanisms, such as baroreceptor and chemoreceptor reflexes, responses to moderate cerebral ischemia, reabsorption of tissue fluids, release of endogenous vasoconstrictors, and renal conservation of water and electrolytes.

- Acute blood loss also induces a number of positive feedback (decompensatory) mechanisms, such as cardiac failure, acidosis, central nervous system depression, aberrations of blood coagulation, and depression of the reticuloendothelial system.

- The outcome of acute blood loss depends on the gains of the various feedback mechanisms and on the interactions between the positive and negative feedback mechanisms.

ADDITIONAL READINGS

Bengel FM, Ueberfuhr P, Karja J, et al: Sympathetic reinnervation, exercise performance and effects of β-adrenergic blockade in cardiac transplant recipients, *Eur Heart J* 25:1726, 2004.

Buckwalter JB, Clifford PS: Autonomic control of skeletal muscle blood flow at the onset of exercise, *Am J Physiol* 277:H1872, 1999.

Calbet JAL, Jensen-Urstad M, van Hall G, et al: Maximal muscular vascular conductances during whole body upright exercise in humans, *J Physiol* 558:319, 2004.

Clark MG, Wallis MG, Barrett EJ, et al: Blood flow and muscle metabolism: A focus on insulin action, *Am J Physiol* 284:E241, 2003.

Clifford PS: Skeletal muscle vasodilatation at the onset of exercise, *J Physiol* 583:825, 2007.

Evans RG, Ventura S, Dampney RA, Ludbrook J: Neural mechanisms in the cardiovascular responses to acute central hypovolaemia, *Clin Exp Pharmacol Physiol* 28:479, 2001.

Foëx BA: Systemic responses to trauma, *Br Med Bull* 55:726, 1999.

Hickner RC, Fisher JS, Ehsani AA, et al: Role of nitric oxide in skeletal muscle blood flow at rest and during dynamic exercise in humans, *Am J Physiol* 273:H405, 1997.

Kulecs JM, Collins HL, Dicarlo SE: Postexercise hypotension is mediated by reductions in sympathetic nerve activity, *Am J Physiol* 276:H27, 1999.

Laughlin MH, Korthuis RJ, Duncker DJ, et al: Control of blood flow to cardiac and skeletal muscles during exercise. In Rowell LB, Shepherd JT, editors: *Handbook of Physiology, Section 12: Exercise: Regulation and Integration of Multiple Systems*, Bethesda, Md, 1996, Oxford University Press.

Michelini LC, Morris M: Endogenous vasopressin modulates the cardiovascular responses to exercise, *Ann N Y Acad Sci* 897:198, 1999.

O'Sullivan SE, Bell C: The effects of exercise and training on human cardiovascular reflex control, *J Auton Nerv Syst* 81:16, 2000.

Potts JT: Exercise and sensory integration. Role of the nucleus tractus solitarius, *Ann N Y Acad Sci* 940:221, 2001.

Prabhakar NR, Peng YJ: Peripheral chemoreceptors in health and disease, *J Appl Physiol* 96:359, 2004.

Prior BM, Yang HT, Terjung RL: What makes vessels grow with exercise training? *J Appl Physiol* 97:1119, 2004.

Putnam RW, Filosa JA, Ritucci NA: Cellular mechanisms involved in CO_2 and acid signaling in chemosensitive neurons, *Am J Physiol* 287:C1493, 2004.

Rowland TW: The circulatory response to exercise: Role of the peripheral pump, *Int J Sports Med* 22:558, 2001.

Squires RW: Exercise therapy for cardiac transplant recipients, *Prog Cardiovasc Dis* 53:429, 2011.

Tipton CM: The autonomic nervous system. In Tipton CM, editor: *Exercise Physiology: People and Ideas*, New York, 2003, Oxford University Press, pp 189–254.

Tschakorsky ME, Hughson RL: Ischemic muscle chemoreflex response elevates blood flow in nonischemic exercising human forearm muscle, *Am J Physiol* 277:H635, 1999.

CASE 13-1

HISTORY

A 23-year-old male track star decided to enter the Boston Marathon. He had only run in short distance events, up to 10 K (6.21 miles), before entry in the marathon. At the 15-mile mark, he was leading the race, but he was soon passed by one of his competitors. This inspired him to make a strong effort to retake the lead, but he was unable to increase his speed. At the 20-mile mark he began to feel faint, and within the next mile he became sick to his stomach and somewhat disoriented, and he finally staggered and fell to the ground, exhausted.

QUESTIONS

1. When the runner was at the 17-mile mark, what limited him from achieving his goal of retaking the lead?

  a. His leg muscles were unable to use more oxygen.
  b. His respiratory system was unable to saturate the arterial blood with oxygen.
  c. He had inadequate vasoconstriction in the splanchnic regions and in the inactive muscles.
  d. His cardiac output became inadequate.
  e. His arteriovenous oxygen difference was decreased.

2. At the time of his collapse, which of the following did *not* occur?

  a. His body temperature fell.
  b. His heart rate reached a maximal level.
  c. His skin blood vessels constricted.
  d. His blood pH decreased.
  e. His blood pressure decreased.

CASE 13-2

HISTORY

A 47-year-old woman had an acute episode of severe abdominal pain, and she suddenly vomited a large amount of bloody material. Her husband called for an ambulance to take her to the hospital. The emergency room physician learned that the patient had had frequent, severe episodes of upper abdominal pain over the past 6 weeks. Physical examination revealed that the patient's skin was very pale and cold, her heart rate was 110 beats/min, and her blood pressure was 85/65 mm Hg. Examination of the patient's blood revealed that the hematocrit ratio (the ratio of red blood cell volume to whole blood volume) was 40%. The physician made the tentative diagnosis of a bleeding peptic ulcer.

QUESTIONS

1. The patient's skin was pale and cold because:

  a. the arterial baroreceptors reflexly induced the parasympathetic nerves to the skin to release acetylcholine.
  b. the arterial chemoreceptors reflexly induced the parasympathetic nerves to the skin to release vasoactive intestinal peptide.

   c. the arterial chemoreceptors reflexly induced the parasympathetic nerves to the skin to release neuropeptide Y.
   d. the arterial baroreceptors reflexly induced the sympathetic nerves to the skin to release nitric oxide.
   e. the arterial baroreceptors reflexly induced the sympathetic nerves to the skin to release norepinephrine.
2. The patient's arterial blood pressure, 85/65 mm Hg, indicates that:
   a. the patient's left ventricle was pumping an abnormally low cardiac output and low stroke volume.
   b. the patient's left ventricle was pumping more blood than her right ventricle.
   c. the patient's left ventricle was pumping an abnormally low cardiac output but a normal stroke volume.
   d. the patient's left ventricle was pumping a normal cardiac output and an abnormally low stroke volume.
   e. the patient's left ventricle was pumping less blood than her right ventricle.
3. If the patient's bleeding had stopped before she arrived at the hospital, which of the following changes would be expected in the patient's blood 1 hour after she had arrived at the hospital?
   a. The individual red blood cells would be larger than normal.
   b. The hematocrit ratio would be reduced.
   c. The lymphocyte count would be abnormally high.
   d. The plasma albumin concentration would be increased.
   e. The plasma globulin concentration would be increased.

APPENDIX

■ ■ ■ ■ ■ ■ ■ ■ ■ ■ ■ ■ ■ ■ ■ ■ ■

CASE STUDY ANSWERS

CASE 1-1

1. **b** is correct. The circulation time will be shortened because some blood passes through the shunt (short circuit).

CASE 2-1

1. **c** is correct. When the extracellular K^+ concentration increases, the Nernst equation indicates that the transmembrane potential will become less negative.

2. **d** is correct. When the extracellular K^+ concentration increases and depolarizes the membrane, the rate of rise of the action potential is diminished because some Na^+ channels are inactivated by the persistent depolarization.

3. **d** is correct. The Purkinje fibers are automatic fibers, and they generate action potentials at a low frequency whenever they are not depolarized by action potentials that originate in higher-frequency pacemaker sites.

4. **a** is correct. When ventricular pacing at 75 beats per minute was discontinued, spontaneous pacemaker activity in the ventricles was suppressed for several seconds because the preceding period of artificial pacing had hyperpolarized the ventricular pacemaker cells (Purkinje fibers).

CASE 3-1

1. **c** is correct because the PR interval, which indicates the time for conduction from atria through the AV node and ventricular conducting system to the ventricle, is normal.

2. **e** is correct because the QT interval measures the duration of the average ventricular action potential.

3. **a** is correct because heart rate can be taken from either the R-R or the P-P interval when conduction is normal.

4. **d** is correct because there is greater activation of repolarizing K channels when heart rate increases.

CASE 4-1

1. **d** is correct. The murmur is characteristic of mitral stenosis.

2. **c** is correct. The pulse is totally irregular.

3. **b** is correct. A "loop" diuretic like furosemide would relieve the excessive preload and allow the cardiac output to improve and the edema and ascites to subside.

4. **b** is correct. The elevated left atrial pressure would be transmitted back to the wedged catheter (wedge pressure).

5. **c** is correct. 300 mL O_2/min /[(18 − 8) mL O_2/100 mL blood] = 3000 mL/min = 3 L/min.

CASE 5-1

1. **d** is correct. A decrease in arterial pressure would reflexly increase sympathetic activity and thereby increase the neuronal release of norepinephrine.

2. **d** is correct. The ACh released from vagal fibers acts on muscarinic receptors on SA node automatic cells, and these receptors interact very quickly with specific K^+ channels because no second messenger intervenes.

3. **a** is correct. The cardiac responses to vagal stimulation develop and decay rapidly, but the responses to sympathetic stimulation develop and decay very slowly. Hence respiratory dysrhythmia is mediated almost entirely by the vagus nerves, and this dysrhythmia would be abolished by a potent muscarinic antagonist.

4. **a** is correct. Heart rate increases during inspiration in this dysrhythmia, and this increase is mediated mainly by a reduction in vagal activity.

5. **e** is correct. Acetylcholinesterase is abundant in atrial tissues, and especially in the SA and AV nodes.

CASE 6-1

1. **b** is correct. $(P_a - P_v)/Q$—that is, $[(100 - 80) + (80 - 10)]/300$—equals 0.30 mm Hg/mL/min.

2. **d** is correct. The left $([100 - 10]/500)$ and right $([100 - 10]/300)$ vascular resistances were 0.18 and 0.30 mm Hg/mL/min, respectively, and the reciprocals of those resistances were 5.56 and 3.33 mL/min/mm Hg, respectively. Hence the reciprocal of the sum (8.89 mL/min/mm Hg) of these reciprocals equals 0.11 mm Hg/mL/min.

3. **a** is correct. The pressure difference across the plaque (100 − 80 mm Hg), divided by the flow past the plaque (300 mL/min), equals 0.066 mm Hg/mL/min.

CASE 7-1

1. **a** is correct. The mean arterial pressure in the systemic and pulmonary vascular beds depends on the outputs of the left and right ventricles and the systemic vascular resistances. Over any substantial time interval, the outputs of the two ventricles are equal, but the systemic vascular resistance far exceeds the pulmonary vascular resistance.

2. **c** is correct. When the arterial pressure rises, the arteries become less compliant (as does a balloon), and also the arterial compliance decreases with age.

CASE 8-1

1. **d** is correct. $1[(44 - 8) - 0.7(23 - 3)] = 22$.

2. **c** is correct. Portal-caval shunt (portal vein to inferior vena cava) could reduce the high venous pressure in the mesentery by allowing mesenteric blood to bypass the high vascular resistance in the liver. This would aid in eliminating the ascites.

3. **b** is correct. Albumin is small enough (low molecular weight) to exert the main osmotic force of plasma and large enough to remain within the vascular compartment.

CASE 8-2

1. **e** is correct. The albumin concentration in the patient's blood is low because of the loss of albumin from the burned tissues. This results in a decreased plasma oncotic pressure, and that plus the loss of fluid from the damaged microvessels leads to a decreased blood volume and an increased red blood cell concentration. Therefore a plasma transfusion, which supplies albumin plus saline without red blood cells, is the most effective treatment.

2. **d** is correct. The small diameter (or radius) of the capillaries is responsible for the low wall tension, according to the law of Laplace, whereby T (wall tension) = P (pressure) × r (radius of capillary). The low wall tension protects against capillary rupture.

CASE 9-1

1. **b** is correct. The arterioles are maximally dilated secondary to the inadequate blood flow that causes the local release of vasodilator metabolites.

2. **d** is correct. The ankle-brachial index is taken from the ratio of systolic pressure in the dorsalis pedis artery to that in the brachial artery (112 mm Hg/140 mm Hg = 0.80).

3. **a** is correct. Use of tobacco is believed to be a contributing factor to the cause and exacerbation of thromboangiitis obliterans.

CASE 10-1

1. **c** is correct. The blood loss would decrease the central venous pressure, and this reduction in cardiac preload would reduce the cardiac output.

2. **a** is correct. A drug that improves cardiac contractility would increase cardiac output, a change that would tend to increase the arterial blood volume. Hence, if total blood volume remains constant, the venous blood volume would decrease. Consequently, the central venous pressure would decline.

3. **e** is correct. Gravity acts to pool blood in the compliant, dependent veins, and hence the pressure in the foot veins increases. The redistribution of the venous blood volume causes the central venous volume and pressure to diminish. The consequent reduction in preload decreases the cardiac output.

4. **b** is correct. When the heart rate is abnormally high (250 beats/min), cardiac filling is inadequate, and therefore stroke volume and cardiac output are decreased.

CASE 11-1

1. **d** is correct. Two factors operate in bradycardia. At the slower rate, more time is spent in diastole, thereby decreasing coronary resistance (less extravascular compression). However, at the slower rate the heart uses less oxygen and fewer vasodilator metabolites are present, permitting greater expression of basal tone (coronary constriction). The end result is the algebraic sum of these two opposing factors.

2. **a** is correct. The coronary vessels are maximally dilated as a result of the accumulation of vasodilator metabolites consequent to an inadequate oxygen supply to the myocardial cells. If any vasoconstriction occurred, it would be transient.

3. **b** is correct. Endothelin is a powerful vasoconstrictor.

4. **e** is correct. With exercise, a denervated heart increases stroke volume more than heart rate to meet the required cardiac output. Any increase in heart rate must come from release of epinephrine and norepinephrine from the adrenal medulla.

CASE 12-1

1. **a** is correct. The hepatic fibrosis increases the hepatic vascular resistance, and therefore the pressure in the vessels downstream to the liver is elevated. Consequently, the balance of Starling forces in the splanchnic capillaries favors the movement of fluid out of the capillaries and into the abdominal cavity.

CASE 12-2

1. **b** is correct. The murmur, the high right ventricular systolic pressure with a normal right atrial pressure, the elevated Po_2 of the right ventricular blood, and the absence of cyanosis indicated a left-to-right shunt through an interventricular septal defect.

CASE 12-3

1. **d** is correct. The ankle-brachial index (ABI) is the ratio of systolic blood pressure in the dorsal pedal artery to that in the brachial artery. The ratio (70 mm Hg/140 mm Hg) yields an ABI of 0.5.

CASE 13-1

1. **d** is correct. The patient's heart became unable to pump enough blood per unit time owing to a decrease in stroke volume and hence in cardiac output.

2. **a** is correct. The patient's body temperature reached an alarmingly high level because of inadequate heat loss via the skin (vasoconstriction secondary to decrease in blood pressure) in the presence of the great heat production in the active muscles.

CASE 13-2

1. **e** is correct. The hypotension would act via the arterial baroreceptors to activate the sympathetic nerves to the skin. The consequent release of norepinephrine would constrict the cutaneous arterioles, and the skin temperature would drop.

2. *a* is correct. The abnormally low mean arterial pressure (about 72 mm Hg) would signify an abnormally small cardiac output. The low mean arterial pressure could not have been caused by arterial vasodilation because the baroreceptor reflex response to a low mean arterial pressure would be vasoconstriction, not dilation. The low pulse pressure (20 mm Hg) would signify an abnormally small stroke volume.

3. *b* is correct. The decrease in capillary hydrostatic pressure draws interstitial fluid into the plasma compartment and thereby dilutes the red cell component of whole blood.

INDEX

Page numbers followed by *f* indicate figures; *t*, tables; *b*, boxes.